Chronic Diseases and Health Care

Stephen J. Morewitz

Chronic Diseases and Health Care:

New Trends in Diabetes, Arthritis, Osteoporosis, Fibromyalgia, Low Back Pain, Cardiovascular Disease, and Cancer

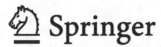

Stephen J. Morewitz
morewitz@earthlink.net

e-ISBN   0-387-28779-5
ISBN   978-1-4419-3953-1   e-ISBN   978-0-387-28779-9

Printed on acid-free paper.

Printed in the United States of America.   (BS/EB)

9 8 7 6 5 4 3 2 1

springer.com

Preface

CHRONIC DISEASES AND HEALTH CARE: New Patterns of Diabetes, Arthritis, Osteoporosis, Fibromyalgia, Low Back Pain, Cardiovascular Disease, and Cancer.

Twenty-five million Americans are victims of chronic disease, and approximately two-thirds of all deaths each year are due to cardiovascular disease (including stroke), cancer, and diabetes. This book evaluates new trends in epidemiology, health care costs, risk factors, treatment and rehabilitation outcomes, stress and coping strategies, social support, disability, patient education, and self-management for seven prevalent chronic diseases. Case studies from a clinical psychologist's private practice and the research literature are used to clarify the issues underlying chronic diseases and health care.

There are many questions still to be addressed in the field of chronic disease and health care. What is the prevalence of chronic diseases? What are the health care costs associated with these conditions? What are the major risk factors and health care disparities that contribute to the development of chronic diseases? How have these risk factors and health care disparities changed over time? What impact do chronic diseases have on disability, quality of life, and health care disparities? How do individuals cope with the stresses of chronic diseases? What are the most effective forms of social support? What are the most effective treatments and rehabilitation programs for chronic diseases? How can patient education and self-management activities be improved to help patients and their families better understand and treat their conditions?

Chapter One analyzes the latest trends in the epidemiology of the seven chronic diseases. Disparities in socioeconomic status, race/ethnicity, gender, and age and their impact on chronic diseases are stressed in this chapter. Health care planners can use these analyses to improve primary and secondary health care prevention activities through more effective uses of health care resources.

Chapter Two examines the latest information on health costs that can point to a more efficient means of reducing the rising health care costs.

In Chapter Three, Dr. Mark L. Goldstein, a clinical psychologist, uses composite case studies from his practice to illustrate the problems that patients may have in coping with chronic diseases.

In the remaining four chapters, each of the seven chronic diseases is evaluated in terms of five major issues. First, the latest trends in risk factors and health care disparities associated with each chronic condition are explored. Second, the impact of each disease on disability, quality of life, and health care disparities are analyzed. Third, the processes of stress, coping and social support are described. Fourth, latest information on treatment and rehabilitation outcomes are discussed. Finally, new trends in patient education and self-management are presented.

Stephen J. Morewitz
January 2006

Acknowledgments

I would like to thank Mrs. Myra Kalkin Morewitz and Dr. Harry A. Morewitz for their advice and support. I also want to thank Bill Tucker, Public Health Editor at Springer, and Anna Tobias, Psychology Associate Editor at Springer, who have been supportive as well as thorough and thoughtful.

Contents

1

Chronic Diseases: Epidemiology and Health Care Disparities

Chronic diseases, with their prolonged span of pain and suffering, are a major cause of disability and death. The 25 million Americans, who are victims of chronic diseases, are unable to work, experience a decreased quality of life and find themselves subject to significantly increased direct and indirect medical costs. In the United States, cardiovascular disease (including stroke), cancer, and diabetes make up about 2/3rds of all deaths annually (Eyre, et al., 2004; CDC, National Center for Chronic Disease Prevention and Health Promotion, p. 1, http://www.cdc.gov/needphp/overview. htm).

These conditions are the result of complex interactions among environmental, social, and genetic factors (Quadrilatero and Hoffman-Goetz, 2003). Health care problems such as: smoking, overweight, obesity, poor nutrition, sedentary lifestyles, and genetics are some of the many factors associated with chronic diseases.

Racial, ethnic, gender, age, and socioeconomic disparities in health care may be risk factors for chronic diseases and also exacerbate the impact of these conditions. Chronic health problems, such as diabetes and cardiovascular disease, pose a particularly severe burden on disadvantaged minority groups, including

1

African-Americans, Hispanics, and Native-American Indians, women, and disadvantaged socioeconomic groups. For instance, in the United States, African-Americans suffer a disproportionate stroke-burden and African-American stroke survivors have greater functional impairment than white stroke survivors (Ruland and Gorelick, 2005; MMWR Morb Mortal Weekly Report, 2005).

In the United States cardiovascular disease is the overall leading cause of death. Smoking, obesity, poor nutrition, physical inactivity, and genetic factors increase the risk of cardiovascular disease burden. In 2000, among U.S. adults, ages 25 to 44 years, heart disease was the leading cause of death among non-Hispanic Black adults and the 5th leading cause among Hispanics. Among adults in the 45 to 64 year age group, heart disease was the 2nd leading cause among Non-Hispanic Blacks, and the 2nd leading cause among Hispanics.

Gender differences in cardiovascular disease and its treatment have been documented. Several investigations have shown that women with coronary heart disease have a poorer prognosis as compared to men (Horsten, et al., 2000). Women are less likely than men to have invasive treatment of coronary heart disease although the prevalence of angina is increasing in women (Philpott, et al., 2001).

Socioeconomic factors are also related to coronary artery disease risk factors, coronary morbidity, and mortality in various developed countries such as the United States (Horne, et al., 2004; Sonmez, et al., 2004; Rutledge, et al., 2003). Low socioeconomic status has been linked to coronary artery risk factors, such as higher body mass index and waist-to-hip ratios, cigarette smoking, sedentary behavior, and higher risk for hypertension (Rutledge, et al., 2003). Patients with coronary artery disease who reside in lower socioeconomic status neighborhoods have been found to have an increased risk of death or myocardial infarction (Horne, et al., 2004).

Cancer is the second leading cause of death in the United States and is expected to become the leading cause of death during the next decade (Stewart, et al., 2004). In addition to genetic factors, lifestyle choices such as smoking, obesity, poor nutrition, alcohol use, a sedentary lifestyle, socioeconomic status, and environmental/ occupational exposures can be related to cancer morbidity and mortality. Ethnic and racial disparities in cancer have been documented. Cancer was the leading cause of death among Non-Hispanic Blacks and Hispanics in the 45 to 64 year age group (Centers for Disease Control and Prevention, 2001).

Ethnic and racial disparities in diabetes have been a prevalent pattern in the United States. In 2001, diabetes was the 4th leading cause among Non-Hispanic Blacks, and the 5th leading cause among Hispanics (Centers for Disease Control and Prevention, 2001). Obesity, sedentary lifestyles, and poor nutrition contribute significantly to the diabetes disease burden.

Arthritis, osteoporosis, fibromyalgia, and low back pain also have a major adverse impact on society because of the chronic, disabling nature of these prevalent disorders. Lifestyle, occupational, and genetic factors increase the risk of certain types of arthritis, other rheumatic conditions, and musculoskeletal disorders. One study estimated that in 1997, there were 2.5 million hospitalizations with any-listed arthritis diagnosis and 744,000 hospitalizations with the principal diagnosis of arthritis (Lethbridge-Cejku, 2003).

Gender disparities in arthritis have been documented, with women having a greater risk of developing the disease and suffering higher levels of disability than men. Inequalities in health and access to arthritis care may be related to age, geography, and socioeconomic deprivation. For example, one study of access to knee joint replacements for people in need in the United Kingdom discovered that older and low socioeconomic status persons were less likely to access knee joint replacement services (Yong, et al., 2004).

The epidemiology of these diseases is detailed below.

Trends in Diabetes

Adult type 2 diabetes mellitus (also known as non-insulin-dependent diabetes mellitus or NIDDM) and other abnormalities involving glucose intolerance emerged as an epidemic in the 20th century and continues unchecked into the 21st century (Engelgau, et al., 2004; Shaw and Chisholm, 2003). In 1995, there were an estimated 135 million persons with diabetes worldwide, and the World Health Organization estimates that this number will grow to 300 million by 2025 (Pradeepa and Mohan, 2002). The geographical regions with the largest potential increases in diabetes are Asia and Africa (Amos, et al., 1997).

In the United States, the number of individuals with diabetes is predicted to increase 165%, from 11 million in 2000 to 29 million in 2050 (Boyle, et al., 2001). One investigation reported that between 1988 and 1994, the prevalence of the metabolic syndrome (a constellation of risk factors, including impaired glucose regulation, insulin resistance, raised arterial pressure, raised plasma triglyceride, and central obesity) increased among U.S. adults, aged 20 and older, especially among women. Ford, et al. (2004) found that the increase in the prevalence of the metabolic syndrome was due to increases in high blood pressure, waist circumference, and high triglycerides. The increase in the prevalence of the metabolic syndrome is likely to produce future increases in the prevalence of diabetes and cardiovascular disease.

Age disparities in diabetes have been found. The greatest percent increase in diagnosed diabetes is projected to be among those persons 75 years and older (271% increase in women and 437% increase in men) (Boyle, et al., 2001). It is projected that the fastest growing ethnic/racial group with diagnosed diabetes will be African-American males (363% increase between 2000 and 2050), followed by African-American females (217% increase), White males (148% increase), and White females (107% increase).

The rise in the prevalence of type-2 diabetes is associated with an increase in the prevalence of obesity. One report estimates that there are at least 1.1 billion adults who are overweight and 312 million who are obese (James, 2004). Another study estimated that the prevalence of obesity (a body mass index greater or equal to $30 \text{kg}/\text{m}^2$) among United States adults in 2000 was 19.8% and the prevalence of diabetes was 7.3% (Mokdad, 2001).

Of particular concern is that children and adolescents have some of the same risk factors as adults, and there is a growing epidemic of type 2 diabetes among children and adolescents. Duncan, et al. (2004) discovered that among adolescents in the United States, especially overweight adolescents, there was a significant increase in the incidence of the metabolic syndrome. Based on an initial sample of 2,165 adolescents, aged 12 to 19 years, the authors reported an increased prevalence of the metabolic syndrome in both sexes, although it was more prevalent in adolescent males than females. An increased prevalence of the metabolic syndrome was discovered in all three major racial and ethnic groups.

Trends in Arthritis, Osteoporosis, Fibromyalgia, and Low Back Pain

In the United States, arthritis, other rheumatic conditions, and musculoskeletal disorders are the leading cause of disability and impaired quality of life. In 2001, seventy million U.S. adults were afflicted with arthritis and other rheumatic conditions (MMWR Morb Mortal Wkly Rep, 2003). Age disparities in arthritis have been found, with older persons being at greater risk for developing arthritis and other rheumatic diseases. Given the projected growth of the older population, it is expected that the number of older persons with arthritis will double in the next 25 years (Leveille, 2004).

Rheumatoid arthritis, an inflammatory condition that usually affects multiple joints, is a painful, disabling disorder that can lead to joint destruction with major adverse economic, physical, and social effects (Woolf and Pfleger, 2003; Dai, et al., 2003). Rheumatoid arthritis affects 0.3 to 1.0% of the general population and is more prevalent among women and in developed nations (Woolf and Pfleger, 2003). Rheumatoid arthritis occurs in 1% of the adult population worldwide (Markenson, 1991).

Another type of arthritis, osteoarthritis, is characterized by the loss of joint cartilage, which can result in pain and disability primarily in the knees, hips, and ankles (Woolf and Pfleger, 2003; Felson, 2004). Osteoarthritis afflicts 9.6% of men and 18% of women over the age of 60. It is the leading cause of pain and disability among the elderly and is the 3rd leading cause of life-years lost due to disability (March and Bagga, 2004; Carmona, et al., 2001). Because of increases in life expectancy and the aging of populations, osteoarthritis is expected to become the 4th leading cause of disability by 2020 (Woolf and Pfleger, 2003).

Forty-four million women and men, ages 50 years or older, develop osteoporosis and osteopenia (Hansen and Vondracek, 2004). Osteoporosis, a condition involving low bone mass and microarchitectural deterioration, significantly increases the risks of fractures of the hip, vertebrae, and distal forearm (Woolf and Pfleger, 2003). The most serious fracture is that of the hip since it is related to a 20% mortality rate and a 50% permanent disability rate. Gender disparities in osteoporosis are well known with women having a higher prevalence of the disease and related impairment, than men.

Fibromyalgia has been described as a disorder of endocrine stress responses. The disease consists of a collection of symptoms that have no identifiable cause, although the set of symptoms are clearly considered a distinct disease (Cymet, 2003). Some research indicates that psychosocial stress is implicated in the etiology of the disease and exacerbates the pain symptoms (Dedert, et al., 2004). This controversial pain syndrome has increasingly become a major source of disability claims (Wolfe and Potter, 1996). Gender disparities in fibromyalgia have been found, with women having higher rates of the disease and impairment than men.

The most prevalent musculoskeletal disorder is low back pain, a leading cause of disability (Ozguler, et al., 2004; Ehrlich, 2003a; Ehrlich, 2003b). Almost everyone suffers from low back pain at some point in their life, and at any given time, it is estimated that 4% to 30% of the population suffers from low back pain (Woolf and Pfleger, 2003). Another estimate is that the annual prevalence of low back pain is between 15% and 45% (Ozguler, et al., 2004).

Trends in Cardiovascular Disease

Despite enhanced patient care, greater public awareness, and extensive use of medical innovations, cardiovascular disease remains the leading cause of death in the United States (MMWR, 2001). Lifestyle and socioeconomic factors are major contributors to cardiovascular disease and associated mortality and morbidity. Cigarette smoking causes over 400,000 deaths annually and is a major cause of coronary heart disease (Burns, 2003). Obesity, a sedentary lifestyle, and socioeconomic status factors are also major risk factors for cardiovascular disease morbidity and mortality.

Trends in Cancer

According to the American Cancer Society, 1,368,000 new cases of cancer and 563,700 deaths are expected in the United States in 2004. Among men, cancer incidence rates stabilized between 1995 and 2000, while cancer incidence rates continued to increase between 1987 and 2000 among women. Among men, cancer death rates have continued to decrease from three sites (lung and bronchus, colon and rectum, and prostate), while among women, cancer death rates have continued to decrease from two sites (female breast and colon and rectum) (Jemal, et al., 2004).

Large ethnic and racial disparities occur in the prevalence of cancer. African-American men and women have the highest rates of cancer mortality: 40% and 20% higher mortality rates from all cancers than White men and women, respectively (Jemal, et al., 2004).

It is estimated that 172,570 new cases of lung cancer (both small cell and non-small cell) and 163,510 lung cancer-related deaths will occur in the United States in 2005 (National Cancer Institute, MedNews, www.meb.uni-bonn.de/cancer.gov). In the United States, breast cancer is the most prevalent cancer in women (Harwood, 2004). It is projected that in 2005, more than 215,000 women in the United States will be diagnosed with invasive breast cancer, and more than 40,000 will die from the disease (Eneman, et al., 2004). In western countries, colorectal adenocarcinoma is the second cause of death due to cancer (Pasetto, et al., 2005). It is projected that more than one million cases of skin cancer will be diagnosed in 2005. Of these cancers, about 80% will be basal cell carcinoma, 16% squamous cell carcinoma, and 4% melanoma (Tung and Vidimos, The Cleveland Clinic, www.clevelandclinicmeded. com).

2

Health Care Costs

Chronic health problems account for a substantial part of health care costs. Annually, three diseases, cardiovascular disease (including stroke), cancer, and diabetes, make up about $700 billion in direct and indirect economic costs (Eyre, et al., 2004). The costs of these chronic diseases are increased due to acute and chronic complications and co-morbidities. Furthermore, co-morbidities associated with chronic disorders can worsen disease outcomes and increase health care costs (Mikulis, 2003; Peter, et al., 2004). One study of the costs of dialysis for end-stage renal disease revealed higher costs for patients with diabetes or cardiovascular disease (Peter, et al., 2004).

The lack of health insurance for more than 45 million people in the United States limit access to prompt diagnosis and treatment and increase morbidity, mortality, and health care costs. As a result, many people who do not have access to regular health care, will not take advantage of preventive health services, will delay in obtaining in health care, and will rely on expensive emergency care services for primary care medical conditions. As a result of these socioeconomic disparities, health care costs are higher than they would be if the people had access to and used a regular source of health care.

The malpractice crisis in the U.S., with its escalating malpractice insurance rates, increasing numbers of malpractice claims, and greater emphasis on practicing defensive medicine, has had adverse effects on the health care system. The costs of hospital and physician services have increased, thus resulting in an increase in the costs of employer-provided health insurance, which in turn, has reduced the number of workers and their families covered by employer-provided health insurance (Rubin and Mendelson, 1994). Rubin and Mendelson (1994) estimated that comprehensive medical malpractice reform on a systemwide basis could produce $41 billion in savings over five years.

The rapid aging of the U.S. population results in higher direct and indirect health care costs because of the large numbers of older patients who suffer from multiple chronic, disabling diseases which require expensive, long-term treatment and rehabilitation (Berto, et al., 2002; Daviglus, et al., 2004).

Daviglus et al. (2004) found that the increasing prevalence of overweight and obesity in the U.S. population increases the direct and indirect costs of health care since these conditions are related to an increased incidence of costly chronic disorders, such as diabetes, cardiovascular disease, cancer, and arthritis. They evaluated the relationship between body mass index in young adulthood and middle age and Medicare expenditures associated with cardiovascular disease and diabetes in older age. Using data from the Chicago Heart Association Detection Project in Industry and Medicare data, they reported that overweight and obesity among young and middle-aged adults resulted in subsequently higher Medicare charges in later life. The total average annual Medicare charges for non-overweight, overweight, obese, and severely obese men were $7,205, $8,390, $10,128, and $13,674, respectively.

Inadequate "health literacy" is a major contributor to the rising costs of health care. "Health literacy" refers to the ability to read, comprehend, and act on health information. Andrus and Roth (2002) noted that up to 48% of English-speaking patients have insufficient health literacy. Such patients have communication problems which may lead to adverse outcomes (American Medical Association, 1999). Patients with inadequate health literacy are more likely to report poor health status, have less understanding about their health problems, use preventive and clinical services less, have poorer compliance rates, poorer health status, and are more likely to be hospitalized for their health conditions than more literate individuals (Andrus and Roth, 2002; Williams, et al., 2002; American Medical Association, 1999).

Other factors that increase health costs are: cultural and ethnic obstacles to health care provider/patient communication, the practice of defensive medicine which results in the use of unnecessary procedures and hospitalizations, inappropriate or inadequate diagnostic and treatment procedures, unnecessary hospitalizations, and excessive length of hospital stays (Rizzo and Simons, 1997).

Technological innovations in diagnostic, therapeutic, and health care information technologies such as electronic medical records and telemedicine offer the potential of reducing health care costs (Hersh, et al., 2001). However, more research is needed to determine the cost reductions associated with the use of these technologies.

The costs related to specific chronic disorders are evaluated below.

Diabetes

Diabetes costs make up one of every four Medicare dollars and one of every seven health care dollars spent in the United States for a total of $98 billion each year (http://www.diabetesliving.com). The direct annual medical cost of diabetes-related blindness per patient is $2,000 (http://www.diabetesliving.com). The overall cost is expected to increase to $48 million per year because of the approximately 24,000 new cases of diabetes-related blindness projected to occur each year. Diabetes is also the leading cause of kidney failure and is involved in 40% of all new dialysis patients. Because the annual cost per patient for dialysis is $45,000, new cases of kidney failure increase the cost of diabetes by more than a billion dollars per year.

In addition, diabetes is the most frequent cause of lower limb amputations, with an annual loss of 56,000 limbs. The cost per amputation is $29,500, resulting in a $1.5 billion escalation in the cost of diabetes each year. Overall, diabetic patients incur a total annual per capita medical expenditure of $10,071 compared to $2,669 for persons without diabetes.

Arthritis, Osteoporosis, Fibromyalgia, and Low Back Pain

Arthritis and other rheumatic conditions and musculoskeletal disorders place a huge economic burden on society in terms of direct medical costs as well as the social costs associated with disability and social impairment. It is estimated that the social and economic costs of arthritis accounts for 1 to 2.5% of the gross national product of developed countries (Reginster, 2002). In the United States, the total cost of arthritis and other rheumatic disorders was $116.3 billion in 1997, with $51.1 billion in direct costs and $65.2 billion in indirect costs (MMWR Morbidity Mortal Wkly Rep, 2003). The total costs related to arthritis and other rheumatic disorders ranged from $163 million in Wyoming to $11.3 billion in California.

Michaud, et al. (2003) found that for patients with rheumatoid arthritis, the mean total annual direct costs of medical care in 2001 was $9,519, with the costs of drugs being $6,324, and that of hospitalization was $1,573. For patients receiving biologic therapy, the mean total annual direct costs were $19,016.

The costs of rheumatoid arthritis care may be associated with the patient's level of work disability and other health status. In a study of medical care costs for 1,471 rheumatoid arthritis patients in Japan, Hashimoto, et al. (2002) showed that work disability, physical disability, and rate of functional decline were strong predictors of total out-of-pocket medical care costs.

For osteoarthritis, a review of clinical trial outcome research showed that total hip replacement and total knee replacement were the most efficacious and cost-effective treatments. Total hip replacement and total knee replacement surgery have an estimated cost per quality-adjusted life-year (QALY) of $7,500 and $1,000, respectively. Other cost-effective treatments include exercise and strength training for knee osteoarthritis (less than $5,000 per QALY), knee bracing, and use of Capsaicin or Glucosamine Sulfate (less than $1,000 per QALY). The researchers found that measurement of the cost-effectiveness of non-specific and COX-2 inhibitor non-steroidal anti-inflammatory drugs were influenced by treatment-related deaths and very sensitive to the discounting of lost life-years (Segal, et al., 2004).

With the increase in the prevalence of arthritis and related conditions, the direct and indirect costs of arthritis will also grow (Reginster, 2002). For example, the numbers and rates of hip and knee replacements for older persons increased significantly between 1982 and 1999, but the length of hospitalization for both types of surgeries declined (Millar, 2002).

More than 1.5 million osteoporosis-related fractures occur annually (Orsini, et al., 2005) and the aging population will increase the social and economic costs of osteoporosis on the United States health care system (Burge, et al., 2003). One study evaluated commercial claims involving osteoporosis patients with and without a concurrent fracture and a control group of non-osteoporosis patients enrolled in U.S. plans (Orsini, et al., 2005). The results showed that osteoporosis patients with concurrent fracture had total health care expenditures that were more than twice those of osteoporosis patients who did not have a concurrent fracture ($15,942 vs. $6,476) and almost 3 times those of the control patients ($15,942 vs. $4,658).

The costs of osteoporosis in the United States have also been estimated for individual states. Burge, et al. (2003) found that Florida, with its large over-65 population, had an estimated 86,428 osteoporotic fractures that cost more than $1 billion in the year 2000. It is estimated that by 2025, the incident osteoporotic fractures will rise to 151,622, costing more than $2 billion. In California, it was estimated that osteoporosis was responsible for over $2.4 billion in direct health care costs in 1998 and more than $4 million in lost productivity associated with premature death (Max, et al., 2002).

The costs of fibromyalgia add to the overall costs of health care because of the extensive use of health services made by fibromyalgia patients. Penrod, et al. (2004) found that, in Canada, the average 6-month direct cost among women with primary fibromyalgia was $2,298 (Canadian dollars), with the indirect costs being $5,035. Medications ($758 Canadian dollars), complementary and alternative medicine ($398 Canadian dollars) and diagnostic services ($356 Canadian dollars) made up the largest components of direct cost.

The researchers also showed that co-morbid conditions and disability associated with fibromyalgia were important contributors to the direct costs.

Low back pain poses a huge cost to society because of the costs of medical treatment, lost productivity, and non-monetary costs, such as the reduced ability to perform usual activities (Ozguler, et al., 2004; U.S. Agency for Health Care Policy and Research, 1994). It is estimated that 80% of adults suffer at least one episode of low back pain during their lifetimes (Humphreys, et al., 2002; Koes, et al., 1996). Persons who have low back pain and degenerative joint disease make up 4.9% of all adult physician visits. The annual direct medical costs associated with low back pain are more than $25 billion (Humphreys, et al., 2002).

Cardiovascular Disease

Cardiovascular disease, associated coronary heart disease, and atherothrombotic disease cause a major economic and social burden on society. The direct medical cost of cardiovascular and circulatory diseases was estimated to be $151 billion in 1995 (Lightwood, 2003).

Hypertension, a risk factor for cardiovascular disease and diabetes, is one of the most commonly diagnosed chronic medical problems and creates a major economic and social burden on Americans. Mullins, et al. (2004) show that uncontrolled hypertension significantly increases health care costs. They discovered that when compared to the costs of the care of controlled hypertensive patients, the average total annualized costs for emergency department visits and hospitalizations for uncontrolled hypertensive patients was greater by 9.3% and 28.0%, respectively.

Resource utilization and costs associated with clinical care for stroke patients have a significant impact on health care costs (Doedel, et al., 2004). In 2004, stroke accounted for an estimated $53.6 billion in direct and indirect health care costs (MMWR Morbidity and Mortality Weekly Report, 2005).

Various factors may escalate health care costs for patients with cardiovascular disease or those who are at risk for the disease. Based on a longitudinal study of patients with hypertension, Berto, et al. (2002) found that the average total cost per patient is likely to increase due to age and co-morbidities.

Cancer

In the United States, the economic burden of cancer in 2002 was estimated to be $172 billion, which included $61 billion in direct medical costs (United States DHHS, 2003). The most prevalent types of cancer pose the greatest economic burden. One report estimated that colorectal cancer, the second leading cause of cancer death in the United States, and the third most prevalent cancer throughout the world, accounted for $5.3 billion in direct and indirect costs in the United States in 2000 (Redaelli, et al., 2003; Giovannucci, 2003). The economic impact of cancer is expected to worsen greatly as survival from cancer improves and as the U.S. population ages. Over the next decades, public sector programs, such as Medicare and Medicaid, will have the challenging tasks of paying for comprehensive cancer care with limited fiscal resources (United States DHHS, 2003). More research is needed to determine how economic factors influence clinical outcomes for cancer patients and how to best use cancer prevention, screening and treatment strategies.

3

Living with a Chronic Disease

Mark L. Goldstein
Chicago School of Professional Psychology

People diagnosed with chronic diseases must adjust to the demands of the illness itself, as well as to the treatments for their condition. The illness may affect a person's mobility and independence, and change the way a person lives, sees him or herself, and/or relates to others (The Cleveland Clinic, 2003). There are dramatic reductions in physical, psychological, and social well-being. A certain amount of sadness is normal, but in some instances, a chronic disease may actually cause depression, anxiety, anger, sleep disorders, and/or substance abuse.

Chronic illnesses have been found to be consistently associated with an increased prevalence of depressive symptoms and disorders (Anderson, et al., 2001). In some cases, depression appears to result from specific biologic effects of the chronic medical illness, particularly in Parkinson's disease, multiple sclerosis, and cerebrovascular disease. In other cases, the association between depression and chronic disease appears to be mediated by behavioral mechanisms, in that the limitations on activity imposed by the illness lead to gradual withdrawal from formerly enjoyable activities (Prince, et al., 1998).

Depression also increases the overall burden of illness in patients with chronic illness. For example, a study by Unutzer, et al. (2002) revealed an association between depression and mortality resulting from cardiovascular disease. Other studies have shown that depression is associated with a poorer prognosis and more rapid progression of chronic illnesses, including diabetes (deGroot, et al., 2001) and ischemic heart disease (Glassman, et al., 1998).

Anderson, et al. (2001) studied patients with both Type 1 and Type 2 diabetes from 39 studies and concluded that diabetes doubled the odds of developing depression. The odds of depression were significantly higher in women than in men, a pattern that mirrors the female preponderance of depression in epidemiological studies of the general population.

According to the Cleveland Clinic (2003), the risk of getting depression in the general population is 10–25% for women and 5–12% for men, but it is much higher for those with chronic diseases—25–33%. For example, the rate of depression for those with Parkinson's disease and multiple sclerosis is 40%. The rate of depression is even higher for those with coronary heart disease, who have suffered a heart attack; 40–65% of these individuals will develop depression. For those who suffer a stroke, 10–27% will develop depression. Sullivan (1992) found that patients with chronic low back pain had a prevalence of major depression three to four times greater than the normal population.

More significantly, psychosocial factors, particularly depression, appear to impact the development and progression of such chronic diseases as coronary heart disease and HIV/AIDS (Schneiderman, et al., 2001). All too often, patients and family members overlook the symptoms of depression, assuming that feeling depressed is normal for someone dealing with a serious, chronic disease. Furthermore, symptoms of depression are also frequently masked by other medical conditions, resulting in treatment for the symptoms, but not the underlying cause of the depression. Some chronic illnesses, for example, multiple sclerosis, have both a biological and an environmental component to the depression, further complicating diagnosis and treatment.

Common symptoms of depression include depressed mood, loss of interest or pleasure in daily activities, significant weight loss or gain, sleep disturbances, problems with concentration and/or memory, apathy, lack of energy or fatigue, feelings of worthlessness or guilt, and recurrent thoughts of death or suicide.

Suicidal ideation among individuals suffering from chronic illnesses has not been widely studied, although rates of completed suicide are believed to be elevated in this population relative to the general population (Fisher, et al., 2001). The literature on suicide suggests that chronic pain patients are at greater risk for depression than the general population. Fishbain (1991) reviewed 18 studies relating to the association of chronic pain and suicide. These studies indicated that suicide ideation, suicide attempts and suicide completion are commonly found in individuals with chronic pain. In addition, a number of controlled studies and suicide completion rate studies indicated that chronic pain might be a suicide risk factor. Furthermore, a review of central pain patients by Gonzales (1995) revealed that the risk of suicide is significant in patients with poorly controlled pain. Penttinen (1995) uncovered a relationship between back pain and suicide among Finnish farmers, while Fishbain, et al. (1991) studied patients in a pain center and found that the completed suicide rate for chronic pain patients was significantly higher than that of the general population.

Smith, et al. (2004) studied the role of sleep onset insomnia and pain intensity in individuals with chronic musculoskeletal pain, and the evidence of suicidal ideation in these individuals. They discovered that chronic pain patients with self-reported insomnia with concomitant high pain intensity were more likely to report passive suicidal ideation, independent from the effects of depression severity. In another study, Stenager, et al. (1994) found that among suicide attempters, 52% suffered from a disease and 21% were on daily analgesics for pain.

DeLeo and Spanthonis (2003) reviewed epidemiological studies of suicide in the elderly. Their review revealed that assisted suicide and euthanasia in the elderly have been associated with the desire to escape chronic physical pain and suffering caused by illness, and to relieve mental anguish and feelings of hopelessness and depression. Roscoe, et al. (2003) found that poorly controlled pain was a factor in seeking assistance in dying. In this study, Dr. Jack Kavorkian's patients were studied and the most common diagnoses were amyotrophic lateral sclerosis or multiple sclerosis, inadequately controlled pain, and a recent decline in health. Magni, et al. (1998) found that rates for thoughts about death, wishing to die, suicidal ideation, and suicide attempts were two to three times more frequent in those with chronic pain compared with those without chronic pain. Furthermore, oncology patients with concomitant pain and depression were significantly more likely to request assistance in committing suicide as well as actively taking steps to end their own lives (Emanuel, et al., 1996).

Although depression is the most commonly reported psychological symptom by patients with chronic diseases, many patients also report anxiety symptoms as well. Reich, et al. (1983) evaluated several studies of patients from pain clinics and found that depression and anxiety were common. Linton and Gotestam (1985) studied the relationship between pain, anxiety, mood, and muscle tension in chronic pain patients and found that psychological variables were related to the experience of chronic pain, but that there was a high degree of variability among individuals. In another study, Hadjistavropoulos, et al. (2002) evaluated 65 patients with chronic pain and the role of anxiety in pain. They found that health anxiety played a role in pain behavior.

Although patients with chronic illnesses may complain about depression and anxiety, they may also exhibit signs of increased irritability, lower frustration tolerance and bouts of anger. This may be the result of sleep disturbance and/or a component of depression. Individuals with chronic illnesses, particularly those with pain conditions, often have sleep disorders. For example, fibromyalgia sufferers were found to have abnormalities on sleep studies and were reported to be deficient in deep, non-dream sleep. In addition, they were also found to have an unusual persistence of alpha activity during sleep.

Difficulty with sleep can complicate matters for the chronically ill, in that it impairs their social, educational, and occupational functioning and make them vulnerable to accidents and susceptible to other health problems. Sleep disorder also impair the person's ability to cope with the stress that the chronic condition causes.

There is also an increased risk of substance abuse, whether alcohol, illegal drugs and/or prescribed medications in people with chronic diseases. At times, self-medication may be a means of coping with pain and/or depression. In other instances, the use of alcohol or drugs may assist a person in getting to sleep, although alcohol and many drugs, including marijuana, in fact, interfere with adequate sleep and interfere with the REM sleep in particular.

Traditionally, individuals with chronic illnesses have been treated with medication, notably anxiolytics for the anxiety and stress and antidepressants for depression. Furthermore, the analgesic properties of antidepressants have been well established. Tricyclic antidepressants have been commonly prescribed for the treatment of many chronic pain syndromes, especially neuropathic pain. Current research suggests that the analgesic effect of antidepressants is mediated by the blockade of reuptake of Serotonin and Norepinephrine. The resulting increase of the levels of these neurotransmitters enhances the activation of descending inhibitory neurons (King, 1981). Tricyclic antidepressants have been the most effective in relieving neuropathic pain (Gruber, et al., 1996). The efficacy of serotonin reuptake inhibitors has been variable and inconsistent. For example, Paroxetine (Paxil) was not found to be beneficial in a study of patients with diabetic neuropathy (Sindrup et al., 1990). Yet, Floxetine (Prosac) was found to be equal to Amitriptyline (Elavil) in significantly reducing the pain in patients with rheumatoid arthritis (Rani, et al., 1996). Venlafaxine (Effexor), Nefazodine (Serzone), Mirtazapine (Remeron) and other antidepressants have also been studied with variable results.

In addition, psychotherapy has been utilized as an adjunctive treatment approach with chronically ill patients. Although individual counseling has been widely used for many years, there has been an increase in family involvement and family therapy in recent years in the treatment of patients with chronic diseases. The role of the family in the development and perpetuation of chronic pain conditions has drawn considerable empirical attention (Kerns and Otis, 2003). Although family systems and family stress theories have been the major models in the family therapy literature, these perspectives have had a limited impact on advancing an understanding of family relationships in the context of chronic illness.

Moore and Chaney (1985) were the first to report on the effi-cacy of a treatment approach utilizing the spouse of the person experiencing pain. In their study, they compared a patient only group with a couples group. Both groups received education, problem solving skills training, relaxation training, and assertive-ness training. Both treatment groups improved significantly, in comparison to a control group. Other more recent studies testing the efficacy of cognitive-behavioral, operant conditioning, and coping skills training with arthritic, myofacial, and other chronic pain conditions were effective. However, adding couples, family or spouse involvement did not improve outcome.

Saarijar, et al. (1991) published a series of papers on couples treatment for chronic pain disorders from a family systems per-spective. However, no significant differences were found between the experimental and control groups on measures of pain and pain-related disability.

There has also been an effort to develop a cognitive-behavioral transactional model of family functioning that attempts to integrate aspects of family stress theory and the behavioral perspective on chronic pain (Kerns, et al., 2003). In a more recent article, Kerns and Otis (2004) have further delineated their ideas for the utilization of an integrated family systems model with chronic pain patients.

Case Studies

Cases studies help to illustrate some of the coping mechanisms of persons with chronic diseases. The following two case studies also clarify some of the social, family, and occupational impair-ments of persons with chronic diseases.

Case 1

Rita is a 51-year-old Caucasian female, married with two chil-dren. She had worked as a high school teacher prior to having chil-dren and then worked as a substitute teacher for a number of years after her children were attending school full time. Approximately seven years ago, she was diagnosed with multiple sclerosis (MS), initially presenting with visual problems, including double vision, and muscle weakness. She also experienced muscle twitching and tingling at times. Rita was diagnosed and treated by a neurologist who specialized in patients with MS. She would have periodic exacerbations, which were initially responsive to medication. On two occasions, Rita was hospitalized briefly. As the disease progressed, she stopped working and began to do less around the home, including shopping and cooking. Rita also began to do less with her children, both of whom were still home and in school. Prior to the illness, Rita had been very involved with her family, particularly her children, serving as room parent for each for a number of years, serving as a Parent/Teacher Organization officer on several occasions and coaching her children's athletic teams.

Her neurologist, due to concerns about depression, referred her to a psychiatrist three years ago. Rita complained about fatigue, often slept 12–14 hours per day, had constant somatic complaints including lower back pain, withdrew from friends and family and experienced anhedonia. Prior to the referral to the psychiatrist, she had been taking steroids for exacerbations and Cylert for fatigue. Her psychiatrist initially prescribed Prozac, and subsequently prescribed Serzone, Welbutrin, Zoloft, and Paxil. Rita was also referred to a clinical psychologist for counseling.

Despite medication and counseling, her depression continued. In counseling, Rita complained about weight gain (a common side effect from steroid therapy), feeling useless and chronic pain. She also became increasingly angry—with her family and physicians. Her neurologist prescribed pain medication and she became increasingly dependent on pain medication. Over the next year, Rita began to get various physicians (internist, neurologist, rheumatologist) to prescribe pain medication, leading to abuse of medication. She ultimately had a psychotic episode induced from medication overdose and was hospitalized and detoxed. Rita's husband withdrew from her, while her two children took over many of the household chores and catered to her. Eventually, the entire family became involved in family therapy and each of the family members also had individual counseling to help with coping. At the present time, counseling continues. Medication is now prescribed by only one physician, and all treatment providers have monthly phone contact. Rita's depression remains, but has lessened. Her chronic pain has also lessened, but flares up at times.

Case 2

Frank is a 49-year-old Caucasian male, married with one adult child. After completing high school, he worked as an apprentice electrician before becoming a union electrician. Three years ago, Frank was injured at work when he fell off a ladder and his leg landed on a "horse." He subsequently developed Complex Regional Pain Syndrome-I (CRPS-I) (formerly known as Reflex Sympathetic Dystrophy or RSD), resulting in chronic pain in one foot and leg. Frank saw a specialist at a teaching hospital and was ultimately hospitalized and given intravenous antibiotic therapy, but without success. Another specialist suggested implanting an electrical stimulation block, which he declined. Prior to the accident, Frank could best be described as a workaholic, typically working 50–55 hours per week and never missing a day due to illness.

As the pain continued, Frank began to compensate when he walked, ultimately resulting in the necessity of back surgery. He became increasingly angry, often yelling at his wife and son. In addition, Frank became significantly depressed and frustrated. He consulted with a number of surgeons, seeking to have his leg and foot amputated. No physician would perform such an operation, resulting in an exacerbation of his depression and anger. His primary care physician referred him to a psychiatrist, but he disliked the way the medication made him feel and he discontinued antidepressant medication as a result. Finally, his physician referred him to a clinical psychologist for counseling. The focus of therapy was primarily on pain management and coping strategies, and secondarily, on support. Early in treatment, Frank's wife called and said that Frank had a shotgun in his mouth and was threatening suicide. Frank refused to admit himself to a psychiatric hospital, but agreed to go to a rehabilitation hospital, where he learned biofeedback and self-hypnosis. Although he continues to be in chronic pain, he is no longer suicidal. Furthermore, Frank volunteers in his community for several organizations, giving him a new purpose in his life. His anger continues, but to a far lesser degree. In counseling, he has focused on anger management, which has significantly helped control his anger.

4

Diabetes Mellitus

Persons with diabetes mellitus and lesser abnormalities of glucose tolerance are at risk of developing cardiovascular disease and the metabolic syndrome, a constellation of metabolic and vascular abnormalities, including central obesity, insulin resistance, hyper-insulinemia, glucose intolerance, hypertension, dyslipidemia, hypercoagulability, and increased risk of coronary and cerebral vascular disease (Hamdy, 2005; McVeigh and Cohn, 2003; Schulze, et al., 2004). Individuals with type 2 diabetes mellitus have a 2- to 4-fold increased risk of coronary heart disease (CHD) and a 4-fold increase in mortality from CHD. In addition, there is an increased risk of cardiovascular mortality before the development of type 2 diabetes (Haffner and Cassells, 2003). It is thought that the increase in cardiovascular disease and fatal coronary heart disease is due to hypertension, hyperglycemia, hyperinsulinemia, dyslipidemia, inflammation, and the prothrombotic state (Grant, 2005; Eckel, et al., 2002).

Studies in apparently healthy persons have also emphasized the role of inflammatory and atherothrombotic mechanisms that may have relevance to persons with diabetes mellitus (Dandona, et al., 2003; Balagopal, et al., 2005; Grant, 2005). Because most diabetes-related deaths are due to cardiovascular disease, management strategies must involve both reducing coronary heart disease risk factors and improving traditional diabetic risk factors, such as glycemic control, and non-traditional risk factors, such as inflammatory and atherothrombotic aspects of diabetes (Grant, 2005; Gavin, 2004).

A discussion of the risk factors for and complications of type 2 diabetes are discussed below.

Genetic Factors

Type 2 diabetes has a major genetic basis. However, the molecular process is not well understood, but it is believed that the mode of inheritance is probably polygenic. Penetrance is influenced by environmental factors (Shaw, et al., 1999). Investigations have demonstrated that a history of parental diabetes is directly related to an increased chance of developing type 2 diabetes (Wei, et al., 1999).

Although family aggregation of type 2 diabetes has been established, Shaw, et al. (1999) note that little is known about the prevalence of diabetes in the relatives of persons with diabetes compared to the general population. They evaluated the relative risks of hyperglycemia, obesity, and dyslipidemia in the relatives of patients with type 2 diabetes using a sample of 139 first degree relatives of 90 index cases with type 2 diabetes and a control population from Oxfordshire, England. The results indicated that there is a major familial aggregation of hyperglycemia and obesity in the relatives of index cases. These relatives also had higher fasting plasma insulin concentrations and lower high density lipoprotein (HDL)-cholesterol levels than individuals in the general population. The investigators recommend that first degree relatives of probands with type 2 diabetes should be targeted for screening and intervention to improve the metabolic status of these individuals.

Mohan, et al. (2003) evaluated the effects of family history of diabetes, obesity, and lifestyle factors on glucose intolerance on a population in the southern part of India and found that these factors have a synergistic impact on increasing diabetic risks. Individuals who came from higher socioeconomic status backgrounds and had a positive family history of diabetes had a five times greater prevalence of glucose intolerance (diabetes + impaired glucose tolerance) when compared to those with lower socioeconomic status and no family history of diabetes. The investigators note that lifestyle factors and family history of diabetes have a synergistic impact on increasing diabetic risks.

Age

Age disparities have been identified among persons with type 2 diabetes, hypertension, and hyperlipidemia (Pontiroli and Galli, 1998; Wei, et al., 1999). For example, one investigation showed that age above 50 years predicted low levels of HDL-cholesterol (Devroey, et al., 2004). Gavin (2004) noted that the highest rate of type 2 diabetes occurs at 60 years of age and older.

However, the fastest growing segment of the population with type 2 diabetes is under the age 39. These results point to the need to target older adults as well as other high-risk age groups, such as children and adolescents, who have sedentary lifestyles, poor nutritional habits, and additional risk factors for obesity, type 2 diabetes, hypertension, hyperlipidemia, and cardiovascular disease.

Gender

Gender is not consistently linked to increased diabetic risk factors. Research has found that African-American women with type 2 diabetes have a higher risk of cardiovascular morbidity and mortality compared to African-American males and whites with type 2 diabetes. Gaillard, et al. (1998) suggest that it is possible that there is a greater clustering of pre-existing cardiovascular disease risk factors among African-American females than among African-American males and whites. They evaluated possible gender differences in cardiovascular risk factors based on a sample of 84 healthy first-degree relatives of African-American patients with type 2 diabetes (42 males and 42 females matched for age and waist-to-hip circumference ratio). The findings revealed that African-American females had higher body mass index, % body fat, mean fasting and 2-hour postprandial serum glucose, and insulin levels than among African-American males.

Another study, however, showed that male gender was associated with the risk factors for diabetes (Devroey, et al., 2004). The
authors reported that being male was related to a low level of high-
density lipoprotein and a high level of triglycerides.

Ethnic/Racial Disparities

In the United States, disparities in risks for chronic diseases
occur among certain disadvantaged racial and ethnic groups
(Bolen, et al., 2000). For example, racial and ethnic differences in
diabetic risk factors and the prevalence of diabetes have been
reported. Using data from the 1997 Behavioral Risk Factor Surveillance System, Bolen, et al. (2000) showed that African-Americans, Hispanics, and American-Indians or Alaska Natives were
more likely than whites to report diabetes, obesity, no leisure-time
physical activity, and fair or poor health. There is also higher prevalence of insulin resistance among Mexican-Americans and American-Indians, and higher triglyceride levels among the Japanese
(Kuller, 2004).

Studies have revealed racial and ethnic disparities in diabetic
complications. Based on a longitudinal cohort study of 429,918
veterans with diabetes, Young, et al. (2003) reported that African-
Americans and Native-Americans were more likely than whites to
develop early diabetic nephropathy. Moreover, African-Americans,
Hispanic, Asians, and Native-Americans were more likely to
develop end-stage renal disease. In terms of African-American/
white disparities, these differences may be due to a higher susceptibility to type 2 diabetes in African-Americans or that the risk
factors for type 2 diabetes have a more profound impact in African-
Americans.

Socioeconomic Disparities

It is not clear what accounts for the ethnic and racial disparities in type 2 diabetes. Many of the reported ethnic and racial
differences in risk factors and disease in the United States may be
a function of disparities in socioeconomic status and inadequate

utilization of preventive and clinical health services (Kuller, 2004). In fact, various studies reveal that lower socioeconomic status is associated with the early development of diabetes (Gaillard, et al., 1997). Research has shown that risk factors for diabetes and coronary heart disease have increased in low-educational status groups.

Cirera, et al. (1998) evaluated the link between socioeconomic status factors and cardiovascular risk using a random sample of 3,091 adults. They discovered that low educational attainment is related to a greater prevalence of arterial hypertension in both women and men and overweight in women. In addition, higher educational status is positively associated with leisure-time physical activity in men and women.

Based on two successive coronary risk surveys in an urban Asian Indian population, one study found that over a seven year period, obesity, diabetes, LDL-cholesterol, low HDL- cholesterol, and triglycerides increased in this population (Gupta, et al., 2003). Three risk factors, smoking, diabetes, and dyslipidemia increased more in persons with low educational attainment.

Stelmach, et al. (2005) assessed the impact of education, income, and other factors on risk factors for cardiovascular disease among 2,000 men and 2,000 women in Lodz, Poland. He found that low education is a major predictor of the metabolic syndrome.

In some studies, however, high socioeconomic status has been linked to an increased risk of diabetic and cardiovascular risk factors. As noted previously, Mohan, et al. (2003), discovered that individuals with high socioeconomic status and a family history of diabetes had a five times greater prevalence of glucose intolerance than individuals from lower socioeconomic status backgrounds with no family history of diabetes.

In two successive coronary risk surveys in an urban Indian population, higher educational level was shown to predict smoking in women (Gupta, et al., 2003). A study in Southern Spain, based on 1,514 men and 1,577 women, also showed that high educational level is linked to cigarette smoking in women (Cirera, et al., 1998).

Based on a sample of 260 in Karachi, 157 low-income children and 103 middle-income children, Hydrie, et al. (2005) evaluated dietary habits, body mass index, physical activity and other risk factors. They discovered that both low-income and middle-income children had increased diabetic risk factors. For example, children from both the low-income and middle-income groups had poor dietary habits, e.g. a diet low in fruits, vegetables, and milk and high in fat content. However, children from the middle-income group had more risk factors for diabetes.

Psychosocial Factors

A number of psychological, social, and occupational conditions are thought to increase the incidence of diabetes (Kumari, et al., 2004; Stelmach, et al., 2005). Feelings of control over the environment may be predictive of diabetes incidence. A prospective occupational cohort investigation of 10,308 civil servants, aged 35 to 55 years, from the Whitehall Study revealed that depression was associated with diabetes incidence and impaired glucose tolerance (Kumari, et al., 2004). The investigators also found that an imbalance in effort-reward on the job was related to incidence of diabetes in men.

Likewise, Stelmach, et al. (2005) note that low levels of perceived control over the environment, e.g., having unfulfilled work, receiving little reward for effort and having unfulfilled needs on a daily basis predict the constellation of metabolic abnormalities known as the metabolic syndrome, e.g., abdominal obesity, high blood pressure, hypertriglyceridemia.

Overweight and Obesity

According to Perry (2002), the global epidemic of type 2 diabetes is mainly caused by the globalization of sedentary and Western lifestyles and culture. There is increasing evidence of synergistic interactions among diet, obesity, physical inactivity, smoking, and excessive alcohol use in causing glucose intolerance and type 2 diabetes (Perry, 2002). It is estimated that up to 75% of the risk of type 2 diabetes is due to obesity (Costacou and Mayer-Davis, 2003).

Overweight and obesity (body mass index of $30 \, kg/m^2$, including abdominal or central obesity or greater or equal to 102 cm for men and greater or equal to 88 cm for women) increase the risk of type 2 diabetes and other chronic diseases (Koh-Banerjee, et al., 2003). Being overweight and obese is recognized as major risk factors for type 2 diabetes, hyperlipidemia, hypertension, and cardiovascular disease (Borissova, et al., 2004; Ruland, et al., 2005).

One report by Borissova, et al. (2004) noted that the changes in insulin sensitivity, insulin-receptor binding and beta-cell secretion in individuals with III degree obesity are similar to those in type 2 diabetic patients, suggesting that III degree obesity may be a risk factor for type 2 diabetes. Another study found that individuals with a body mass index greater or equal to 27 kg/m2 had an increased risk of developing type 2 diabetes (Yamagishi, et al., 2003).

The duration of obesity, including central obesity, also has been found to be associated with an increased risk of type 2 diabetes (Nkondjock and Receveur, 2003; Wannamethee and Shaper, 1999). Therefore, it is important to emphasize prevention of obesity in children and adolescents (Pontiroli and Galli, 1998). Diabetes prevention programs have been found to be effective in lowering the risks of type 2 diabetes. Investigations have shown that the reduction in central adiposity, through exercise and diet, is associated with decreases in diabetes and hypertension in various populations. Okosun, et al. (1998) discovered that lifestyle modifications aimed at reducing waist size, such as moderate to vigorous physical activity and diet, produced substantial reductions in the prevalence of diabetes and hypertension in African-origin populations.

Physical Activity

A sedentary lifestyle, which fosters low cardiorespiratory fitness, has been associated with an increased risk for impaired fasting glucose and type 2 diabetes among children, adolescents, and adults (Major, et al., 2005; Eisenmann, 2004). Regular physical activity protects against diabetes and cardiovascular disease possibly by controlling risk factors, such as hypertension and obesity. It is also an independent preventive factor for diabetes and cardiovascular disease.

It is estimated that more than 90% of cases of type 2 diabetes could be prevented by following a healthy lifestyle that included moderate to vigorous physical activity for at least a half hour per day, good nutrition, weight control, and smoking cessation. One investigation evaluated the relationship between prolonged television watching and type 2 diabetes using data from a large prospective cohort study (Hu, 2003). Hu (2003) reported that prolonged television watching is related to an increased risk for type 2 diabetes. Among men, watching television more than 40 hours per week was associated with almost a threefold increase in developing type 2 diabetes compared to those who watched television 1 hour per week.

Major, et al. (2005) studied physical activity in 118 postmenopausal women, and found that higher intensity physical activity is related to a healthier metabolic profile and higher energy expenditure was associated with lower body mass index and lower accumulation of visceral adipose tissue. After controlling for visceral adipose tissue accumulation, higher engagement in physical activity was related to favorable systolic blood pressure, HDL-cholesterol, and insuln sensitivity.

Eisenmann (2004) notes that physical activity levels are reduced during adolescence, and while aerobic fitness remains stable in boys, it gradually declines among adolescent girls. These declining physical activity levels, along with inadequate weight control and poor nutritional intake, contribute to an increased prevalence of overweight, obesity, and type 2 diabetes in children and adolescents, especially among certain ethnic groups (Gavin, 2004; Eisenmann, 2004; Wabitsch, et al., 2003).

Some interventions involving exercise training and other lifestyle changes have been found to be effective in managing glycemic control and improving cardiovascular risk factors among individuals with type 2 diabetes (Lim, et al., 2004). Physical activity also decreases insulin resistance and delays the development of diabetes (Gohlke, 2004).

Diet and Nutrition

Researchers have focused on the role of diet and nutrition in the development of type 2 diabetes (Harding, et al., 2004; van Dam, 2003). Although there are controversies about the relationship between the amount and types of dietary fat and carbohydrates and the risk of type 2 diabetes, studies have demonstrated that alterations in nutrition and physical activity can improve insulin sensitivity and protect against type 2 diabetes (Steyn, et al., 2004; Hu, et al., 2001). It is estimated that more than 90% of cases of type 2 diabetes could be prevented by a diet high in cereal fiber and polyunsaturated fatty acids and low in trans-fatty acids and glycemic load, avoidance of overweight and obesity, participation in moderate to vigorous physical activity for a half hour a day, non-smoking, and moderate consumption of alcohol (Perry, 2002).

Harding, et al. (2004) demonstrated that increased polyunsaturated fat and decreased saturated fat were related to a reduced risk of type 2 diabetes. Steyn, et al. (2004), in their review of clinical trials, noted that high-saturated fat intake and intrauterine growth retardation may increase the risk of type 2 diabetes. The investigators suggest that non-starch polysaccharides, omega-3 fatty acids, low glycemic index foods, and breast-feeding exclusively may protect against the disease. Data from cohort studies and trials indicate that higher consumption of whole grain food and exchanging unsaturated fat for saturated fat and trans fatty acids may reduce the risk for type 2 diabetes (Fung, et al., 2002; Hu, et al., 2001).

Other studies are assessing the impact of fish consumption on risk for type 2 diabetes. Based on an ecological study of 41 countries in five continents, Nkondjock and Receveur (2003) showed that a high consumption of fish and seafood was associated with a reduction in the risk of type 2 diabetes in populations with a high prevalence of obesity.

In addition to studying nutrition in persons with type 2 diabetes, the dietary habits among individuals with type 1 diabetes have been investigated. One investigation in Italy assessed dietary habits and nutritional biomarkers, such as plasma levels of albumin, iron, lipids, homocysteine, vitamin B9 and vitamin B12 and urinary outputs of nitrogen, sodium, and potassium in 38 type 1 diabetic patients, 76 relatives, and 95 controls. The researchers found a number of health problems in the sample. Forty-five percent of the controls were overweight. The proportion of caloric intake obtained from total fat and cholesterol did not conform to accepted guidelines. In only 27% of all participants were intakes of total dietary fiber acceptable. In addition, estimated daily intakes of water-soluble vitamin B9 and fat-soluble vitamin D and vitamin E were below accepted standards. The researchers conclude that deprivation of both vitamin B9 and vitamin E could have an adverse impact on endothelial function because these antioxidants have been found to influence nitric oxide and eicosanoid signaling (Matteucci, et al., 2005).

Metabolic Abnormalities as Risk Factors for Diabetes

A variety of metabolic disorders, including impaired glucose tolerance, insulin resistance, hyperinsulinemia, hyperglycemia, hyperlipidemia, and high tryglericides increase a person's risk of developing type 2 diabetes. Epidemiologic and prospective trials show a connection between impaired glucose tolerance (and/or impaired fasting glucose) and the onset of type 2 diabetes and cardiovascular disease (Irons, et al., 2004; Costa, et al., 2002).

Insulin resistance, which is a major part of the insulin resistance syndrome, and hyperinsulinemia are major risk factors for type 2 diabetes (Nishimura, et al., 2005; Cettour-Rose, et al., 2005). Insulin-resistant persons are also at risk for acquiring cardiovascular disease (Wheatcroft, et al., 2003).

In the pre-insulin dependent diabetes mellitus state, hyperinsulinemia can occur for 5 to 8 years (Borissova, et al., 2004; Suehiro, et al., 2005). Obese individuals are at risk of developing hyperinsulinemia. Elevated plasma nonesterified fatty acid concentrations are responsible for peripheral and hepatic insulin resistance and may cause hyperinsulinemia in obese patients (Wuesten, et al., 2005).

Various molecules/factors, including GLUT-4 (glucose transporter) receptor, tumor necrosis factor-alpha (TNF-alpha), interleukins-6 (IL-6) daf genes and PPARs (peroxisome proliferators-activated receptors) influence the onset of the insulin resistance syndrome and related conditions (Das, 2005). However, the ways in which these molecules/factors interact and the mechanisms by which they trigger the insulin resistance syndrome are not understood.

Enormous attention has been given to PPARs, which are members of the nuclear hormone receptor superfamily of ligand—

activated transcription factors (Zhang, et al., 2005; Terauchi and Kadowaki, 2005). Three PPAR isoforms, PPAR-alpha, -beta/delta, and -gamma, have been discovered, and now it is known that these receptors help to regulate adipogenesis, lipid metabolism, insulin sensitivity, inflammation, and blood pressure. These receptors serve as lipid sensors that regulate the expression of gene arrays, resulting in a modulation of major metabolic events (Berger, et al., 2005).

The three PPAR isoforms have separate expression patterns and influence glucose metabolism based on the need of a specific tissue. PPAR-alpha potentiates fatty acid catabolism in the liver and is the molecular target of the lipid-lowering fibrates. PPAR-gamma plays an important role in adipocyte differentiation and hypertrophy, and mediates the functions of the insulin sensitizing thiazolidinediones. PPAR-delta may be significant in influencing body weight and lipid metabolism in fat tissues (Terauchi and Kadowaki, 2005).

Two PPARs, PPAR-alpha and PPAR-gamma, are related to activation by different ligands. However, a new class of agents, dual alpha-gamma PPAR activators has the potential to activate both receptors. The dual alpha-gamma PPAR activators may influence two cardiovascular risk factors, diabetes and dyslipidemia, by having an effect on glucose and lipid metabolism (Liu, et al., 2005).

Studies suggest that PPAR activity plays a role in causing the metabolic syndrome, which consists of a cluster of metabolic and vascular abnormalities, including central obesity, insulin resistance, hyperinsulinemia, glucose intolerance, hypertension, dyslipidemia, hypercoagulability, and increased risk of coronary and cerebral vascular disease (Zhang, et al., 2005; Hamdy, 2005). The metabolic syndrome is produced through the interaction of lifestyle, genetic, and hormal factors (McVeigh and Cohn, 2003).

This cluster of metabolic and vascular abnormalities, which is highly prevalent, is a major determinant of cardiovascular mortality in developed and developing countries. The elements of the metabolic syndrome and the accelerate phase of atherogenesis are frequently silent (McVeigh and Cohn, 2003).

Abnormally high levels of lipids or hyperlipidemia and triglycerides have been recognized as risk factors for diabetes (Pontiroli and Galli, 1998; Wei, et al., 1999). One investigation of

760 obese individuals revealed that those with hyperlipidemia were older, had a longer duration of obesity, and were more likely to experience impaired glucose tolerance and type 2 diabetes (Pontiroli and Galli, 1998). Another study demonstrated that high triglyceride levels and other factors were associated with the risk of type 2 diabetes (Wei, et al., 1999).

The endothelium is believed to have an essential role in maintaining vascular homeostasis. This process depends on a balance between the production of nitric oxide, superoxide, and other vasoactive substances (Wheatcroft, et al., 2003). Endothelial impairment, an early marker in the etiology of atherosclerosis, has been found in obese, non-diabetic persons (Hamdy, 2005). It has also been identified in patients with type 2 diabetes and in persons at risk for type 2 diabetes, including those with impaired glucose tolerance and normoglycemic first-degree relatives of patients with type 2 diabetes. Endothelial dysfunction and increased arterial stiffness develop early in the onset of diabetic vasculopathy, and they are both strong predictors of cardiovascular risk (Woodman, et al., 2005).

Endothelial dysfunction mostly reflects decreased amounts of nitric oxide (NO), which is an essential endothelium-derived vasoactive factor that has vasodilatory and anti-atherosclerotic functions. Various conditions, such as oxidative stress, dyslipidemia, and hyperglycemia are believed to be the major causes of endothelial impairment in type 2 diabetes (Woodman, et al., 2005). Endothelial impairment can be measured by various methods, including ultrasonographic measurement of flow-mediated vasodilation of the brachial artery and plethysmography measurement of forearm blood flow responses to vasoactive agents.

Adipocytes, a complex and active endocrine tissue, have secretory products that regulate metabolic and vascular biology. The adipocytes' secretory products include free fatty acids and several cytokines (e.g., leptin, adiponectin, tissue necrosis factor-alpha, interleukin-6, and resistin). It is believed that these adipocytokines are the missing link between insulin resistance and cardiovascular disease. Lifestyle interventions are designed to enhance endothelial and/or adipose tissue functions in order to reduce the risks of cardiovascular disease in persons with either the metabolic syndrome or type 2 diabetes (Hamdy, 2005).

Cardiovascular Disease as a Risk Factor for Diabetes

Persons with cardiovascular disease are at increased risk of developing diabetes. There is a very strong link between diabetes and cardiovascular disease. The conditions develop together more commonly than separately. Risk factors for diabetes and insulin resistance, such as hypertension, hyperinsulinemia, hyperglycemia, and lipid abnormalities, have been broadened to include inflammation and thrombotic factors (Grant, 2005).

Normal High Blood Pressure and Hypertension

Researchers have identified high normal blood pressure and hypertension as risk factors for type 2 diabetes. Based on a study of 7,594 Japanese men, aged 35 to 60 years, Hayashi, et al. (1999) reported that Japanese men with high normal blood pressure and hypertension had a higher relative risk of developing develop type 2 diabetes than those with normal blood pressure. Even among lean men (body mass index less than 22.7kg/m^2), those with high normal blood pressure had an increased relative risk of acquiring type 2 diabetes. Among persons with diabetes, there is a higher risk for renal and cardiovascular disease with blood pressures greater than $130/80 \text{mm Hg}$ (Bakris, 2004).

Inflammatory and Prothrombotic Factors

Inflammation and prothrombotic (coagulation and thrombolytic) processes are known risk factors for the development of both diabetes and cardiovascular disease. Prospective studies reveal that diabetic patients have a high prevalence of both inflammatory cells and thrombosis in coronary plaques compared to control groups (Grant, 2005). These reports also show that C-reactive protein (CRP), a known inflammatory marker, and other inflammatory markers, such as TNF-alpha and interleukin-6 and interleukin 18, are related to an increased risk of diabetes and cardiovascular disease (Grant, 2005; Godefroi, et al., 2005; Hung, et al., 2005).

Research is underway to investigate whether hyperinsulinemia associated with glucose intolerance increases cardiovascular

risk directly or whether its impact is mediated by impaired fibrinolysis and hypercoagulability. Using data from the Framingham
Offspring Study, Meigs, et al. (2000) found that hyperinsulinemia
is related to fibrinolysis and hypercoagulability in persons with
normal glucose tolerance. Hyperinsulinemia is mainly related to
impaired fibrinolysis in persons with glucose intolerance. The
researchers conclude that cardiovascular risks related to hyperinsulinemia and glucose intolerance may be partly mediated by a
greater potential for acute thrombosis.

There is limited information about the prevalence of elevated
CRP in the adult population and the factors related to this inflammatory marker of increased cardiovascular disease risk. Based on
a sample of employed adults participating in a worksite cardiovascular screening program, Godefroi, et al. (2005) reported that
25% of the participants in a sample of employed adults participating in a worksite cardiovascular screening program, had elevated
levels of CRP. They found that women, obese persons, and individuals with increasing heart rate and higher serum triglyceride
levels were more likely to have elevated CRP levels, than did
members of the control group. Regular exercise and lower total
cholesterol levels were related to lower CRP levels.

Although obesity is related to increased cardiovascular risk,
the pathways have not been fully delineated (Rosito, et al., 2004).
Since thrombosis is a major component of cardiovascular disease,
a chronic inflammatory process may place obese persons at risk for
metabolic and cardiovascular complications of obesity (Skurk and
Hauner, 2005; Kiortsis, et al., 2005). Fatty tissue synthesizes and
secretes a variety of products known as adipokines that may trigger
these metabolic and cardiovascular complications (Skurk and
Hauner, 2005).

Researchers have analyzed the association between obesity
and a prothrombotic state in different populations. Using data on
3,230 participants in cycle 5 of the Framingham Offspring Study,
Rosito, et al. (2004) discovered that body mass index was related
to four hemostatic factors, (fibrinogen, factor VII, PAI-1, and tPA
antigen) in both men and women and two hemostatic factors (VWF
and viscosity) in women. Similar relationships between waist-to-
hip ratio and the hemostatic factors were found. The authors
conclude that the association between body mass index and

waist-to-hip ratio and hemostatic factors and impaired fibrinolysis indicates that obesity is a cardiovascular risk which is partly mediated by a prothrombotic state.

In the future, it might be possible to prevent obesity-related metabolic and cardiovascular complications by altering the fatty tissue secretions. Current research findings indicate that weight reduction and certain anti-inflammatory substances reduce the metabolic and cardiovascular complications of obesity. However, Skurk and Hauner (2005) point out that there is no causal relationship between the secretory activity of adipocytes and obesity complications.

Inflammatory markers and insulin resistance also appear to be affected by sex steroids. Researchers have evaluated inflammatory markers, insulin resistance, and regional body fat distribution during the menstrual cycle. Blum, et al. (2005) showed that concentrations of highly sensitive CRP and sex hormone-binding globulin changed significantly during the menstrual cycle. In their study of the menstrual cycle in 8 normal and 9 overweight women, they discovered that highly sensitive CRP was negatively related to sex-hormone globulin concentrations while it was positively associated with estimates of insulin resistance and central accumulation of body fat. These investigators conclude that in regularly menstruating women, sub-clinical inflammation is closely related to sex steroids, insulin resistance, and body fat distribution.

Cigarette Smoking

Smoking is the cause of 50% of all avoidable deaths, and a number of investigations have revealed that cigarette smoking increases the risk of type 2 diabetes (Gohlke, 2004; Hu, et al., 2001). For example, based on a prospective study of 84,941 female nurses, Hu, et al. (2001) demonstrated that current smoking was one of the predictors of type 2 diabetes. In a prospective cohort study of 1,266 Japanese male office workers, aged 35 to 59 years, Nakanishi, et al. (2000) showed that the number of cigarettes smoked daily and the number of pack-years of exposure was positively associated with the development of impaired fasting glucose and type 2 diabetes.

Among persons with diabetes, smoking is also linked to an increased risk of cardiovascular disease mortality and microvascular complications. Gulliford, et al. (2003) reported that diabetics who smoked had worse health status, but were less likely to be referred to a hospital or treated for their hypertension than non-smoking diabetics.

Alcohol Consumption

Light to moderate alcohol consumption may actually protect against the development of type 2 diabetes. Wannamethee, et al. (2003) used a prospective study of 109, 690 women in the 25 to 42 age group, and discovered that light to moderate alcohol use was related to a lower risk of type 2 diabetes among women, aged 25 to 42 years.

Hu, et al. (2001) showed that abstinence from alcohol was related to an increased risk of type 2 diabetes in a cohort of 84,941 female nurses. However, moderate and heavy alcohol use may be related to an increased risk of type 2 diabetes (Waki, et al., 2005).

Using data from the Japan Public Health Center prospective study on cancer and cardiovascular diseases, Waki, et al. (2005) evaluated risk factors for type 2 diabetes in middle-aged Japanese. In Japanese lean (body mass index less than or equal to $22 \text{kg}/\text{m}^2$), moderate and high alcohol use was related to the incidence of diabetes. Tsumura, et al. (1999) also found that heavy alcohol use (greater or equal to $50.1 \text{ml}/\text{day}$) among lean men (body mass index less than or equal to $22.0 \text{kg}/\text{m}^2$) was associated with an increased risk of type 2 diabetes.

Diabetes, Disability/Quality of Life, and Health Care Disparities

Individuals with diabetes have an increased risk of disability and diminished quality of life. Gender, age, socioeconomic, and ethnic/racial disparities in diabetes exacerbate disability. Researchers have investigated the prevalence of physical limitations among adults with diabetes and have found that persons with diabetes have a higher percentage of physical limitations compared to those without diabetes. Using the population-based 1997–1999 National Health Interview Survey of U.S. adults, 18 years or older, one investigation showed that persons with diabetes had some physical limitation among all age groups compared to non-diabetics (Ryerson, et al., 2003). However, these differences in physical limitation declined with increasing age. In the 18 to 44 age group, 46% of the persons with diabetes had physical limitations when compared to 18% of those without diabetes. Eighty-five percent of the diabetics 75 years and older reported physical limitations compared to 70% of those who did not have diabetes. After controlling for various demographic factors, diabetics had a greater chance of having a physical limitation compared to non-diabetics.

Diabetes can produce significant physical limitations in some high-risk populations. For example, a study of 338 stable, insulin-treated veterans with type 2 diabetes with an average age of 65.1 years showed that almost three-quarters of them reported limited physical activity (Murata, et al., 2003).

Persons with diabetes have higher rates of work disability compared to those without diabetes. Mayfield, et al. (1999) examined the rate of work disability, hours worked per week, work-loss days, and wages in individuals with diabetes using the National Medical Expenditures Survey, a population-based survey of the U.S. non-institutionalized population. Work disability was defined as a self-report of being unable to work because of an illness or disability for 2 or more quarters in 1987. The investigators discovered that 25.6% of the persons with diabetes reported work disability, while only 7.8% of those without diabetes reported work disability. In regard to work-loss days, diabetics reported more work-loss days than non-diabetics. Persons with diabetes at all ages had significantly lower average earnings than persons without diabetes. Diabetics in 1987 had $4.7 million loss of earnings because of work disability.

Other investigations have found different rates of work disability. Songer, et al. (1989), in a case-control study of 158 persons with insulin-dependent diabetes mellitus and 158 matched non-diabetic siblings, found that 13% of the individuals with insulin-dependent diabetes mellitus were unable to work because of disability. Persons with insulin-dependent diabetes mellitus were more than 7 times likely to report work disability than the non-diabetic siblings. Insulin-dependent diabetics also were less likely to be employed full-time compared to the matched non-diabetic siblings (55% vs. 73%), and this was associated with work disability.

Murata, et al. (2003) analyzed the rate of self-reported work disability in a sample of 338 stable, insulin-treated veterans with type 2 diabetes. The authors found that 53% of the insulin-treated veterans with type-2 diabetes viewed themselves as disabled for work.

Persons with diabetes also report more job discrimination than those without diabetes. Songer, et al. (1989) discovered that individuals with insulin-dependent diabetes mellitus were more likely to be refused a job at some time in their lives compared to their non-diabetic siblings (56% vs. 42%). Persons who disclosed their diabetes during job interviews were more likely to report job refusal than their non-diabetic siblings (64% vs. 42%).

Various demographic, socioeconomic, psychosocial, and disease-related factors may influence disability and quality of life among persons with diabetes. Age disparities in diabetes may affect disability and quality of life in diabetics. Older individuals with diabetes are at increased risk of becoming disabled and having reduced quality of life. Mayfield, et al. (1999), using data from the population-based National Medical Expenditures Survey, discovered that work disability rates were higher for older persons. Likewise, a sample of persons, aged 65 years and older, in Madrid showed that having diabetes was related to disability (Valderrama-Gama, et al., 2002).

Drawing on a sample of 437 persons with type-2 diabetes, Senez, et al. (2004) used two quality of life questionnaires, to evaluate factors that might influence quality of life in type 2 diabetics. The authors found that age negatively affected the quality of life of persons with type 2 diabetes.

In addition to age, gender disparities in disability and quality of life among persons with diabetes have been found. According to Mayfield, et al. (1999) work disability among diabetics was higher for women compared to men. Araki, et al. (1995), in their study of elderly diabetics, found that older women had more disease burden than elderly men. Senez, et al. (2004) also reported that women diabetics had a poorer quality of life than their male counterparts.

Gender differences may exist in the prevalence of foot pain and associated impairment among diabetics. These gender disparities may be due to a variety of factors, including differences in footwear, body weight, hypertension, and lower extremity disease. Using the population-based National Health Interview Survey, one investigation analyzed possible gender differences in hypertension and toe pain in insulin-taking diabetics (Morewitz, et al., 2002). The results indicated that female insulin-taking diabetics were more likely to have toe pain and stiffness than male insulin-taking diabetics, after controlling for possible predictor variables.

In another study, Mullins, et al. (2002) explored possible gender differences in perceived weight impairment and exercise among insulin-taking diabetics. The results showed that male insulin-taking diabetics who felt that their weight impaired their daily activities were less likely to participate in vigorous physical activity. However, there was no association between perceived weight impairment and vigorous physical activity among female insulin-taking diabetics. These gender differences persisted after controlling for possible confounding factors.

Racial and ethnic disparities also are increasingly recognized as predictors of disability and quality of life in individuals with diabetes. African-Americans and Hispanics are especially at risk because of the consistent health disparities found in these populations. Mayfield, et al. (1999) showed that among diabetics, work disability was higher among African-Americans but lower among Hispanics. On the basis of data from the population-based 1992 Health and Retirement Survey, one report demonstrated that among individuals with chronic diseases such as diabetes, African-Americans and Hispanics had worse functional status when compared to whites (Kington and Smith, 1997).

Socioeconomic factors may be a better predictor of disability than racial and ethnic factors. According to Kington and Smith (1997), ethnic and racial disparities in functional status among persons with different chronic diseases were eliminated after controlling for socioeconomic status.

Other research illustrates how socioeconomic disparities predict disability and quality of life in persons with diabetes.

Koster, et al. (2004) studied mobility decline among individuals suffering from one of four chronic conditions (diabetes mellitus, asthma/chronic obstructive pulmonary disease, heart disease, and low back pain). The authors revealed that mobility decline was significantly higher in persons from high socioeconomic backgrounds compared to those from low socioeconomic backgrounds. Very little of the mobility decline in these persons could be explained by their higher disease severity and co-morbidity (Koster, et al., 2004).

One investigation assessed the possible relationship between income disparities and duration of heart problems among non-insulin taking diabetics (Morewitz, 2004a). According to this report, non-insulin taking diabetics with household incomes less than $20,000 had duration of heart problems (19.96 years) that were more than two times the duration of heart problems among non-insulin-taking diabetics with household incomes of $20,000 or more (9.21 years). These findings remained significant after adjusting for possible confounding variables.

Obesity and overweight, sedentary behaviors, alcohol and smoking, some of the same lifestyle factors that increase the risk of diabetes also may increase disability levels and thus impair quality of life in diabetics.

Based on a study of 500 patients with type 2 diabetes, Shera, et al. (2004) showed that obesity, hypertension, poor metabolic control, and duration of diabetes were related to an increased prevalence of microvascular complications.

Overweight and obesity also have been related to diabetic complications in persons with type 1 diabetes. Using retrospective data from 241 type 1 diabetic patients admitted to a metabolic department, one report found that obesity, hypertension, and dyslipidemia are associated with microangiopathy, neuropathy, and coronary artery disease (Kozek, et al., 2003).

One report evaluated the relation between overweight and obesity and disability levels in elderly men with diabetes, cardiovascular disease, and cancer, based on a sample of 4,232 men aged 60 to 79 years (Goya Wannamethee, et al., 2004). The findings revealed that overweight and obesity were related to 60% of the prevalence of insulin resistance, one third of the prevalence of diabetes, and 25% of locomotor disability.

Research is underway to explore attitudes toward weight impairment and obesity among diabetics to better understand and prevent overweight and obesity in these individuals. One report analyzed possible African-American and white differences in perceived weight impairment and desirable body weight in insulin-taking and non-insulin-taking diabetics (Muhl, et al., 2002). The initial analysis revealed that insulin-taking and non-insulin-taking whites who felt that weight impaired their daily activities were more likely to report that they were over their desired weight. In contrast, this association did not hold true for insulin-taking and non-insulin-taking African-Americans. However, after controlling for household income and frequency of vigorous leisure-time physical activity, this association was significant for insulin-taking African-Americans. Among insulin-taking African-Americans, household income and vigorous leisure-time physical activity mediate the association between perceived weight impairment and believing that they are above their desired body weight.

An investigation in the Netherlands assessed health-related quality of life and treatment satisfaction among 1,348 type 2 diabetes patients (Redekop, et al., 2002). The study results indicated that obesity predicted a lower quality of life among these patients.

Another report evaluated the quality of life of patients with 437 type 2 diabetes and discovered that lack of professional or physical activity was one of the conditions that diminished the quality of life (Senez, et al., 2004).

Redekop, et al. (2002) discovered that the presence of complications was related to impaired quality of life. In another investigation, poorly controlled diabetes, the presence of two or more diabetic complications, and management by a diabetes specialist were related to lower quality of life (Senez, et al., 2004).

Social and demographic factors may contribute to lower quality of life and increased disability in persons with diabetes. Older age has been shown to diminish the quality of life in type 2 diabetics (Senez, et al., 2004; Araki, et al., 1995). In a study of 437 patients with type 2 diabetes, one report discovered that older age (over 75 years) predicted lower quality of life (Senez, et al., 2004).

Elderly diabetics who are taking insulin may be at risk for increased disability and reduced quality of life. An investigation of 383 outpatients, over 60 years, in Japan showed that insulin therapy was related to an increased burden on the patients (Araki, et al., 1995). In the study, a low level of activities of daily living or diabetic complications resulted in a greater burden on the patients.

Gender roles, loneliness, and the lack of social support are other factors that may lead to diminished quality of life and disability in diabetics. Senez, et al. (2004), in their study of 437 type 2 diabetics, discovered that being female, diabetic, and lonely led to a diminished quality of life.

A study in Sweden analyzed the health-related quality of life of 457 diabetic patients treated for foot ulcers (Ragnarson, et al., 2000). Their results showed that patients with current foot ulcers reported lower health-related quality of life than patients who had healed without having to undergo an amputation.

Other lower extremity disease is also associated with diminished health-related quality of life and disability. In their investigation, Pinzur and Evans (2003) found that various measures of quality of life (e.g., physical functioning, social functioning, and mental health status) of patients with Charcot foot were lower than a control group.

Do diabetic foot ulcers have the same impact on quality of life as Charcot foot and ankle deformity? Based on a preliminary evaluation of 60 adults with diabetes, Willrich, et al. (2005) discovered that patients with diabetic foot ulcers and Charcot foot and ankle deformity had severely impaired health-related quality of life. The investigators conclude that the negative effects of diabetic foot ulcers or Charcot foot and ankle deformity on health-related quality of life may be as severe as the impact of lower extremity amputations.

One report sought to determine if there were differences in ankle joint pain symptoms among insulin-taking diabetics and non-insulin taking diabetics (Lim, et al., 2002). This population-based survey revealed that insulin-taking diabetics were more likely to have ankle joint pain symptoms (34%) than non-insulin-taking diabetics (26%). These results persisted, after controlling for possible confounding variables.

Ethnic and racial disparities have been identified for lower extremity complications among persons with diabetes. One study of hospitalizations for lower-extremity amputations in California found that Hispanics had a higher proportion of diabetes-related amputations of the lower extremity than did African-Americans or non-Hispanic whites (Lavery, et al., 1996).

Stress, Coping Strategies, and Social Support for Persons with Diabetes

Persons with diabetes can experience severe stress and difficulties in coping with their chronic disease. Dr. Mark L. Goldstein provides a case study to illustrate some of the coping strategies that persons use to deal with their condition.

Case Study

Carl is a 71-year-old married African-American male, with two adult children. He is a retired dentist, having retired four years ago. About ten years ago, he began to experience constant thirst and frequent urination. In addition, he later experienced weight loss and tingling in his hands and feet, followed by impotence. Although he recognized the symptoms as possible diabetes, he did not see a physician for several months.

When Carl did see his physician, he was initially placed on oral medication, but had to utilize insulin injections within six months. In the past two years, he began to lose his vision, although he was initially in denial and refused assistance despite several falls. His wife and family noticed a significant change in temperament, with outbursts of anger not evident before in his behavior. Carl began to sleep during the day, even after he had slept the night before. In addition, he withdrew from friends, including his men's church group. Carl complained about his restrictive diet and "cheated" at times, resulting in increasing medical problems and two brief hospitalizations. Finally, his physician referred him to a psychiatrist, who placed him on antidepressant medication, initially Zoloft and then Effexor. Both medications helped only marginally. He refused to go for counseling, although his wife started psychotherapy herself to cope with her husband.

Approximately six months ago, Carl attempted suicide by ingesting a number of medications. He was hospitalized and prescribed Welbutrin; family and individual therapy was initiated and continues at present. There have been no further suicide attempts and his depression has decreased. Counseling has focused on helping Carl accept his disease. He began using a cane and accepting help from others, including his wife and church members.

Donnelly et al. (2004) evaluated the role of coping strategies and social support in reducing disability, increasing the quality of life, and improving glycemic control among diabetics. Are there certain coping strategies that are more effective than others in helping diabetics to follow self-care practices and deal with the stresses and social disruptions caused by their condition? Skills in planning and preparing meals, foot care, and planning and implementing an effective exercise regimen all require sustained efforts (Donnelly, et al., 2004).

Peyrot, et al. (1999) evaluated the impact of coping styles and other psychosocial resources on glycemic control. They discovered that positive coping styles along with educational attainment and being married were related to increased chronic metabolic control.

Positive locus of control or the belief that people can control their environment may foster important coping strategies that enable diabetics to cope with the stresses of diabetes and minimize or prevent diabetes-related complications. Positive locus of control has been found to be associated with improved outcomes in persons with chronic diseases. However, some studies in diabetics have not found an association between locus of control and improved glycemic control. In a study of 169 diabetics who attended a 4-day outpatient diabetes education program, O'Connor, et al. (1992) reported that the patients' health-related locus of control before attending the program did not predict glycemic control after attending the program.

Attitudes, emotions, personality characteristics, and knowledge about diabetes may influence the diabetics' coping styles and in turn affect their capacity to practice self-care behaviors and achieve glycemic control. Persons with diabetes who have high levels of anxiety, depression, and hostility may be less likely to have positive coping styles. On the basis of 209 patients who attended a 2-day diabetes education program, one report found that attitudes and personality characteristics as well as other psychosocial factors predicted improvements in glycemic control (Dunn, et al., 1990).

Wilson, et al. (1986) evaluated psychosocial predictors of self-care behaviors and metabolic control in 184 non-insulin-dependent diabetics. They discovered that diabetes-specific health beliefs predicted self-care practices including taking medications, self-monitoring, and exercise.

Along with positive coping resources and strategies, social support can help diabetics follow self-care behaviors and attain metabolic control. Social support can involve assistance and encouragement in self-care practices, such as foot care, exercise, weight loss, following diets, self-monitoring, and taking their medications. Social support can involve providing information to help diabetics follow effective self-care practices. Social support also involves emotional aspects such as offering motivational support in coping with the complications of diabetes.

What kinds of social support do persons with diabetes frequently rely on in helping them to cope with their condition? Family members frequently provide assistance in selecting and preparing appropriate food, following self-monitoring activities such as testing blood at home, and support and encouragement in exercising and foot care.

Diabetics who attend diabetes education programs also can gain social support in the form of increased motivation and capacity to follow self-care practices and deal with the psychosocial problems of having diabetes. Persons with diabetes who participate in exercise and weight loss and maintenance programs gain assistance and encouragement in meeting their exercise, weight loss, and weight maintenance goals and may develop attitudes that help them deal with the stresses of their regimen.

With the increased access to the Internet, persons with diabetes increasingly are obtaining different forms of social support from the Internet. Ravert et al. (2004) evaluated 340 public online messages posted by adolescent diabetics. The findings revealed that adolescents with diabetes use online forums for three purposes: 1) social support, 2) information advice, and 3) sharing experiences. The results alsow showed that female adolescents were more likely to visit the public Web-based forums and male adolescents made more requests for information.

How effective are different forms and sources of social support in helping diabetics achieve a good quality of life, normal functioning, and effective metabolic control? Are certain diabetics without social support more at risk than others for having poor metabolic control and associated diabetic complications?

Based on a survey of 138 older Mexican Americans with type 2 diabetes, Wen, et al. (2004) evaluated the role of diabetes-specific family support and other psychosocial conditions in altering patient compliance with diet and exercise recommendations. The authors discovered that a greater degree of perceived family support and self-efficacy were associated with greater self-reported adherence to diet and exercise recommendations. Living with family members was related to greater dietary compliance. The authors recommend that diabetes educators should involve the entire family in managing older patients with type 2 diabetes.

Senez, et al. (2004) discovered that loneliness was associated with diminished quality of life in type 2 diabetics. The researchers also found that the lack of occupational pursuits was associated with reduced quality of life. This may indicate that occupational activities may provide some needed social support and personal gratification for persons with type 2 diabetes.

Elderly diabetics may be especially vulnerable to the lack of social support. An investigation by Araki, et al. (1995) showed that low positive social support and high negative social support were related to greater disease burden in elderly diabetics. Their results illustrate the significance of social support in helping older diabetics cope with the burden of diabetes.

Other studies have analyzed the extent to which different types of social support help to ensure glycemic control among diabetics. One report used a sample of 57 type 1 diabetics and 61 type 2 diabetics to evaluate the association between psychosocial risk factors and glycemic control (Peyrot, et al., 1999). The investigators discovered that stable psychosocial resources, e.g., being married, educational attainment, and positive coping strategies, were related to increased chronic glycemic control.

Wilson, Ary, and Biglan, et al. (1986) analyzed the degree to which social support predicted improvements in metabolic control in non-insulin-dependent diabetics, and they showed that social support was one of the strongest determinants of self-care practices.

A report on 309 diabetic patients who attended a 2-week in-patient diabetes education program evaluated psychosocial pre-dictors of relapse (Akimoto, et al., 2004). The findings revealed that having their food prepared by their spouses, low levels of social support, and not having prior diabetes education increased the probability of relapse.

Treatment and Rehabilitation Outcomes in Persons with Type 2 Diabetes

A significant part of diabetes treatment and rehabilitation is designed to modify lifestyle choices, which result in obesity, dia-betes and cardiovascular disorders. Mobley, (2004) calls these three conditions "diabesity." He notes that an increase in body weight of about 2.2 pounds (1 kg) has been found to increase risks for dia-betes by 4.5%. Conversely, a decrease in body weight of about 5% to 10% enhances control of diabetes.

Restricting calories and increasing physical activity are the most common methods for treating persons at risk for type 2 dia-betes, and they are the initial steps in managing the disease (Hamdy, 2005). Weight loss decreases the risk for diabetes and is one of the desired treatment outcomes for many persons with type 2 diabetes since most of these individuals are overweight, and obesity exacerbates the metabolic and physiologic complications related to diabetes (Norris, et al., 2004a). Weight reduction is com-plicated by the fact that genetics influences obesity, and there does not appear to be one metabolic pathway that determines fat dis-position (White, 2005). Stimulants such as Phentermine (Adipex-P) and Diethylpropion (Tenuate) have been or are being used for weight loss. These medications are used to suppress appetite, but do so only for a short time. Research has shown that they do not produce weight loss on a long-term basis.

After the withdrawal of Fenfluramine and Dexfenfluramine from the market, researchers became interested in Orlistat (Xenical), a medication that suppresses fat absorption. Both Orlistat and Sibutramine (Meridia), a drug that blocks the reuptake of norepinephrine, serotonin, and dopamine, have reduced weight by about 10% over a 1-year period (White, 2005).

O'meara, et al. (2001), in their review of 14 randomized controlled trials (including 3 company submissions) and two economic studies (including one company submission), revealed that Orlistat in most of the trials produced greater weight loss and better weight maintenance compared to patients receiving a placebo. A majority of the trials demonstrated improvement in at least some measures of lipid concentrations, and in 3 trials, the drug reduced blood pressure compared to patients receiving a placebo. At a one-year follow-up, obese patients with type 2 diabetes who received Orlistat had greater weight loss than patients receiving the placebo. Patients in the Orlistat group had a higher incidence of gastrointestinal problems and using Orlistat was related to lower serum levels of fat-soluble vitamins.

Heller (2004) notes that weight control agents, such as Orlistat and Sibutramine, produce weight loss on a short-term basis but have not brought about weight control on a long-term basis. Fluoxetine, Orlistat, and Sibutramine also modestly reduced the patients' glycated hemoglobin levels. Patients on Orlistat experienced gastrointestinal adverse effects; patients on Fluoxetine experienced tremors, somnolence, and sweating, and patients on Sibutramine experienced palpitations.

Other weight loss treatments have had mixed responses (White, 2005). These treatments include Amphetamines, Bupropion (Wellbutrin), some of the selective serotonin reuptake inhibitors (SSRIs), and many over-the-counter and herbal remedies.

In recent years, an anti-convulsant medication, Topiramate (Topamax), has been found to be effective for weight loss in patients with uncomplicated obesity, patients who have experienced weight gain due to psychotropic drugs, patients suffering from binge eating disorder, and patients with migraines (White, 2005). However, the use of Topiramate has resulted in a large number of adverse events, including parasthesias, impaired memory, taste disorder, fatigue, insomnia, problems in concentrating, and dizziness. Investigations with the conventional dosage form were terminated, and new studies are now evaluating slow-release formulations.

Bariatric surgery is another treatment alternative for obesity. Two procedures are the Roux-en-Y gastric bypass and the laparocopic silicone gastric banding technique. Ferchak and Meneghini (2004), in their review of gastric bypass studies, have demonstrated a 99 to 100% prevention of diabetes in patients with impaired glucose tolerance and an 80 to 90% remission of early type 2 diabetes. Studies evaluating the gastric banding procedures have shown a lower median clinical remission of type 2 diabetes (50 to 60%).

Researchers are investigating the effects of a variety of lifestyle and behavioral weight loss interventions in adults with type 2 diabetes (Mobley, 2004; Norris, et al., 2004b; Ferchak and Meneghini, 2004). According to Mobley (2004), randomized controlled clinical trials involving dietary and physical activity interventions have decreased the risk for and delayed the development of the metabolic syndrome (e.g., a constellation of dyslipidemia, hypertension, and central obesity). Four multi-site clinical trials in the U.S., United Kingdom, and Finland since 1977 have shown that lifestyle interventions lead to enhanced metabolic and hypertensive control that have favorable effects on related disease complications (Mobley, 2004). Hamdy (2005) notes that several recent lifestyle interventions have produced improved endothelial function and insulin sensitivity as well as improved serum levels of adipocytokines. These favorable impacts have the potential of reducing the incidence of adverse cardiovascular events.

The Diabetes Prevention Program randomized clinical trial evaluated the impact of Metformin and intensive lifestyle intervention on the metabolic syndrome. At the study baseline, Orchard, et al. (2005) found that 53% of the research subjects had the metabolic syndrome (defined as having three or more conditions, e.g., waist circumference, blood pressure, HDL-cholesterol, triglycerides, and fasting plasma glucose that met criteria from the National Cholesterol Education Program Adult Treatment Panel III). At the end of the study, there was a 41% reduction in the incidence of the metabolic syndrome in the intensive lifestyle intervention group and 17% reduction in the Metformin group compared to the placebo group. The 3-year cumulative incidences of the metabolic syndrome were 51% in the placebo, 45% in the Metformin group, and 34% in the intensive lifestyle intervention group. The authors conclude that intensive lifestyle intervention and Metformin lessened the incidence of the metabolic syndrome.

Ferchak and Meneghini (2004), in their review of lifestyle interventions, including the Diabetes Prevention Program, reported that lifestyle interventions involving obese and glucose-intolerant patients have produced a 50% reduction in the progression of impaired glucose tolerance to diabetes on a short-term basis. They discovered that no lifestyle intervention has produced a complete remission of diabetes. They concluded that weight loss by any means, e.g., bariatric surgery or dietary changes, seems to prevent the progression to type 2 diabetes, at least on a short-term basis.

In a meta-analysis of lifestyle and behavioral weight loss interventions for adults with type 2 diabetes, Norris, et al. (2004b) evaluated randomized controlled trials that sought to achieve weight loss or weight control by using one or more dietary, physical activity, or behavioral interventions and had a follow-up period of at least 12 months. The results of the meta-analysis revealed that weight loss interventions consisting of dietary change, physical activity, or behavioral interventions were linked to only small changes in weight loss. These results occurred because individuals in the control groups often had major weight loss. The researchers suggest that multiple strategies, including very low-calories or low-calorie diets may be beneficial in achieving weight loss in adults with type 2 diabetes.

Moore, et al. (2004) assessed the efficacy of dietary management on adults with type 2 diabetes. The authors reviewed clinical trials that evaluated low-fat/high-carbohydrate diets, high-fat/low-carbohydrate diets, low calorie (1000 kcal daily) and very-low-calorie (500 kcal daily) diets, and modified fat diets. Six of the clinical trials compared dietary advice alone, with dietary advice combined with exercise. Three other investigations compared dietary advice alone, with dietary advice combined with behavioral techniques. All of the clinical trials measured changes in weight and metabolic control, although not all reported the results in their published articles. Other outcome measures assessed included mortality, blood pressure, serum cholesterol, serum triglycerides, maximal exercise capacity, and adherence. The authors conclude that there are no high quality data on the effectiveness of dietary therapy for persons with type 2 diabetes.

However, exercise seems to enhance metabolic control at 6-month and 12-month follow-up periods.

Other studies have reported that lifestyle interventions, including patient education about diet and exercise, facilitate weight loss on a short-term basis, but have not produced weight control over longer periods (Heller, 2004). Lifestyle interventions can facilitate weight maintenance, a redistribution of body composition, and decreased insulin resistance. One investigation of obese adolescents found that participation in a lifestyle intervention resulted in weight maintenance, whereas members of the control group gained weight (Balagopal, et al., 2005). Participants in the lifestyle intervention also had a redistribution of body composition and reduced insulin resistance, compared to those in the control group. Heller (2004) recommends that lifestyle intervention should be continued throughout the course of therapy in order to produce permanent weight control.

The impact of lifestyle interventions on the inflammatory state related to obesity has been studied. A randomized controlled lifestyle intervention in obese adolescents assessed the effects of a lifestyle intervention on inflammatory factors, which are non-traditional risk factors for cardiovascular disease (Balagopal, et al., 2005). The study findings indicated that participation in the intervention resulted in a reduction in three inflammatory factors (C-reactive protein, fibrinogen, and interleukin-6), while the control did not experience a reduction in these inflammatory factors.

When lifestyle interventions are unable to control dyslipidemia and hypertension in persons with the metabolic syndrome, pharmacotherapy is recommended (Rosenson, 2005). Lipid-regulating agents, such as statins (HMG-CoA reductase inhibitors), fibrates (fibric acid derivatives), and fish oils are treatments for diabetic dyslipidemia. Rosenson (2005) notes that statins are the first-line medication for dyslipidemia because of their effectiveness in reducing low LDL-cholesterol and may also enhance HDL-cholesterol and triglycerides. Fibrates and niacin, combined with statins, may also be helpful in lowering triglycerides or increasing HDL-cholesterol.

Clinical trials have demonstrated a 22–24% reduction in the risk of future cardiovascular events in diabetic patients treated with statins (Leiter, 2005). The National Cholesterol Education Program and other guidelines recommend early, aggressive intervention in very-high-risk patients, e.g., patients with both diabetes and car-diovascular disease, regardless of their baseline LDL-cholesterol levels in order to meet a goal of 70 mg/dL for LDL-cholesterol. Leiter (2005) notes that despite the evidence of the value of lipid-lowering medications, a recent survey of diabetes specialists revealed that many diabetic patients are still not treated or are under-treated.

However, the impact of lipid-regulating drugs, fibrates, and fish oils on vascular function has been found to be inconsistent (Woodman, et al., 2005). Intervention trials with positive effects suggest that improvement in vascular function may be influenced by both lipid and non-lipid mechanisms, including anti-inflammatory, anti-oxidative, and direct effects on the arterial wall. Lifestyle interventions, renin-angiotensin-aldosterone system antagonists, and insulin sensitizers have been shown to have pos-itive effects on vascular function in persons with type 2 diabetes. New treatments, such as targeting eNOS and aGEs, are underway, along with lipid-regulating therapies that better lower LDL-cholesterol and raise HDL-cholesterol. Concomitant treatments that target oxidative stress may enhance endothelial impairment in diabetes.

Two or more drugs are generally needed to effectively control hypertension. Agents that block the renin-angiotensin system are very useful because they have been found to reduce the risk of car-diovascular events and end-stage renal disease separate from the lowering of blood pressure (Rosenson, 2005).

Growing evidence indicates that both PPAR-alpha activators, such as the fibric acid class of hypolipidemic drugs and PPAR-gamma agonists, such as antidiabetic thiazolidinediones (TZDs), have been shown to be efficacious in enhancing the metabolic syn-drome (Zhang, et al., 2005). Ongoing studies indicate that PPARs have potential in the treatment of type 2 diabetes, dyslipidemia, and atherosclerosis and may be effective in treating additional problems related to the metabolic syndrome, including obesity (Berger, et al., 2005; Liu, et al., 2005). For example, Liu, et al. (2005) report on a novel series of PPAR alpha/gamma dual agonists for the treatment of type 2 diabetes and dyslipidemia. It is expected that discovering the regulatory mechanisms and transcriptional targets of PPARs will clarify the causes of metabolic diseases and provide a basis for therapy (Terauchi and Kadowaki, 2005).

Interventions should also attempt to reduce cardiovascular risk in patients with microalbuminuria and diabetes or hypertension. Prospective research had demonstrated that microalbuminuria is a predictor of adverse cardiovascular event and all-cause mortality among patients with diabetes or hypertension (Yuyun, et al., 2005).

Frayn (2002) notes that lifestyle interventions that increase physical activity and improve nutrition still offer the best hope for the primary prevention of coronary heart disease. Governmental interventions, instead of just advice from individual physicians, are probably the best way to to achieve these lifestyle goals.

Clinicians are also developing new clinical pathways to improve outcomes in diabetic patients. Clinical pathways refer to attempts by clinicians to define the optimal care process, sequences, and timing of diagnostic and treatment procedures (Cheah, 2000). The goals of clinical pathways are to improve the quality of patient care and minimize the costs of health care for patients. These clinical pathways have goals which are consistent with other quality ssurance approaches, such as total quality management (TQM) and continuous clinical quality improvement (CQI).

Various institutions have implemented diabetes clinical pathways. For example, the Australian Commonwealth Department of Veterans' Affairs has developed a diabetes clinical pathway to improve the diagnosis and treatment of diabetic patients using pre-established clinical criteria for a wide range of patient care outcomes. Their diabetes clinical pathway provides criteria for assessing and treating metabolic control, patient compliance, diabetic complications, exercise, nutritional treatment, patient education, and patient referrals.

Patout, et al. (2001) developed a clinical pathway to standardize lower extremity care for diabetic patients in a medically underserved community. The authors developed a clinical pathway to standardize lower extremity treatment in five areas: injury prevention, warm swollen foot, ulcer, osteomyelitis, and remodeling.

Martinez, et al. (2004) assessed the impact of a clinical pathway for hospitalized patients with the diagnosis of a complicated diabetic foot. They found that patients who were treated after the implementation of a clinical pathway for the diabetic foot had a fewer number of greater amputations and a lower rate of readmissions to the hospital compared to patients who were treated before the implementation of the clinical pathway.

Other clinicians have designed clinical practice guidelines to provide evidence-based guidance for clinicians who treat diabetic patients. For example, Frykberg, et al. (2000) developed a clinical practice guideline for diabetic foot disease using currently available evidence. They presented guidelines on the pathophysiology and treatment of foot ulcers, infections, and the diabetic Charcot foot.

Additional research is needed to evaluate the impact of clinical pathways and clinical practice guidelines on diabetic patient outcomes.

Patient Education and Self-Management among Persons with Diabetes

Diabetes education and self-management programs seek to increase patient compliance with their treatment plans, reduce the serious complications of diabetes, and help patients deal with the difficult problems of lifestyle and behavioral changes that are necessary to achieve metabolic control. Diabetic patient education and self-management programs can help to reduce the chronic complications of diabetes, such as peripheral vascular disease, peripheral arterial disease, lower limb amputations, and atherosclerosis (Jaar, et al., 2004; Strojek, 2003). Diabetes education and self-management interventions can occur in both formal and informal clinical settings.

Effective diabetes education and self-management programs identify and reduce barriers to following treatment and lifestyle recommendations. Individuals with diabetes may face a variety of barriers to following their insulin therapy, oral medications, dietary therapies, weight loss and weight control goals, and physical activity recommendations. Vijan, et al. (2005) discovered that a moderate diet was viewed more difficult to follow than oral agents but less of a burden than insulin. Diabetics considered a strict diet with the goal of weight loss as burdensome as taking insulin. Despite these findings, diabetic patients reported that they complied more with oral agents and insulin than a moderate diet. Patients reported a number of barriers to following dietary therapies, including cost, small portion sizes, social and family support problems, and quality of life and lifestyle issues.

Another obstacle is intensive insulin therapy and some oral anti-diabetic agents may produce weight gain. It is believed that insulin-associated weight gain is related to the anabolic effects of insulin, appetite increases, and reduction of glycosuria. Heller (2004) notes that Metformin along with insulin are used to reduce weight gain among patients with type 2 diabetes. In addition, other new oral therapies and insulin analogs may be useful in reducing insulin-associated weight gain.

What makes up effective diabetes patient education and self-management programs? These activities frequently involve one-on-one advice, informational and counseling sessions, group patient education sessions, self-care skill training and evaluation, and should involve exercise and nutrition components (Ellis, et al., 2004). The content of patient education and self-management activities emphasizes the mechanisms underlying diabetes, its possible short-term and long-term complications, self-care skills, and ways to control diabetes through nutrition, exercise, stress management, oral agents, and insulin therapy.

Some diabetes patient education and self-management programs try to identify and eliminate cognitive problems that impede self-management skills. Patients with low educational levels may be especially at risk for developing life-threatening complications, such as diabetes-related lower extremity amputations. Dangelser, et al. (2003) found that some diabetics have very limited knowledge about their disease and do not engage in preventive behaviors to avoid foot trauma, increasing their risks for lower limb amputations and other chronic complications. Populations with a high prevalence of diabetes are at risk for an increase in the chronic complications of diabetes, including lower limb amputations.

Older persons with diabetes may suffer from mild to severe cognitive impairment, jeopardizing their ability to follow self-care practices. Patient education and self-management programs should customize their interventions to meet the educational needs of diabetics with limited knowledge of their disease and low educational attainment.

Some patients may misperceive the severity of their disease and, as a consequence, fail to engage in appropriate self-management skills. For example, Frijling, et al. (2004) showed that a significant percentage of patients with hypertension or diabetes incorrectly perceive their risk of cardiovascular disease. Diabetic patients may also exaggerate their risks for atherosclerosis (Strojek, 2003). Patient educational and self-management programs should provide greater information about risk factors for diabetic complications to deal with patient misperceptions.

The use of information technology and other innovations in diabetes self-care will increasingly become a major issue in patient education and self-management activities as these technological innovations become widely used (Boukhurs, et al., 2003). Innovations in diabetes care, such as the use of computer programs by patients for the adjustment of insulin doses and patients' use of insulin pumps, require effective patient education. Clinicians will need to assess the patients' readiness to use and benefit from these sophisticated techniques and equipment in their self-care management.

Another important focus of diabetes patient education and self-management interventions is dealing with psychosocial problems associated with living with diabetes. Adolescents with diabetes are especially at risk for having difficulties in dealing with their disease. Diabetes can drastically change the social world of adolescents by forcing them to be different from their friends. The disease requires that they take insulin and follow self-care practices that disrupt their normal daily routines and interactions with friends and family. Having diabetes can be especially devastating to adolescents who are seeking to establish a normal social identity in relationship to their friends, family members, and acquaintances.

Dickinson and O'Reilly (2004), using a sample of 10 adolescent females who were recruited from a diabetes camp, identified five issues that may affect adolescents living with diabetes. First, adolescent females with diabetes face the problem of blending in with the culture of adolescence. Second, they do not want to stand out from their friends and acquaintances and do not want to be watched by their parents and others in authority to ensure that they comply with treatment plans and self-care practices. Third, adolescent females with diabetes are faced with evaluating different strategies and making choices. Fourth, they must grapple with the problem of being tied to a chronic disease and a health care system. Finally, adolescent females with diabetes struggle to overcome conflicts that they are forced to confront on a daily basis. They must adapt to having diabetes and make it manageable in their daily lives.

Patient education and self-care management interventions must consider the psychosocial needs of diabetic adolescents. However, more research is needed to evaluate existing programs and determine their effectiveness. Kyngas (2003) interviewed 40 Finnish adolescents, aged 13 to 17 years, with insulin-dependent diabetes, juvenile rheumatoid arthritis, and asthma to determine the effectiveness of patient education programs in meeting the needs of these adolescents. His findings indicated that patient education interventions had positive and negative aspects.

The negative characteristics were: 1. Some programs tended to be geared more to the needs of the health care providers than to the needs of the adolescents. (For example, sessions were offered when they were convenient for the clinicians and not the adolescents.) 2. The program was not geared to the developmental level of the adolescents. 3. The programs were poorly planned, unsystematic, and did not provide continuity.

Kyngas (2003) believed that the most successful programs are those that: 1. foster an encouraging atmosphere where the clinicians motivated the adolescents, 2. respect their patients' views, and 3. encourage them to express their feelings and ask questions. The most beneficial interventions were planned in advance, focusing on the developmental needs of adolescents. Efficacious programs were ones that offered adolescents self-care skills and provided them with ways to to respond to a variety of problems.

Psychosocial issues may worsen problem-solving skills among diabetics, leading to impaired self-care practices. Hill-Briggs, et al. (2003) used focus groups to evaluate the problem-solving process in urban African-Americans in good diabetes control compared to those in poor diabetes control. They found that individuals in good diabetes control tended to have a positive orientation toward diabetes self-management and problem solving, had a rational problem-solving process, and had a positive transfer of past learning to new situations. In contrast, those persons in poor diabetes control had a negative orientation toward self-care practices, were careless or avoided participating in problem-solving activities, and had a negative transfer of past learning.

In their study, Vijan, et al. (2005) found that patients in urban sites who were mainly African-American reported more problems in communicating with their clinician about dietary therapy and social circumstances as well as more difficulties in following the rigid schedule of a diabetes diet than other groups.

D'Eramo-Melkus, et al. (2004) evaluated the impact of a culturally competent intervention on African-American women who have type 2 diabetes (D'Eramo-Melkus, et al., 2004). The investigators evaluated the feasibility and acceptability of culturally competent patient education materials as well as possible changes in glycemic control associated with this intervention. According to the study findings, African-American women with type 2 diabetes who received the culturally competent program showed significant improvements in their glycemic control. The authors suggest that a culturally appropriate patient education program can increase patient attendance, increase kept appointments, enhance metabolic control and weight goals, and minimize the incidence of emotional problems associated with diabetes. Therefore, patient education and self-management interventions need to incorporate ethnic and cultural issues into their programs to enhance the diagnosis and management of diabetes.

How effective are diabetes patient education and self-management interventions? Ellis, et al. (2004) has demonstrated that diabetes patient education programs modestly improve metabolic control. Based on a meta-analysis of 28 randomized controlled trials of diabetes patient education, they discovered that net glycemic change was .320% lower in the diabetics who received education, when compared to the control groups. A meta-regression was performed to determine which variables in the 28 interventions, most accurately predicted variability in glycemic control. The results indicated that face-to-face delivery, emphasis on cognitive reframing and the use of physical exercise were the best predictors of improvement in glycemic control.

Gilden, et al. (1992) found that a diabetes education program for the elderly that was combined with 18 months of support group sessions produced increased knowledge, quality of life, and better scores on a depression measure than did those who received only the education program or the control group who received neither intervention.

Patient learning can occur both in informal and formal settings, and research is underway to evaluate the usefulness of informal clinical settings in improving patient learning. For example, patient participation in screening clinics may be an effective patient education intervention. Gillard, et al. (2004) evaluated the impact of diabetic eye screening clinics on self-management behaviors and glycemic control over a two-year period involving 3 diabetes disease screenings. They found that patient participation in a diabetic eye screening clinic resulted in an increased use of insulin, increased glucose self-monitoring, and an improved glucose control. These significant positive changes in self-management behaviors and glycemic control occurred, even though the original use of the screening clinics had not been for patient learning. The investigators proposed that significant patient learning can take place in informal settings and should be incorporated into every patient encounter.

Disease management programs have been found to enhance outcomes in diabetic patients. Sidorov, et al. (2000) evaluated the impact of a health maintenance organization-sponsored disease management program on diabetic patients' glycemic control and use of medications. The disease management program included the use of a Steering Committee, clinical guidelines, diabetes patient education, glucose meters and strips, simple reporting of outcomes and clinical leadership support. At 3-month and 1-year follow-ups, patients in the disease management program had significant improvements in their glycemic control (HbA1c). Program participants also increased their use of insulin, Troglitazone, and Metformin. The authors suggest that although glycemic control was accompanied by increases in patients' use of insulin, Troglitazone, and Metformin, the disease management program played a significant role in improving the patients' glycemic control.

More information is needed to determine the extent to which diabetes disease management programs reduce health care costs and use of health care services. One investigation by Sidorov, et al. (2002) evaluated the impact of a diabetes disease management program on health care costs, utilization of services, and metabolic control using a retrospective analysis of 6,779 enrolled health plan patients with diabetes. Two groups of diabetic patients were compared: those enrolled in a disease management program and those not enrolled in the program. According to the study results, diabetic patients in the disease management program had lower average claims per member per month: $394.62 for patients in the program and $502.48 for non-program patients. Diabetic patients in the disease management program also had lower use of in-patient services (mean of 0.12 admissions per patient per year and 0.56 inpatient days per patient per year for patients in the disease management program vs. 0.16 admissions and 0.98 inpatient days for the non-program patients. Patients in the disease program also achieved better metabolic control than those who did not participate in the program. Program participants had lower HbA(1c) levels than non-program participants; 6.7% had a level higher than 9.5% compared to 14.4% of those not in the disease management program.

Research also focuses on the impact of information technology and other technological innovations on patient education and self-care behaviors. A variety of questions are emerging in the field of diabetes patient education and self-management. Which patients can best benefit from sophisticated technological advances, such as the use of computer programs to calculate dietary exchanges, basal-bolus insulin regimes, blood glucose self-monitors, and insulin pumps? How effective is patient access to the Internet in providing useful information to facilitate self-care behaviors and improved patient care outcomes? What are the obstacles to using these technological innovations? What impact do these innovations have on patient education, self-care behaviors, and glycemic control?

Boukhors, et al. (2003) assessed the safety and patient education impact of a computer program used by type 1 diabetic patients to help them adjust their insulin doses to attain tight glucose control. In the investigation, 10 patients were randomized using a crossover design to receive 2 intensive insulin therapy periods, one with the help of an Internet-based computer program and the other without computer assistance. According to the results, patients in the Internet-based computer group followed 89% of the recommendations offered by the computer program. Patients adjusted their insulin doses more frequently when they received computer assistance than when they did not obtain such assistance (98% versus 50%). Patients who had computer assistance showed similar improvements in their glycemic control to those who did not have computer assistance. In addition, the incidence of minor hypoglycemia was similar for patients with and without computer assistance. In terms of patient education outcomes, patients who received computer assistance showed increased knowledge of their disease compared to those who did not receive computer assistance. Quality of life was not affected for patients in either group. The authors conclude that it is feasible and safe for patients to use computer programs to adjust their insulin doses for intensive insulin therapy.

The impact of telemedicine on diabetes patient education also has been evaluated (Izquierdo, et al., 2003). Cherry, et al. (2002) assessed the effects of a web-based patient interface technology as part of a disease management program. The telemedicine program included use of the Health Hero iCare Desktop and the Health Buddy appliance. Patients who used these technologies practiced daily self-management at home, and nurses were alerted if the patients reported abnormalities. The investigators evaluated the impact of this program on quality of life and health care utilization of indigent diabetic patients. The study results indicated that indigent diabetic patients who participated in the telemedicine program showed improvements in quality of life and reductions in health care utilization.

One question in evaluating telemedicine programs is whether telemedicine programs can be offered as effectively as in-person patient education encounters with diabetes patient educators. Using a sample of 56 adults with diabetes, Izquierdo, et al. (2003) assessed whether a telemedicine program was as effective as in-person patient education encounters. Diabetic patients in the telemedicine group were found to be just as effective in enhancing glycemic control as the patients who received education in the in-person encounters. In addition, patients accepted both educational methods equally.

5

Rheumatoid Arthritis, Osteoarthritis, Osteoporosis, Fibromyalgia, and Low Back Pain

Rheumatoid arthritis, oteoarthritis, osteoporosis, fibromyalgia, and low back pain are some conditions that can lead to work disability, increased stress, and reduced quality of life (Carmona, et al., 2001; Gilworth, et al., 2003; Backman, 2004). Researchers have studied persons with these diseases in terms of risk factors, health care disparities, disability levels, occupational factors, stress, quality of life, and coping strategies.

Arthritis Risk Factors and Health Care Disparities

For reasons that are still not well understood, arthritis is more prevalent among women than men. Osteoarthritis and rheumatoid arthritis, and less prevalent diseases that cause arthralgia, are between two and 10 times higher in women than men (Buckwalter and Lappin, 2000). Other investigations have documented that gender, age, socioeconomic, and lifestyle factors predict increased prevalence of arthritis.

Using cross-sectional survey data from the Behavioral Risk Factor Surveillance System, Mili, et al. (2002) showed that the following groups had high prevalence rates of arthritis: older persons, women, individuals with low educational attainment, persons with low income, sedentary individuals, and overweight and obese persons. According to the researchers, high rates of arthritis were also prevalent among groups that had not been previously recognized: separated and divorced individuals, those unemployed or unable to return to work, and current or former smokers.

Similar gender, age, and socioeconomic disparities associated with arthritis have been identified in other countries. Using a representative population survey in South Australia, Hill, et al. (1999) reported that individuals with arthritis had a higher probability of being female, aged, and of lower socioeconomic status compared to persons without arthritis.

Based on a sample of 7,575 Shanghai residents, aged 15 years and older, Shi, et al. (2003) discovered older age, female gender, and obesity may be risk factors for arthritis. The authors recommend weight control and more exercise to reduce the risks of arthritis.

Arthritis, Increased Stress, Disability, and Quality of Life

Individuals who suffer from arthritis and musculoskeletal disorders can experience increased stress, work disability, impaired social and family functioning, and diminished quality of life. An analysis of population-based health and activity limitation surveys showed that arthritis/rheumatism was responsible for over 30% of all disabilities related to mobility and agility (Raina, et al., 1998).

According to the Mini-Finland Health Survey of 7,217 men and women aged 30 years or more, inflammatory arthritis was the best predictor of all types of disability (Makela, et al., 1993). Persons with inflammatory arthritis were at increased risk for having reduced work capacity and a regular need for help in daily activities. Those individuals with inflammatory disease in the 30 to 64 year age group had a higher probability of occasionally needing assistance.

Disability rates are influenced by the number of co-existing chronic diseases. Using data from the National Health Interview Survey, Supplement on Aging, Verbrugge, et al. (1991) reported that the rate of impairment among individuals with arthritis increases with the number of chronic diseases and associated impairments. In their study, long duration of arthritis and recent medical care for the condition predicted disability.

Obesity may be an important determinant of disability among arthritis sufferers. Verbrugge, et al. (1991) discovered that obesity (a body mass index greater than or equal to $30 \, kg/m^2$) predicts disability in persons with arthritis. Low body mass index (less than $20 \, kg/m^2$) also was related to an increased rate of disability among individuals with arthritis.

Persons with musculoskeletal disorders report some of the poorest quality of life, particularly in regard to bodily pain and physical functioning (Reginster, 2002). These persons have complained of lower quality of life than persons with gastrointestinal problems, chronic respiratory conditions, and cardiovascular diseases.

Persons who suffer from arthritis and chronic co-morbidity may be physically inactive and experience higher rates of disability and impaired quality of life (Breedveld, 2004; Kriegsman, et al., 2004). Drawing on data from 2,497 older persons in the Longitudinal Aging Study Amsterdam, Kriegsman, et al. (2004) found that arthritis led to a major decline in physical functioning in persons with diabetes or malignancies. The authors showed that combinations of chronic diseases that both affect physical functioning but through different pathways (e.g., reduced locomotor functioning compared to decreased endurance) may result in more disability than other combination of diseases.

Physical inactivity among those afflicted with arthritis is associated with functional limitations, disability, and increased risk for cardiovascular disease. Kaplan, et al. (2003) investigated older adults with arthritis and identified risk factors for physical inactivity using data from the Canadian National Population Health Survey. Their findings indicated that physically inactive persons with arthritis were more likely to be women, older than 75 years, have functional impairments, be underweight (body mass index less than $25 \, kg/m^2$) or overweight (body mass index over $25 \, kg/m^2$), have high levels of pain, and not have prescription drug insurance.

Arthritis has been found to adversely influence different aspects of a person's quality of life. In one investigation of older adults with arthritis, Dominick, et al. (2004b) showed that patients with osteoarthritis and rheumatoid arthritis reported worse general health, physical health, mental health, reduced participation in activities, pain, and less sleep than controls. Osteoarthritis and rheumatoid arthritis patients also were less likely to report feeling healthy and being full of energy compared to controls.

A variety of demographic, socioeconomic, and psychosocial factors influence disability levels among persons with arthritis (Makela, et al., 1993). Gender may influence the odds of becoming disabled among persons with arthritis and other musculoskeletal problems (van Schaardenburg, et al., 1994). One study of persons, aged 85 years and over, with musculoskeletal disorders revealed that female gender was associated with disability (van Schaardenburg, et al., 1994).

Age factors may affect disability levels among individuals with arthritis and musculoskeletal problems. Verbrugge, et al. (1991) found that older age increases the risks of disability among arthritis sufferers. In an investigation based on data from the Canadian Health and Activity Limitation Survey, Badley and Ibanez (1994) showed that increasing age is a predictor of disability among individuals with musculoskeletal disorders.

Using data from four national surveys, Miles, et al. (1993) evaluated disability among older adults with arthritis. They discovered that among individuals, aged 65–74 years, 20% of individuals with arthritis stated that they had difficulty walking. The percentages of persons with arthritis reporting this disability increased in older age groups.

The elderly are especially vulnerable to high rates of disability since other conditions besides muscuoloskeletal disorders contribute to increased risks of disability (van Schaardenburg, et al., 1994). One report showed that vision problems, cognitive difficulties, and neurological disorders in women and men, aged 85 years and over, were related to other disabilities in addition to musculoskeletal problems.

Racial and ethnic factors are increasingly recognized as predictors of disability in individuals with arthritis and other musculoskeletal problems. Disadvantaged minority groups with various musculoskeletal disorders may be especially at risk of becoming disabled. In their study of arthritis, Verbrugge, et al. (1991) discovered that non-whites with arthritis had higher odds of becoming disabled than whites with arthritis.

Marital status may predict disability among sufferers of arthritis and other musculoskeletal problems. In their investigation, Badley and Ibanez (1994) found that being single predicted disability among persons with musculoskeletal disorders. Likewise, not being married was associated with increased odds of disability in another report (Verbrugge, et al., 1991).

Socioeconomic conditions may affect the degree to which individuals with arthritis become disabled. Low educational attainment among persons with different musculoskeletal disorders may increase their chances of being impaired. Makela, et al. (1993) discovered that a low educational level was an independent predictor of disability among individuals suffering from various musculoskeletal problems. In another study, Badley and Ibanez (1994) indicated that fewer years of education was independently related to disability among individuals suffering from musculoskeletal disorders. Verbrugge, et al. (1991) also reported that lower education predicted impairment among arthritis sufferers.

Arthritis sufferers with low income may be especially at risk of becoming disabled because of their reduced access to health care services and inadequate knowledge about techniques to prevent the disabling effects of arthritis. One report using the population-based 1998 National Health Interview Survey analyzed possible income disparities in arthritis impairment among non-insulin-taking diabetics (Morewitz, 2003a). The findings showed that non-insulin taking diabetics with incomes less than $20,000 were more likely to report that arthritis impaired their daily activities than non-insulin-taking diabetics with incomes of $20,000 or more. The income differences persisted after controlling for possible predictor variables.

Unemployment may increase the risk of disability among sufferers of musculoskeletal disorders. In one investigation, not being employed was an independent predictor of disability among persons with musculoskeletal disorders (Badley and Ibanez, 1994).

Low socioeconomic status is an impediment to accessing and using health care services for musculoskeletal problems. Since early medical treatment can minimize the development of permanent joint and visceral damage in patients with rheumatoid arthritis and other inflammatory diseases, a delay in treatment may result in irreversible impairment (Buckwalter and Lappin, 2000).

Some of the same occupational and lifestyle characteristics that are risk factors for arthritis also may increase disability levels in individuals who suffer from arthritis and related disorders. Repetitive heavy lifting at work, obesity and overweight, smoking, alcohol use, and inadequate nutrition may influence disability rates among persons suffering from arthritis and related disorders.

Individuals with arthritis can experience work instability, the condition under which there is a mismatch between their functional limitations associated with their disease and the demands of their job (Gilworth, et al., 2003). This mismatch may lead to work disability if it is not corrected.

Lower extremity problems also increase the risk of disability among persons with arthritis, diabetes, and associated disorders. In one population-based report, Morewitz, Dintcho, and Lim, et al. (2002) discovered that diabetics and non-diabetics suffering ankle pain, stiffness, and aching in the last 12 months were more likely to have significant decreased physical mobility.

Anxiety and depression may increase the risk of disability in individuals with arthritis and related problems. Zautra and Smith (2001) investigated a study of 188 older women with rheumatoid arthritis and osteoarthritis (n = 101), and discovered that depressive symptoms were related to pain increases in persons with rheumatoid arthritis and osteoarthritis and to increased reactivity to stress and pain in individuals with rheumatoid arthritis.

Ethnic and cultural factors may influence the extent to which individuals with anthritis and lower extremity pain develop anxiety and lower extremity impairment. Using the population-based 1998 National Health Interview Survey, Morewitz, Shamtoub, and Ky, et al. (2002) explored possible ethnic and racial differences in feelings of anxiety and ankle pain and stiffness. According to their results, African-Americans who suffer ankle pain, stiffness, and aching in the previous 12 months were less likely to report anxiety than whites with similar ankle problems.

Researchers are studying the degree to which personality factors and coping strategies influence increased disease severity and disability in arthritis sufferers. Evers, et al. (2003) studied patients with early rheumatoid arthritis and examined the role of personality characteristics, e.g., neuroticism and extroversion, and coping and social support at initial diagnosis as predictors of changes in disease activity. The study results showed that personality characteristics did not predict subsequent disease activity at a 1-year follow-up. However, low levels of social support and extensive use of avoidance coping strategies were linked to increased disease activity at the 3- and 5-year follow-ups.

Below is a discussion of risk factors, quality of life and disability, coping strategies, social support factors, treatment outcomes, and patient education programs for patients with rheumatoid arthritis and other disorders.

Rheumatoid Arthritis

Rheumatoid Arthritis Risk Factors

Genetic, environmental, and social risk factors have been implicated in the etiology of rheumatoid arthritis. Social and environmental factors may influence the development of rheumatoid arthritis even in genetically-related communities. Solomon, et al. (1975) studied two South African black communities, one rural in north-western Transvaal, and the other urban in Johannesburg. They found that blacks in the rural community had a much lower prevalence of rheumatoid arthritis than those in the urban community. The study subjects in the rural community had a mild form of rheumatoid arthritis and lacked the classical features of rheumatoid arthritis, whereas the urban community subjects resembled classical rheumatoid arthritis in the white populations. These results highlight the salience of sociological and environmental factors in the development of rheumatoid arthritis in genetically related communities.

Cigarette smoking is a well-known rheumatoid arthritis risk factor (Stolt, et al., 2003; Harrison, 2002). A study, using 679 persons diagnosed with rheumatoid arthritis and 847 controls, showed that smoking was related to an increased risk of developing seropostive rheumatoid arthritis, but not seronegative rheumatoid arthritis. (Stolt, et al., 2003). In their study, current smokers, and ex-smokers, of both sexes had greater odds of developing seropositive rheumatoid arthritis. Individuals who had smoked for 20 or more years had increased odds of acquiring seropostive rheumatoid arthritis. Smoking 6 to 9 cigarettes a day also was related to an increased risk of developing the disease, and the risks for developing seropostive rheumatoid arthritis continued for 10 to 19 years after quitting smoking.

One study by Krishnan, et al. (2003) evaluated the possible association between gender, smoking, and the risk for acquiring rheumatoid arthritis. Based on a sample of Finnish patients with rheumatoid arthritis, the investigators discovered that in men, a past history of smoking was linked to an increased risk of developing seropostive rheumatoid arthritis. However, among women, smoking history was not associated with an increased risk of the disease.

Researchers have assessed the effects of smoking on the risk of acquiring rheumatoid arthritis among postmenopausal women. Using data from the Iowa Women's Health Study, Criswell, et al. (2002) found that postmenopausal women who were current smokers or who had stopped smoking 10 years or less before the start of the study had an increased risk of acquiring rheumatoid arthritis compared to those postmenopausal women who had never smoked. Their results indicated that the duration and intensity of smoking were related to an increased risk of developing rheumatoid arthritis.

The role of menopause as a risk factor for rheumatoid arthritis needs further investigation (Krishnan, et al., 2003). Epidemiologic data has shown a strong association between hormonal and reproductive factors and the risk of rheumatoid arthritis. Oral contraceptives or estrogen replacement therapy may protect against the onset of the disease. In addition, at least one pregnancy may have a protective effect. Oral contraceptives or estrogen replacement therapy may lead to higher levels of endogenous heat shock proteins, which triggers immunotolerance to subsequent exposure to triggering agents of rheumatoid arthritis.

Some men with rheumatoid arthritis are more likely to have low levels testosterone levels. However, less is known about the levels of other sex hormones (estradiol, estrone, and the adrenal androgen dehydroepiandrosterone) among male rheumatoid arthritis sufferers (Tengstrand, et al., 2003). Based on a study of 101 men with rheumatoid arthritis, one report revealed that subjects had high levels of estradiol and other abnormalities in sex hormones. In these subjects, high concentrations of estradiol were related consistently to joint inflammation. The authors suggest that the high levels of estradiol may be due to an increased conversion of estrone to estradiol (Tengstrand, et al., 2003).

Occupational factors have been linked to the etiology of rheumatoid arthritis. In a study of 422 individuals with rheumatoid arthritis and 858 controls, Olsson, et al. (2004) discovered that the risk for rheumatoid arthritis increased with increasing duration of occupational exposure to vibrations and mineral dust. The findings supported a causal relationship among men and multiple exposures were related to an increased risk of rheumatoid arthritis for most occupations. For example, among farmers, exposure to organic dust was related to an increased risk of rheumatoid arthritis, and multiple exposures predicted an elevated risk of the disease.

Older age and low socioeconomic status, including low educational attainment, are correlated with the incidence of rheumatoid arthritis in the United States (Markenson, 1991). These factors are also associated with a poorer prognosis.

Risk Factors for Rheumatoid Arthritis-Related Disability

Backman (2004) noted that about one third of individuals with rheumatoid arthritis will leave employment prematurely. Prospective cohort studies have shown that 20% to 30% of individuals with early rheumatoid arthritis become permanently work disabled during the first 2 to 3 years of the disease (Sokka, 2003). In addition to causing early retirement, rheumatoid arthritis can cause a significant number of absences from work (Kapidzic-Basic, et al., 2004).

Although rheumatoid arthritis can not be assessed by a single diagnostic measure, a variety of measures can be used to determine disability in patients with rheumatoid arthritis. Various measures, including pain assessment, Ritchie articular index, the number of painful and swollen joints, morning stiffness duration, and index of joint motion, can be used to assess disability in rheumatoid arthritis patients (Kapidzic-Basic, et al., 2004; Pincus and Sokka, 2003).

Kapidzic-Basic, et al. (2004) recommended that assessment of working ability should not be made based on current status of certain measures, such as pain assessment, Ritchie articular index, motion assessment, functional ability, and number of painful and swollen joints. However, clinicians should make their decisions based on the progression of the disease.

Genetic and non-genetic factors may be risk factors for work disability among patients with rheumatoid arthritis (Symmons, 2003; Backman, 2004). Pain, joint destruction, demographic, socioeconomic status, occupational factors, policies related to work accommodation, and psychosocial distress and social support are some of the factors that influence work disability and failure to return to work among persons with rheumatoid arthritis (Backman, 2004; Reisine, et al., 2001).

Rheumatoid factor status, disease activity, joint destruction, deformity, and intense chronic pain are associated with rheumatoid arthritis-related work disability and decreased quality of life (Mullan and Bresnihan, 2003; Scott, et al., 2003). The development of measurable structural joint damage indicates severity of rheumatoid arthritis and future disability (Mullan and Bresnihan, 2003).

However, more research is needed to evaluate the role of pain, joint destruction, and other factors in predicting work disability compared to other risk factors. For example, both joint damage and disability in rheumatoid arthritis increase with disease duration, but the nature of their association is not certain. Scott, et al. (2003) noted that 39 to 73% of patients with early rheumatoid arthritis acquire one or more erosions in their hands and wrists in 5 years. In addition, there is a constant worsening of joint damage during the first 20 years of the disease. With regard to work disability, there is an initial drop in disability in the first years of the disease followed by an increase in disability. Their studies show that in early rheumatoid arthritis, there is either no association or a weak association between joint damage and disability. However, as the duration of rheumatoid arthritis increases, the link between joint damage and disability becomes more prominent. The authors suggest that the rheumatoid factor status and disease activity are the strongest determinants of joint damage and disability.

One investigation of employed patients with early rheumatoid arthritis revealed that high pain intensity and radiographic erosions were only related to work disability in the univariate analysis. In subsequent multivariate analysis, the report found that limited joint motion that interfered with job tasks, but not high pain intensity, predicted work disability (Brauer, et al., 2002).

Based on a longitudinal study with a 5-year follow-up, Maillefert, et al. (2004) discovered that in patients with recent-onset rheumatoid arthritis, early joint narrowing, but not joint erosion, was associated with later disability, as measured by the Health Assessment Questionnaire.

Co-Morbidity as a Risk Factor for Rheumatoid Arthritis-Related Work Disability

Co-morbidities related to rheumatoid arthritis are major risk factors for work disability and other outcomes (Mikulis, 2003). These rheumatoid arthritis-related co-morbidities include anemia, cardiovascular disease, pulmonary disease, infection, osteoporosis, lymphoproliferative malignancy, and peptic ulcer disease (Mikulis, 2003; Wilson, et al., 2004; Shi, et al., 2003).

Certain co-morbidities are prevalent and may result in high levels of disability in rheumatoid arthritis patients. Patients with rheumatoid arthritis may have similar risk factors for cardiovascular disease as persons in the general population. A 2-year study of 13,171 patients with rheumatoid arthritis revealed that rheumatoid arthritis increases the risk of heart failure, which may be reduced by anti-TNF therapies. The investigation also found that patients with rheumatoid arthritis had similar risk factors for heart failure, including hypertension, previous myocardial infarction, diabetes, and advanced age, as those individuals in population-based studies (Wolfe and Michaud, 2004).

Another investigation showed an increased intima-media thickness of the common carotid arteries in rheumatoid arthritis patients without any clinical evidence of cardiovascular disease (Cuomo, et al., 2004). These study results document the prevalence of sub-clinical atherosclerosis in patients with rheumatoid arthritis.

One report showed that the number of vertebral deformities was significantly increased in patients with rheumatoid arthritis compared to population controls (Orstavik, et al., 2004). Another condition, anemia of the type consisting of low serum iron concentrations and inadequate iron stores, is often related to rheumatoid arthritis. In a review of the literature, Wilson, et al. (2004) discovered that improvement in rheumatoid arthritis indicators (swollen, painful, and tender joints, pain, low muscle strength, and low energy levels) was associated with resolution of anemia. However, the authors note that it is not possible to determine if the patients' improvement in quality of life and functional status were due to resolution of the anemia independent of the patients' response to rheumatoid arthritis treatment.

Patients with rheumatoid arthritis have an increased risk of lymphoma, and this co-morbid condition can lead to early work disability and mortality. The underlying cause of this increased risk is unclear, but research indicates that the severity of rheumatoid arthritis may be more likely linked to lymphoma than the risks related to specific treatments, such as TNF-blocking therapies (Baecklund, et al., 2004).

Researchers have assessed the extent to which the number of co-morbidities and the specific types of co-morbidities among patients with arthritis and other chronic diseases result in different levels of decline in physical functioning in older adults. Based on data from the Longitudinal Aging Study, Amsterdam, Kriegsman, et al. (2004) discovered that the number of co-morbidities predicted decline in physical functioning. In addition, individuals with arthritis who also had diabetes or malignancies were more likely to experience decline in physical functioning.

Occupational and Socioeconomic Disparities in Rheumatoid Arthritis-Related Disability

Aspects of the work environment, occupational activities, and socioeconomic factors have been linked to an increased risk of rheumatoid arthritis-related disability (Sokka, 2003; Brauer, et al., 2002). Work settings that do not provide accommodations for workers with rheumatoid arthritis are related to increased work disability for these individuals (Gilworth, et al., 2003; Backman, 2004). A physically demanding job has been identified as a possible risk factor for early work disability among patients with rheumatoid arthritis (Sokka, 2003). Another investigation of 141 employed individuals with early rheumatoid arthritis revealed that working under pressure of time predicted work disability (Brauer, et al., 2002). Individuals with rheumatoid arthritis who suffer fatigue and feelings of poor health may be likely to find their job physically or emotionally demanding.

Workplaces that do not provide social support for workers with rheumatoid arthritis may contribute to their high rate of disability (McQuade, 2002; Backman, 2004). Individuals who experience negative interpersonal relations at work because of their disease may be at risk for increased work disability (Backman, 2004). McQuade (2002) evaluated attitudes toward workers with rheumatoid arthritis based on a study of evaluations of job performance of hypothetical workers with rheumatoid arthritis. The author showed that those with rheumatoid arthritis are viewed as having poorer interpersonal job skills and deserve a poorer overall job rating than paraplegic and healthy workers even though no differences were found in their job commitment or job expertise. He suggests that negative social responses to workers with rheumatoid arthritis disrupt social support for these individuals and increases their chances of being disabled.

A study of 472 employed patients with rheumatoid arthritis found that being self-employed, having a higher prestige occupation, and missing fewer days of work during the baseline years were associated with the ability to remain employed over a 9-year period (Reisine, et al., 2001).

Low Educational Attainment and Work Disability in Rheumatoid Arthritis Patients

Socioeconomic disparities, especially low educational achievement, may increase impairment among rheumatoid arthritis sufferers. Persons with low education attainment may be at risk for early work disability associated with rheumatoid arthritis (Sokka, 2003; Symmons, 2003). Reisine, et al. (2001), in a study of 472 employed patients with rheumatoid arthritis, showed that having higher educational attainment predicted the ability to remain employed over a 9-year period.

In a study of arthritis, another report revealed that patients with early adult-onset arthritis had lower educational attainment relative to a control group (Archenholtz, et al., 2001). More research is necessary to assess the independent effects of low educational attainment in predicting work disability in rheumatoid arthritis patients.

Another investigation of 141 employed patients with early rheumatoid arthritis showed that unskilled, blue-collar workers were at greater risk of experiencing work disability than white-collar professionals and self-employed individuals (Brauer, et al., 2002). Young, et al. (2002) also discovered that manual work was a major predictor of work disability among rheumatoid arthritis patients.

Fatigue, Feeling of Poor Health, and Depression associated with Disability in Rheumatoid Arthritis

In addition to physical discomfort, individuals with rheumatoid arthritis can suffer fatigue, feelings of poor health, and depression associated with the disease (Carr, et al., 2003; Symmons, 2003). Psychological factors can influence the level of pain and disability, resulting in an increased risk of work disability and limited functional status. One investigation, using a sample of 480 long-term disability claimants with rheumatoid arthritis and other major medical problems, showed that about 34% of the sample met the criteria for major depressive disorder (Leon, et al., 2001).

Low Functional Status among Rheumatoid Arthritis Patients

Studies have shown that low levels of functional status in daily activities are related to pain, stiffness, and work disability among individuals with rheumatoid arthritis (Sokka, et al., 2004; Sokka, 2003). Low functional status in these patients is also related to disease flare, fatigue, and feelings of poor health (Carr, et al., 2003). Sokka, et al. (2004), using a sample of 1,095 patients with rheumatoid arthritis and 1,490 community controls, showed that disability in activities of daily living, as measured by the Health Assessment Questionnaire, predicted mortality in patients with rheumatoid arthritis.

Older Age and Disability in Rheumatoid Arthritis

Various investigations have shown that older age may be a risk factor for early work disability among patients with rheumatoid arthritis (Sokka, 2003; Straaton, et al., 1996). Reisine, et al. (2001) used the results of a study of 472 employed patients with rheumatoid arthritis to show that being younger was related to continued employment over a 9-year period. Brauer, et al. (2002), examined 141 employed patients with early rheumatoid arthritis, and discovered that being over 45 years old predicted work disability. Likewise, a study of 218 persons who were unemployed because of arthritis and musculoskeletal disorders showed that older age was one of the barriers to re-employment (Straaton, et al., 1996).

Smoking and Disability in Rheumatoid Arthritis Patients

Among patients with rheumatoid arthritis, smoking may increase levels of pain and disability (Symmons, 2003). In addition, smoking may be linked to poor long-term radiological outcomes among rheumatoid arthritis patients (Symmons, 2003). Smoking may have an adverse impact both on the immune system and sex hormones that in turn may affect the pathogenesis of rheumatoid arthritis (Harrison, 2002). Smoking has been shown to negatively influence disease outcomes in other inflammatory diseases. However, the data on the effects of smoking on persons with rheumatoid arthritis are quite new and, according to Harrison (2002), the findings have been inconsistent.

Diet and Work Disability in Patients with Rheumatoid Arthritis

Dietary patterns among patients with rheumatoid arthritis may affect their levels of pain and disability (Symmons, 2003). Dietary factors, along with physical activity, can modify cytokines in rheumatoid arthritis and other inflammatory diseases (Robinson and Graham, 2004).

A prospective study found that excessive consumption of meat and total protein and lower consumption of fruit, vegetables, and vitamin C are linked to an increased risk of developing inflammatory polyarthritis or rheumatoid arthritis (Choi, 2005).

Several investigations have reported that the predominantly plant-based Mediterranean-style diet or its main components may protect against the development or worsening of rheumatoid arthritis (Choi, 2005; Wahle, et al., 2004).

Olive oil is a non-oxidative dietary substance that helps to modulate the oxidative and inflammatory processes underlying rheumatoid arthritis, cardiovascular disease, and, to a lesser extent, various cancers. Wahle, et al. (2004) point out that the antioxidant effects of olive oil may be due to both its high oleic acid content and its content of various plant antioxidants, especially oleuropein, hydroxytyrosol, and tyrosol. They also believe that olive oil's high content of oleic acid, in combination with a proportionately reduced intake of linoleic acid, promotes increased conversion of alpha-linolenic acid to the longer-chain n-3 polyunsaturated fatty acid, which may be useful in treating inflammatory diseases.

A diet that includes fish and evening primrose oils may reduce the inflammatory process in rheumatoid arthritis, although these effects are mild compared with standard drug treatment (Cleland, et al., 2005; Mera, 1994). Fish oil, a rich source of a beneficial long chain n-3 polyunsaturated fatty acid, has been used as an anti-inflammatory agent in the treatment of inflammatory diseases of joints and other organs and tissues. The n-3 polyunsaturated fatty acid metabolizes to mediators that control cardiovascular homeostasis and inflammation. Cleland, et al. (2005) also suggest that fish oil, combined with traditional medications, can be helpful in controlling the symptoms of rheumatoid arthritis on a long-term basis. Another important benefit of the n-3 polyunsaturated fatty acid is that it can lower the increased cardiovascular risks, which are inherent in rheumatoid arthritis.

Sundrarjun, et al. (2004) evaluated the impact of a low n-6 polyunsaturated fatty acid diet (which is pro-inflammatory) supplemented with fish oil (rich in n-3 polyunsaturated fatty acid) on inflammatory factors in patients with rheumatoid arthritis. They investigated patients who received a low n-6 polyunsaturated fatty acid diet supplemented with n-3 polyunsaturated fatty acid and found that these patients had a decrease in two inflammatory factors, C-reactive protein and soluble tumor necrosis factor receptor p55.

Barriers to Employment among Rheumatoid Arthritis Patients

Persons with arthritis may face discrimination and other barriers when they try to re-enter the workforce or maintain their employment. Many companies lack policies related to work accommodation for employees with rheumatoid arthritis (Backman, 2004). Small companies may be more likely to not have work accommodation policies because of the costs involved in modifying their workplace to accommodate persons with handicaps due to rheumatoid arthritis.

Stress, Coping Strategies, Social Support, Rheumatoid Arthritis Patients

Living with rheumatoid arthritis involves learning to deal with pain, reduced physical functioning, fatigue, mobility loss, reduced independence, and uncertainty and role losses during periods of exacerbation and remission (Melanson and Downe-Wamboldt, 2003).

Varying levels of pain, stress, and other factors may determine disease activity and other outcomes in patients with rheumatoid arthritis (Barlow, et al., 2003). It is not surprising that pain levels among rheumatoid arthritis patients have been found to be associated with low levels of satisfaction with social support (Minnock, et al., 2003)

Personality characteristics, perceptions of illness-associated stress, and feelings of anxiety and depression may increase the vulnerability of persons with rheumatoid arthritis. A study by Evers, et al. (2003) showed that one personality characteristic, neuroticism, was related to anxiety and depressive symptoms at 3-year and 5-year follow-ups of these victims.

Based on a sample of 122 women with rheumatoid arthritis, Lambert, et al. (1990) showed that hardiness (one's resistance to stress, anxiety & depression) was positively related to the women's psychological well-being, the number of persons in their social support system, and their satisfaction with social support.

The quality of a person's social roles may influence psychological well-being among rheumatoid arthritis sufferers. In a study of 156 women with rheumatoid arthritis, Plach, et al. (2003) discovered that role quality had a significant positive impact on the women. In their study, women in poor health with high role quality were less depressed than those in poor health who also had poor role quality. Moreover, women who had significant pain and high role quality felt that they had more purpose in life than women who reported substantial pain and poor role quality.

Melanson and Downe-Wamboldt (2003) assessed perceptions of illness-associated stressors in older persons with rheumatoid arthritis. A majority of individuals viewed their physical disabilities as their illness-related stressors. These persons tended to use direct coping strategies to cope with the stress related to rheumatoid arthritis.

Other coping strategies, both positive and negative, are thought to influence disease activity, psychological well-being, and other outcomes among persons with rheumatoid arthritis. Evers, et al. (2003), in a prospective study of 78 patients with recently diagnosed rheumatoid arthritis, discovered that one type of coping strategy, avoidance coping, predicted increased disease severity at 3-year and 5-year follow-ups.

Sinclair (2001), using a sample of 90 women with rheumatoid arthritis, found that negative cognitive distortions, also known as catastrophizing, were linked to adverse psychosocial and physical effects. The author discovered 4 determinants of catastrophizing: pessimism, passive coping with pain, venting, and feeling helpless over arthritis.

Social support may buffer the negative impact of stress on psychosocial well-being (Olstad, et al., 2001). Research has shown that social support can enable rheumatoid arthritis sufferers to cope with their painful and disabling symptoms and improve their psychological adjustment. Situational stressors can increase negative mood, and perceived social support, through increased situational control, can help reduce these stress-induced negative mood changes (Atienza, et al., 2001).

Lack of social support from families and friends may contribute to high rates of work disability, emotional distress, and poor quality of life among patients with rheumatoid arthritis (McQuade, 2002). Evers, et al. (2003) reported that poor social support was related to increased disease severity at a 3-year follow-up among early rheumatoid arthritis sufferers. Another investigation by Griffin, et al. (2001) evaluated the impact of negative responses from significant others on patients with rheumatoid arthritis. In their study, patients who perceived irritation or anger from significant others were more likely to cope by venting negative emotions and had increased negative affect and higher disease activity over time.

Different types of social support may influence psychological well-being in persons with rheumatoid arthritis. For example, one investigation, using a sample of 158 rheumatology arthritis patients at a hospital rheumatology clinic, compared the impact of diffuse (e.g., friends and acquaintances) and intimate social relationships (Fitzpatrick, et al., 1988). Their findings indicated that more diffuse social relationships were more strongly related to psychological well-being than intimate relationships.

Using a sample of 54 rheumatoid arthritis patients, Doeglas, et al. (1994) found that daily emotional support was correlated with psychological well-being, while problem-oriented emotional support was not related to some aspects of psychological well-being.

Lambert, et al. (1990) used a sample of 122 women who were rheumatoid arthritis patients to investigate the impact of hardiness, social support, and illness severity on psychosocial status. The authors discovered that patient satisfaction with social support, hardiness, and duration of morning stiffness predicted psychosocial well-being.

Treatment and Rehabilitation Outcomes in Rheumatoid Arthritis Patients

In the last decade, the treatment of rheumatoid arthritis has changed significantly, with emphasis now on early, aggressive intervention in order to prevent disability and irreversible joint damage. Research has focused on the impact of different treatment strategies on patient outcomes. According to Quinn and Emery (2003), research indicates that aggressive early treatment may weaken rheumatoid arthritis disease activity.

Machold, et al. (2003), in their study of patients with early rheumatoid arthritis, found support for these findings. Based on a one-year follow-up study of 182 patients, they showed that patients who received treatment very early appeared to have less severe radiological progression. However, the authors note that direct comparisons with patients in other studies were not possible due to the different patient selection methods used in these reports.

A 3-year follow-up investigation of 866 patients with early rheumatoid arthritis revealed that despite early treatment with conventional drug treatment, most patients had radiological erosions by 3 years (Dixey, et al., 2004). Quinn and Emery (2003) suggest that more research is needed to clarify the underlying mechanisms and their effects on the disease process and disability.

A number of disease-modifying anti-rheumatic drugs (DMARDs) are used to control the effects of rheumatoid arthritis. The goal of treatment is to prevent joint destruction, improve quality of life, and prevent or reduce work disability with the fewest side effects. Clinical research has demonstrated the efficacy of Methotrexate, Etanercept, Infliximab, Gold, Hydroxychloroquine, Leflunomide, and Sulfasalazine (Blumenauer, et al., 2002). Four other drugs (Penicillamine, Cyclosporine, Azathioprine, and Corticosteroids) have greater toxicity and are only recommended if less toxic drugs do not work. Blumenauer, et al. (2002) feel that additional research is needed to evaluate the cost effectiveness of these drugs in preventing long-term complications of rheumatoid arthritis.

Based on data from the North American Cohort of Patients with Early Rheumatoid Arthritis, it was shown that Methotrexate was prescribed for more than half of the patients in the database. The results of the Early RA Treatment Evaluation Registry reveal that Methotrexate was the first DMARD prescribed in 83% of the patients (Sokka, et al., 2003).

Since rheumatoid arthritis has been related to excess mortality, researchers have evaluated the extent to which treatment with Methotrexate is associated with changes in mortality rates (Singer,

2003). Singer (2003) evaluated the mortality rates among 588 rheumatoid arthritis patients who received Methotrexate and 652 patients who did not receive the drug. The results showed that the mortality rate was significantly lower among patients treated with Methotrexate.

Based on a sample of 497 rheumatoid arthritis patients, Yelin, et al. (2003) evaluated whether participating in Etanercept clinical trials was associated with higher employment rates (current employment status and number of hours per week of work). The researchers discovered that having participated in the Etanercept trials was linked to higher rates of employment and a greater number of hours per week of work among all patients who were employed at the time of being diagnosed with rheumatoid arthritis. The authors believe that a randomized trial is now needed to determine the association between Etanercept treatment and employment outcomes.

An investigation by Donnelly and Cooke (1982) evaluated the combined effect of ACTH (gel) and D-Penicillamine on functional disability of patients with rheumatoid disease. Based on a sample of 48 patients who were treated with a combination of D-Penicillamine and ACTH (gel) over a 6-year period, the authors showed that 77% of the patients had rapid remission of the disease within one month as reflected in their ability to return to full employment. By the end of three years, 71% had remission of the disease and 89% had been classified as either Steinbrocker functional class I or II. The side effects were very low except for kidney toxicity in 10% of the patients and skin rash, dysgeusia, and thrombocytopenia in only one patient. None of the patients had any gastrointestinal upset.

Puolakka, et al. (2004) compared the impact of a combination of DMARDs and single-DMARD therapy on the prevention of work disability in patients with early rheumatoid arthritis. Based on data from the Finnish Rheumatoid Arthritis Combination Therapy trial, 195 patients with recent-onset rheumatoid arthritis were randomly assigned to receive combination therapy (Sulfasalazine, Methotrexate, Hydroxychloroquine) and Prednisolone or single-DMARD therapy with or without prednisolone. The drug treatment strategy was no longer restricted after two years. After a 5-year follow-up, the authors discovered that the combination therapy produced a significantly lower duration of cumulative days of work disability than those receiving the single therapy. The authors conclude that aggressive treatment with combination-DMARD therapy improves 5-year work disability outcomes in patients with early rheumatoid arthritis.

Based on information from focus groups at 5 clinical centers in different geographical areas, Carr, et al. (2003) discovered that rheumatoid arthritis patients considered not only physical outcomes such as pain and disability important, but also rated fatigue, general feelings of wellness, and disease flare-ups as important outcomes. Patient satisfaction with treatment was associated with effective health provider-patient communication, access to therapy, and the effectiveness of therapy. Patients' perceptions of treatment efficacy were associated with a reduction of symptoms. However, the magnitude of the symptom reduction varied depending on the patients' disease stage. Patients with early rheumatoid arthritis considered even small reductions in symptoms important, while patients with long disease duration viewed large changes as significant.

Vocational assessment and intervention should take place early in the course of rheumatoid arthritis. However, more research is needed to study the impact of vocational assessment and rehabilitation on work retention and return-to-work rates among patients with the disease (Backman, 2004; de Buck, et al., 2002). In a review of the literature, Backman (2004) discovered that only 6 uncontrolled investigations showed a positive impact of vocational rehabilitation on patients with rheumatoid arthritis.

de Buck, et al. (2002) reviewed the literature between 1980 and May 2001 and identified 6 uncontrolled evaluation studies of the effectiveness of vocational rehabilitation programs for patients with chronic rheumatic diseases. Follow-up periods ranged from 2 to 84 months. Their analysis revealed that 5 of the 6 studies had significant beneficial effects on vocational status, such as work disability, sick leave, and retraining. For example, the findings showed that 15 to 69% of the patients participating in the vocational rehabilitation programs returned to work successfully. However, the authors caution that it is difficult to evaluate program effectiveness because of the methodological differences and deficits in these studies.

Hakkinen, et al. (2003) drew on an experimental group of 35 patients in a strength training program and 35 control patients, and showed that strength training increased the muscular strength of patients in the experimental group. However, increased muscular strength was not associated with enhanced physical functioning. Moreover, improved muscular strength did not reduce the rate of early retirement among rheumatoid arthritis patients.

Investigators have studied the effects of stress management and mutual support on various outcomes in rheumatoid arthritis patients. Some stress management programs are designed to achieve a variety of goals: improving pain, health status, disability, coping strategies, depression, feelings of helplessness, self-efficacy, and life satisfaction. In one evaluation of stress management, Parker, et al. (1995) randomly assigned rheumatoid arthritis patients to 1 of 3 conditions: a stress management program, an attention control group, or a standard care control group. Both the stress management and attention control interventions were both 10 weeks in duration and were both followed by a maintenance phase of 15-months duration. These interventions reduced the patients' pain and feelings of helplessness, and improved their self efficacy coping techniques and health.

Shearn and Fireman (1985) evaluated the impact of a 10-week stress management program and 10-week mutual support program on disease activity, disability and psychosocial status in 105 rheumatoid arthritis patients. Patients were assigned to 1 of 3 conditions: stress management, mutual support, or control group. Patients in the intervention groups exhibited more improvement in joint tenderness than the control patients. However, there were no significant differences between the intervention patients and the control group on other disability and psychosocial outcomes.

Osteoarthritis

Osteoarthritis Risk Factors

Using epidemiological research on family history and family clustering, studies of twins and investigation of rare genetic disorders, Spector and MacGregor (2004) have found evidence that genetic factors can be important determinants of osteoarthritis. They suggest that genes may function differently in women and men, at different sites of the body and on different aspects of the disease within body sites. Research on twins shows that between 39% and 65% of radiographic osteoarthritis of the hand and knee in women is due to genetic factors. About 60% of hip osteoarthritis and 70% of spine osteoarthritis have genetic determinants. These results indicate that half of the variation in susceptibility to osteoarthritis in the population can be based on genetic factors. Chromosomes 2q, 0q, 11q, and 16p have been some of the chromosomes linked to osteoarthritis. Genes associated with osteoarthritis include VDR, AGC1, IGF-1, ER alpha, TGF beta, CRTM (cartilage matrix protein) CRTL (cartilage link protein), and collagen II, IX, and XI.

Above average body weight and obesity are major potentially modifiable risk factors for the onset of osteoarthritis (March and Bagga, 2004; Felson, 2004). Using data from the Canadian Community Health Survey, Wilkins (2004) reported that for both women and men, obesity was significantly associated with subsequent arthritis. This is likely because excessive body weight puts abnormal pressure and stress on the joints during movement and at rest (Spineuniverse.com).

Joint injury is another important potentially modifiable risk factor for osteoarthritis (March and Bagga, 2004; Felson, 2004). Individuals with abnormal joint anatomy or alignment, prior joint surgery, joint instability, problems in joint or muscle innervation, or inadequate muscle strength may be at increased risk of osteoarthritis (Buckwalter and Lane, 1997).

Certain occupations and job conditions have been linked to an increased risk of osteoarthritis (Croft, et al., 1992; Thelin, et al., 2004). Croft, et al. (1992) tested the hypothesis that farmers have a high risk of hip osteoarthritis compared to persons in primarily sedentary occupations. Using a sample of 167 male farmers, aged 60–76, and 80 controls from mostly sedentary occupations, the authors found hip osteoarthritis was more prevalent among farmers than among the controls. No particular type of farm was linked to a higher risk of hip osteoarthritis. The authors suggest that heavy lifting may be responsible for the excess incidence of the disease in farmers.

In a study of 427 farmers with hip joint arthritis, Thelin, et al. (2004) evaluated possible occupational risk factors for the disease. The results indicated that certain job conditions were associated with an increased risk of hip joint osteoarthritis. Farmers who milked more than 40 cows daily had an elevated risk of the disease compared to those who did not participate in dairy production. Farmers who worked more than hours per day in animal barns over a long duration had an increased risk of acquiring hip joint osteoarthritis, compared to those who did not work with animals. Farmers who worked in large farm areas had a reduced risk of developing the disease compared to farmers who worked in smaller areas.

Age has been implicated as a risk factor for the development of this disease. Although it can develop at any age, the condition increases greatly with age (De Filippis, et al., 2004). The highest incidence of osteoarthritis has been found for those between 40 and 50 years of age.

A combination of increasing risk factors, such as older age, obesity, and joint injury, is likely to increase the prevalence of osteoarthritis and the need for total jont replacement surgery (March and Bagga, 2004; De Filippis, et al., 2004). Hip osteoarthritis is associated with weight, genetic factors, gender previous injury, occupational factors, and increasing age (De Filippis, et al., 2004). Knee osteoarthritis has been found to be correlated with weight, lifestyle habits, and physical activity. Bone marrow edema, synovitis and joint effusion have been identified as risk factors for the onset of symptoms of osteoarthritis.

Choi (2005) evaluated possible dietary factors in the progression of osteoarthritis symptoms. It is thought that antioxidant vitamins halt the progression of knee osteoarthritis. However, recent randomized controlled investigations have found that antioxidant vitamins, such as vitamin E, vitamin C, beta-carotene, and retinol were ineffective in halting the progression of knee osteoarthritis symptoms.

Osteoarthritis-Related Disability

Osteoarthritis can be a very painful and disabling disease. Increased pain is associated with an increase in the number of patients' visits to doctors, use of analgesics or anti-inflammatory medications, and undergoing arthroplasty (Dominick, et al., 2004). The social and occupational burden of osteoarthritis can have significant community-wide effects. One representative study of the Finnish population found that people with hip and knee osteoarthritis had a significant impact on the community in terms of reduced working capacity and a continuing need for assistance in daily activities (Makela, et al., 1993).

Osteoarthritis pain and disability can worsen over time. In one prospective observational study of 2,437 patients reporting hip and/or knee symptoms in 40 general practices, pain and disability generally worsened over a 7-year period (Peters, et al., 2005). However, of those patients with initial hip and knee pain, 35% and 29%, respectively, reported improvement in their pain levels due to treatment.

Co-Morbid Conditions and
Osteoarthritis-related Disability

Co-morbid conditions occur frequently among patients with osteoarthritis, and these diseases increase their risk for disability (Breedveld, 2004; Singh, et al., 2002). Kadam, et al. (2004), in a case-control study of 11,375 osteoarthritis patients and 11,780 matched controls seen in 60 general practices, revealed that co-morbidity was extensive among osteoarthritis patients compared to controls. Osteoarthritis patients reported prevalent co-morbid musculoskeletal disorders that included arthropathies, upper limb sprain, and synovial and tendon disorders. In terms of prevalent non-musculoskeletal co-morbid conditions, osteoarthritis patients reported having gastritis, phlebitis, diaphragmatic hernia, ischemic heart disease, and intestinal diverticula.

Based on a review of 1,000 patients who underwent hip osteoarthritis surgeries, Marks and Allegrante (2002) discovered that 55% of the patients had at least one co-morbid problem such as hypertension or heart disease. Those patients with two or more co-morbid conditions had a higher degree of functional disability before and after surgery than those without co-morbid health problems.

Occupational Risk Factors for Osteoarthritis-related Disability

Researchers have identified occupations that are potentially linked to increased risks for osteoarthritis-associated disability (Rossignol, et al., 2003; Kirkhorn, et al., 2003). Based on the results of the 1998 French National Survey on Health Impairment and Disability, Rossignol, et al. (2003) discovered that blue- collar workers with osteoarthritis had the highest total work disability, while agricultural workers with the disease had the highest partial disability.

Kirkhorn, et al. (2003) studied agriculture-related osteoarthritis among Wisconsin farm operators and farm workers and found that the ability to perform farm duties is greatly affected by arthritis. Arthritis made up 10% to 12% of the disability referrals to state and national agricultural work programs known as AgrAbility programs. Occupational factors have been related to increased risk of disability among persons with osteoarthritis, and ergonomic improvements will help to prevent osteoarthritis among agricultural workers.

Rossignol, et al. (2003) suggest that the increasing evidence that osteoarthritis is etiologically associated with occupational factors indicates that osteoarthritis should no longer be considered an inevitable disease in older populations.

Osteoarthritis of the Lumbar Spine and Disability

Osteoarthritis of the lumbar spine has the same changes in cartilage loss, joint instability, and osteophytosis as that of osteoarthritis in the extremities. Borenstein (2004) questioned whether the osteoarthritis-related degeneration of the lumbar facet joints is a source of disabling chronic back pain. Single photon emission computed tomography scans of the axial skeleton reveal osteoarthritis-related painful facet joints, which may benefit from local anesthetic injections. Borenstein (2004) concludes that osteoarthritis of the lumbar spine does cause low back pain.

Sleep Disorders

Some patients with osteoarthritis experience sleep disorders, including alpha EEG sleep and sleep-related breathing disorders and periodic limb movement disorders (Moldofsky, 2001). Sleep disturbances and associated psychological distress can decrease work performance and the ability to return to work among patients with osteoarthritis and other arthritic disorders.

As noted previously, sleep disturbance occurs among osteoarthritis sufferers and is especially common in older persons (Baird, et al., 2003; Wilcox, et al., 2000). There may be differences in the degree of sleep disturbance depending on the person's social setting. Baird, et al. (2003) evaluated older women with osteoarthritis who lived in homes in the community, in assisted living arrangements, and in long-term care settings. The results showed that women living in homes in the community had more sleep disturbance, pain, negative emotions, and moved more slowly, compared to those in assisted living and long-term care facilities.

Access to Health Care

Certain individuals, such as those without insurance will have difficulty accessing health care for treatment of their osteoarthritis. In their study of agricultural-related osteoarthritis, Kirkhorn, et al. (2003) found that problems in accessing health care have been linked to increased risk of osteoarthritis-related disability. They discovered that the ability to perform agricultural jobs was influenced by the severity of their osteoarthritis and the availability of access to health care. The authors conclude that improving access to health care for diagnosing and treating osteoarthritis can reduce disability levels.

Stress, Coping, and Social Support for Individuals with Osteoarthritis

Individuals with osteoarthritis and other chronic health problems use a broad range of coping strategies to cope with their conditions and related stresses. Aldwin and Yancura (in press) suggest that people use five general types of coping strategies in dealing with stressful situations: 1) problem-focused coping, 2) emotion-focused coping, 3) social support, 4) religious coping, and 5) making meaning. Problem-focused coping consists of cognitions and behaviors, including seeking information and thinking about alternatives to solving a stressful problem. Emotion-focused coping involves a range of strategies such as avoidance and withdrawal and suppression of one's emotions in order to maximize problem-focused strategies. Social support and religious coping are strategies that use both problem-focused and emotion-focused strategies. Social support may involve advice, direct aid, emotional support, or justification for one's actions or perceptions. Religious coping may consist of prayer, advice, or direct aid.

Aldwin and Yancura (in press) point out that these coping strategies are not mutually exclusive. For example, individual may use coping strategies that involve suppressing and expressing emotions sequentially to deal with the same stressful problem.

In their exploratory study involving a series of focused groups, Iwasaki and Butcher (2004) identified similar stress-coping strategies used by middle-aged and older women and men with arthritis: 1) staying active and busy, 2) physical activity, including exercise, 3) learning about arthritis, 4) social support and friendship, 5) spiritual coping, 6) acknowledging stress, 7) helping others, and 8) leisure time. The participants in their study identified two overall coping strategies that cross-cut all the above strategies: being active and having control over one's life.

With increasing age, adults experience personal and social losses. Osteoarthritis, the most prevalent form of arthritis in the elderly, is the most significant cause of disability and impairment in daily activities in this population (Tak and Laffrey, 2003).

In a study of 101 older women with osteoarthritis, Zautra and Smith (2001) found that symptoms of depression were related to increased arthritic pain and negative affect. The level of functional disability, perceived stress, perceived control, quality of life, social support, treatment impact, co-morbidities, and other factors may significantly influence the ability of individuals to cope with osteoarthritis. Individuals with osteoarthritis who have poorer functional ability may be more likely to experience chronic stress, decreased quality of life, and develop dysfunctional coping strategies.

Treatment and Rehabilitation Outcomes in
Osteoarthritis Patients

There are limited high quality studies available to compare the relative efficacy of different treatments of osteoarthritis (Segal, et al., 2004). Analgesics and non-steroidal anti-inflammatory medications are frequently used to treat osteoarthritis symptoms (Breedveld, 2004; Dominick, et al., 2004). Breedveld (2004) notes that non-steroidal anti-inflammatory drugs can have serious gastrointestinal side-effects, and he recommends that patient's gastrointestinal tolerability should be considered when designing new therapies.

Clinical trial results indicate that total hip replacement and total knee replacement surgery are the most effective osteoarthritis treatments, are very cost-effective, and improve the quality of life (Segal, et al., 2004). Total hip replacement surgery has an estimated cost per quality-adjusted life year (QALY) of $7,500, and total knee replacement surgery has an estimated cost per QALY of $10,000. Exercise and strength training for knee osteoarthritis (less than $5,000/QALY), knee bracing and Capsaicin or Glucosamine Sulfate treatment ($1,000/QALY) were other highly cost-effective treatments.

Clinical pathways and continuous quality improvement techniques have been developed to improve outcomes for patients with total hip replacement, hip fracture, and knee replacement. Healy, et al. (1998) evaluated the impact of a clinical pathway and hip implant standardization program on the quality and cost of total hip arthroplasty. Based on a sample of 206 unilateral total hip arthroplasty operations, the authors showed that initiation of the clinical pathway and hip implant standardization program reduced hospital length of stay and hospital cost without causing adverse short-term outcomes.

Lin, et al. (2002) used a sample of 122 patients in Taiwan to assess the effects of a clinical pathway on total knee arthroplasty outcomes. The researchers showed that the implementation of a clinical pathway reduced hospital length of stay by 24% and hospital costs by 16%. In addition, the initiation of the clinical pathway reduced the number of unnecessary procedures. Clinical outcomes and complication rates were not affected by the implementation of the clinical pathway. The researchers conclude that use of clinical pathway can reduce consumption of health care resources and hospital costs without having an adverse impact on quality of care.

Intra-articular injection of hyaluronic acid has been used in the treatment of knee osteoarthritis, however its efficacy has not been resolved. Based on a meta-analysis of 20 blinded, randomized, controlled trials, Wang, et al. (2004) supported the efficacy and safety of intra-articular injection of Hyaluronic Acid for knee osteoarthritis. The investigators point out that more research is needed to assess the efficacy of different types of Hyaluronic Acid product on knee osteoarthritis in patients with different clinical conditions and in different patient populations.

Weight reduction to achieve normal body weight is an important goal in the rehabilitation of individuals with osteoarthritis. In a study of 126 obese patients with bilateral knee osteoarthritis Huang, et al. (2000) analyzed the effects of weight reduction and electrotherapy. Participants were assigned to 3 groups based on their stage of knee osteoarthritis. Each group was then assigned to one of three therapies conditions: 1) weight reduction, 2) weight reduction and electrotherapy, and 3) electrotherapy. The results indicated that patients assigned to the first two groups did better than the third group in terms of pain reduction, weight reduction, speed of ambulation, and functional status. The researchers also reported that significant pain reduction in the first two groups was achieved when the weight reduction was more than 15% and 12%, respectively, of the patient's initial body weight. The authors suggest that weight reduction is one practical approach to rehabilitation for patients suffering from knee osteoarthritis.

Exercise (both therapeutic and recreational), alone or combined with weight reduction, can reduce pain, improve functioning and reduce the risk for disease related morbidity in patients with osteoarthritis (Roos and Dahlberg, 2004; Huang, et al., 2000). Exercise increases the osteoarthritis patients' flexibility and muscular conditioning and an additional benefit can be derived from aerobic exercise which enhances their cardiovascular functioning.

More research is needed to determine both the positive and negative health effects of exercise and physical activity on cartilage (Roos and Dahlberg, 2004). Cartilage adapts to loading like bone and muscle. Moderate loading of the cartilage seems to help prevent and treat osteoarthritis (Roos and Dahlberg, 2004; Buckwalter and Lane, 1997). However, if the loading of the cartilage is too high, e.g., repeated knee bendings several hours daily, there may be an increased risk for osteoarthritis (Roos and Dahlberg, 2004). Exercise and sports that produce high levels of impact and torsional loading of joints increase the risk of degeneration of articular cartilage, resulting in osteoarthritis (Buckwalter and Lane, 1997).

Roos and Dahlberg (2004) propose that too high or too low mechanical loading can reduce the proteoglycan content of cartilage, suggesting that either high levels of competitive sports or physical inactivity are risk factors for osteoarthritis. They recommend three strategies to prevent and treat osteoarthritis: 1) regular loading of the cartilage, 2) maintaining strong muscles, and 3) achieving and maintaining normal body weight.

Similarly, Buckwalter and Lane (1997) propose that moderate regular activity does not increase the risk of osteoarthritis and improves strength and mobility in older persons and in individuals with mild and moderate osteoarthritis. They recommend that people with joint or muscle problems and abnormal anatomy receive an evaluation before undertaking exercise. Patients should participate in exercises that reduce the intensity and frequency of impact and torsional loading loading of joints and use sports equipment that reduces joint impact loading.

Clinical research has focused on the effects of physical activity on osteoarthritis at different body sites, such as the lower extremity, knee, or hip osteoarthritis (Hughes, et al., 2004; Penninx, et al., 2001).

A randomized controlled trial by Hughes, et al. (2004) evaluated the outcome of a facility-based training and home-based adherence for older adults with lower extremity osteoarthritis. Older adults were randomly assigned to receive either an experimental (n = 80) training program (range of motion, resistance training, aerobic walking, and education-group problem solving regarding their ability to exercise and adhere to the program activities) or a wait-list control group (n = 70). Based on evaluations at 2- and 6-months follow-up periods, the researchers discovered the individuals in the exercise training program experienced beneficial results compared to those in the control group. The participants showed a 45.8% increase in exercise adherence and a 13.3% increase in a 6-minute distance walk with associated decreases in lower extremity stiffness at 2- and 6-month follow-ups. Individuals in the training group also had a significant increase in efficacy to adhere to the exercise regimen over time at the 6-month follow-up. Individuals in the wait-list control group, in contrast, declined in their exercise efficacy and adherence levels and exhibited no change in other measures.

Based on a review of findings from randomized controlled trials and observational research, the Philadelphia Panel found that therapeutic exercise was useful for knee osteoarthritis (Philadelphia Panel, 2001).

Using a 2-center, randomized controlled trial, Penninx, et al. (2001) assessed the effects of physical exercise in older persons with knee osteoarthritis. The study originally relied on a sample of 439 persons in the community, aged 60 years and older, who had knee osteoarthritis. From this sample, 250 persons who were initially free of disability in activities of daily living (e.g., dressing, bathing) were randomized to one of three groups: 1) an aerobic exercise program; 2) a resistance exercise program, or 3) an attention control group. The researchers discovered that the incidence of disability in activities of daily living was lower in the exercise groups (37.1%) compared to the attention control group (52.5%). Individuals who participated in resistance exercise and aerobic exercise programs had lower relative risks of disability in activities of daily living, compared to the attention control group. Those persons who had the highest adherence to the exercise regimen had the lowest disability in activities of daily living. The authors conclude that aerobic and resistance exercise may be useful in preventing disability and increasing autonomy in older persons with knee osteoarthritis.

Osteoporosis

Risk Factors for Osteoporosis

Osteoporosis may be idiopathic or secondary to other conditions, such as long decreased level of estrogen at menopause, prolonged calcium insufficiency, duration of Androgen deprivation therapy, steroid use, thyrotoxicosis, rheumatoid arthritis, and bone demineralization caused by hyperparathyroidism (Schacht, 2000; Hay, 1991). Most research on osteoporosis has emphasized post-menopausal women, but various other patient populations are at risk for osteoporosis. Patients taking medications that produce bone loss and those with health conditions that cause bone loss include patients with anorexia nervosa, organ transplantation, chronic obstructive pulmonary disease, and inflammatory bowel disease (Hansen and Vondracek, 2004). Osteoporosis can cause pain and disability, especially in the lower back, pathologic frac-tures, loss of stature, and different deformities (Tanvetyanon, 2005). The disease can have a major impact on quality of life (Hansen and Vondracek, 2004)

A major risk factor for osteoporosis is low bone mineral density (Journal of Bone Mineral Research, December 2002; Nevitt, et al., 1999). Research has shown that low bone mineral density increases the risk of fractures in women. Incident vertebral frac-tures are more prevalent in women than men because women's spine bone mineral density is lower than men's at any age (Journal of Bone Mineral Research, December 2002).

Postmenopausal women, since they have decreased levels of estrogen, have an increased risk of suffering from osteoporosis, indicating that hormones play a role in the etiology of the disease (Hay, 1991). Patients on long-term steroid therapy have a greater chance of developing osteoporosis (Tanvetyanon, 2005).

The most important dietary factor associated with osteoporo-sis is calcium (Mera, 1994). Calcium is essential for promoting peak bone mass and in reducing bone loss later in life. It has been suggested that excessive dietary salt intake also may be an impor-tant risk factor in the development of osteoporosis. However, in their review of the available data, Cohen and Roe (2000) con-clude that high salt intake is not related to an increased risk of osteoporosis.

Other lifestyle factors, such as smoking and drinking alcohol have been found to increase the risk of developing osteoporosis (Tanvetyanon, 2005). Valtola, et al. (2002) evaluated the data from the Kuopio Osteoporosis Risk Factor and Prevention Study, a population-based prospective cohort study of 11,798 women, aged 47–56 years, to determine risk factors for fractures and low bone density among middle-aged women in Finland. In their 5-year follow-up, the investigators identified several lifestyle factors that were related to an increase in the risk of ankle fractures. Middle-aged women with a body mass index of 25–30 kg/m^2 had a higher risk of ankle fractures compared to those with a body mass index less than 25 kg/m^2. Women who used three or more prescribed drugs had a higher rate of ankle fractures than those who did not use prescription medicine. The researchers also found that smoking had a dose-response effect on the rate of ankle fractures. Women who smoked 20 or more cigarettes per day had a higher rate of ankle fractures than those who smoked 1 to 19 cigarettes per day.

On the other hand, the European Prospective Osteoporosis Study, based on 3,173 men and 3,402 women from 28 European centers, did not show that lifestyle factors were related to an increased risk of vertebral fractures (Roy, et al., 2003). The authors reported that none of the lifestyle variables investigated, including smoking, alcohol consumption, physical activity, or drinking milk, were consistently related with an incident vertebral fracture. The study did report that age at menarche 16 years or older was related to an increased probability of developing a vertebral fracture.

Older adults and individuals who have sedentary lifestyles or who are immobilized have a greater risk of developing osteoporosis (Tanvetyanon, 2005). Older age is associated with an increased risk of vertebral fractures (Journal of Bone Mineral Research, April 2002). According to the results of the European Prospective Osteoporosis Study, age was associated with a significant increase in the incidence of vertebral fractures in both women and men over the age of 50 years.

Vertebral fractures are the most common osteoporotic fracture (Nevitt, et al., 1999). The presence of vertebral deformity increases the risk of spinal fractures and may increase the occurrence of other types of fractures (Hasserius, et al., 2003; Ismail, et al., 2001). Using the results of the European Prospective Osteoporosis Study, Ismail, et al. (2001) reported that among women, the number of prevalent deformities predicted incident hip fractures, but it only weakly predicted other limb fractures and did not predict distal forearm fractures. Among men, the authors discovered that the number of prevalent vertebral deformities was associated with a non-significant trend toward an increased rate of hip fractures, but it was not related to an increased risk of incident limb fractures among men.

Using data from the European Prospective Osteoporosis Study, Lunt, et al. (2003) reported that the characteristics of the prevalent vertebral deformity, including their shape and location in the spine may influence the risk of a subsequent vertebral fracture. The relative risks for vertebral fractures were higher if the anterior and mid-heights, and posterior of the prevalent vertebral deformity were reduced.

An investigation of 6,082 women, ages 55–80 years, revealed that women with prevalent vertebral fractures in any location had a higher chance of new fractures in the upper spine than in the lower spine (Nevitt, et al., 1999). The same situation exists for individuals with a prior vertebral fracture and low bone density (Tanvetyanon, 2005).

Patients with a major depressive disorder may be at increased risk of developing osteoporosis. Patients with a major depressive disorder have an increased chance of having hypercortisolism and its resistance to dexamethasone suppression. Based on a sample of 31 patients with major depressive disorder and 17 healthy male volunteers, Vrkljan, et al. (2001) evaluated whether cortisol levels were related to a severe type of osteoporosis, and found that individuals with elevated cortisol levels predicted the development of a strong type of osteoporosis. They suggest that patients with a long history of a major depressive disorder may be at risk for developing a severe type of osteoporosis.

Osteoporosis, Disability, and Quality of Life

Osteoporosis is associated with substantial pain, kyphosis (increased convexity in the curvature of the thoracic spine), restricted range of motion, and associated disability and decreased quality of life (Gold, 1996). Paier (1996) found that women who had postmenopausal vertebral fractures faced major challenges to their ability to function normally and retain their independence. These women face continuous pain, role losses, increased dependence, alterations in physical appearance, isolation, feelings of vulnerability and low-self-esteem, decreased quality of life, and a questionable future. The severity of the impairments associated with osteoporotic fractures is reflected in one study that found an increased mortality rate in both women and men who had a prevalent vertebral deformity (Hasserius, et al., 2003; Gold, 1996).

Pain and disability levels may vary depending on the location of the fractures. Hip fractures frequently result in substantial pain and disability. Prospective population-based data on 909 women, aged 55–81 years, from the Fracture Intervention Trial revealed that hip fractures produced the greatest percentage of women with days confined to bed (94%) or days with limited activity (100%) (Fink, et al., 2003).

Vertebral fractures are the most prevalent osteoporotic fracture and cause major back pain, disability, and reduced quality of life (O'Neill, et al., 2004; Fink, et al., 2003). The results from the Fracture Intervention Trial showed that older women with lumbar vertebral fractures had the highest mean number of days confined to bed (25.8 mean bed days) and the highest mean number of days with limited activity (158.5 mean limited activity days) (Fink, et al., 2003).

Women with new vertebral fractures have a significant chance of suffering back pain, limitations in functioning, and impairment in quality of life (Cockerill, et al., 2004; Nevitt, et al., 2000). In a prospective analysis of older women, Ross, et al. (1994) demonstrated that back pain and disability associated with new vertebral fractures were greater in magnitude than for prevalent fractures. Using data from 569 postmenopausal Japanese-American participants in the Hawaii Osteoporosis Study, Huang, et al. (1996) discovered that the odds of physical disability doubled for each recent vertebral fracture. Recent vertebral fractures resulted in poor scores in functional reach tests and walking speed tests. The authors also note that the physical impairments associated with vertebral fractures may persist for several years.

Prospective data from 2,260 women, aged 50 years and older, from the European Prospective Osteoporosis Study revealed that women with both a prevalent fracture and an incident fracture were much more likely to be physically impaired (O'Neill, et al., 2004). These women suffered major impairments in independent living.

One risk factor for disability may be the degree of vertebral deformity. With a sample of 2,992 white women, aged 65–70 years, researchers demonstrated that vertebral height ratios that fell four standard deviations below the normal mean were related to major pain, disability, or loss of height (Ettinger, et al., 1992).

Fink, et al. (2003) found that in the Fracture Intervention Trial, women, aged 55 to 81 years, suffered major disability after fractures of their thoracic vertebrae, humerous, distal forearm, ankle, and foot. They believe that more research needs to be done to evaluate disability outcomes resulting from osteoporotic fractures at non-hip, non-vertebral skeletal sites.

In addition to fractures, co-morbid health problems are associated with an increased risk of disability. One population-based investigation of 12,192 women, aged 47 to 56 years, discovered that fractures were related to long-term work disability independent of other health problems (Honkanen, et al., 1998).

Stress, Coping, and Social Support for Individuals with Osteoporosis

Persons with osteoporosis can face a significant amount of stress due to the disabling nature of their painful disease. In an investigation of 115 older women living with osteoporosis, Roberto (1988) discovered that women were likely to feel more stress after being diagnosed with the condition than before the diagnosis. A number of factors, such as pain symptoms, role losses, and other disease-related impairments impacted their perceptions of stress.

Osteoporotic individuals, especially those with osteoporotic fractures, can suffer anxiety, depression, social withdrawal, and feelings of social isolation due to their chronic pain symptoms, changes in physical appearance, loss of roles, and other disabilities (Gold, 2001; Paier, 1996). Gold (1996) noted that many persons with osteoporosis, especially those in the early stages of their condition, are anxious about the possibility of developing future fractures and the resulting physical deformities. Over time, individuals with osteoporosis who suffer hip or multiple vertebral fractures are at increased risk of developing depression. Unless these physical, social, and psychological problems are addressed, these patients will have a significant decline in physical health, psychosocial functioning, and quality of life.

To cope with the disease-related pain, impairment, and anxieties, osteoporotic individuals may use a variety of coping strategies on a short-term and long-term basis (Roberto, 1988). Using a sample of 286 older adults with osteoporosis or osteoarthritis, Gignac, et al. (2000) evaluated the adaptation to physical illness and impairment. Their results showed that these persons employ varied coping techniques, including compensating for role losses, improving performance, limiting activities, and obtaining assistance from others.

Treatment and Rehabilitation Outcomes in Osteoporosis Patients

Ideally, the treatment of osteoporosis should prevent fractures by normalizing bone mass and bone micro-architecture (Brixen, et al., 2004). Until recently, the main pharmacological treatment for osteoporosis patients consisted of medications that inhibited bone resorption and decreased fracture risk (Dobnig, 2004; Borgstrom, et al., 2004; Uebelhart, et al., 2003). Among these medications, the Bisphosphonate family is most widely known and used by physicians (Uebelhart, et al., 2003). Second- and third- generation Bisphosphonates, such Alendronate and Risedronate, are available as weekly tablets. This simple dosage schedule, according to Uebelhart, et al. (2003), has promoted patient compliance and has reduced the incidence of gastrointestinal side effects. These medications have been used to treat women with postmenopausal osteoporosis and men with osteoporosis. They have been shown to increase bone mineral density and reduce the rates of fractures. Physicians also use intravenous Bisphosphonates, such as Zoledronate, Ibandronate, and Pamidronate, in instances in which patients have intolerance to oral medications or have bone metastases.

Raloxifene, which is part of the selective estrogen modulators (SERM's) family, inhibits bone resorption, and in postmenopausal women, it has been shown to increase bone mineral density and reduce the rate of vertebral fractures (Uebelhart, et al., 2003). There is also evidence that Raloxifene reduces the incidence of breast cancer in postmenopausal women (Borgstrom, et al., 2004; Uebelhart, et al., 2003). In their Swedish study, Borgstrom, et al. (2004) reported that Raloxifene, compared with no treatment, is cost effective in treating postmenopausal women who are at risk of vertebral fracture.

Teriparatide, the recombinant 1–34 fragment of human parathyroid hormone, promotes bone formation, increases bone mineral density, and restores bone architecture (Brixen, et al., 2004; Debiais, 2003). In a randomized trial of 1,637 postmenopausal women with osteoporosis, Teriparatide was found to reduce the relative risk of both vertebral and appendicular fractures (Brixen, et al., 2004). In addition, the treatment increased bone mineral density in the lumbar spine and hip by 9.7% and 2.6%, respectively.

In another investigation, a sample of 146 postmenopausal women with osteoporosis were randomized to receive either injections of Teriparatide (n = 73) or oral Alendronate (n = 73) (Body, et al., 2002). The results showed that Teriparatide increased bone mineral density at most sites and reduced the rate of non-vertebral fractures compared to Alendronate. Patients tolerated both therapies despite transient mild asymptomatic hypercalcemia that occurred in patients taking Teriparatide.

According to Lippuner (2003), there are conflicting data about the efficacy of Calcitriol, Fluoride or insufficient data regarding calcium, Clodronate, Etidronate, hormone replacement therapy, Pamidronate, Strontium, Tiludronate, and vitamin D.

Researchers have investigated the effects of discontinuing Teriparatide therapy. Brixen, et al. (2004) reported that bone mineral density of the lumbar spine is reduced by about 2–3% after $2\frac{1}{2}$ years. However, this reduction can be prevented with Bisphosphonate therapy. Lindsay, et al. (2004), in a follow-up to the Fracture Prevention Trial, discovered that postmenopausal women sustained vertebral fracture risk reduction 18 months after discontinuing therapy.

Fibromyalgia

Risk Factors for Fibromyalgia

Fibromyalgia is a chronic pain condition of the musculoskeletal system that the American College of Rheumatology classifies as widespread pain and tenderness (Giesecke, et al., 2003; Blumenstiel and Eich, 2003). The etiology of fibromyalgia is still not fully understood (Blumenstiel and Eich, 2003). The condition has been classified as either primary fibromyalgia (idiopathic in origin) or secondary fibromyalgia, which develops along with other conditions, such as ankylosing spondylitis, trauma, or surgery (Borenstein, 1995; Waylonis and Perkins, 1994). The condition may be caused by a number of genetic, central nervous system, muscular, and psychological factors (Blumenstiel and Eich, 2003). Because the etiology is not well understood and clinical measurements do not always correlate with patients' self-reported disability, fibromyalgia is a controversial disorder. This controversy is intensified by the fact that psychosocial factors are related to this pain syndrome and individuals with this disease may seek compensation for disability (Goldenberg, 1999; Wolfe and Potter, 1996).

Arnold, et al. (2004) discovered that fibromyalgia and reduced pain thresholds aggregate in families, and the disease co-aggregates with major mood disorders in families. These findings suggest that genetic factors may be a cause of fibromyalgia and pain sensitivity. Moreover, patients with mood disorders and fibromyalgia may share some of the same genetic factors. Other studies have found that the condition is frequently associated with psychological problems (Kissel and Mahnig, 1998; Aaron, et al., 1997).

Martinez, et al. (2003) reported that intense physical activity, physical trauma, climate changes, and genetic factors were thought to trigger painful episodes. They found that stressful events, emotional difficulties, climate changes, and the time of day were factors that modulated pain symptoms in fibromyalgia patients.

According to Blumenstiel and Eich (2003), there are a number of different psychological conditions that may cause fibromyalgia. These conditions include: personality traits, traumatic events, conflict, and somatoform disorders. Kissel and Mahnig (1998) found that psychological problems precede the onset of the disease in about 70% of patients.

Giesecke, et al. (2003) report that fibromyalgia patients vary in their clinical symptoms, and their symptoms are influenced by various biologic, psychological, and cognitive conditions. Based on a sample of 97 persons meeting the American College of Rheumatology criteria of fibromyalgia, the researchers showed that there are three distinct types of patients. One group of patients has extreme tenderness but has no related psychological and cognitive factors. A second group has moderate tenderness and normal mood. The third group of fibromyalgia patients is influenced significantly by mood and cognitive factors.

Wolfe and Michaud (2004) found fibromyalgia to be associated with rheumatoid arthritis. In a study of 11,866 patients with rheumatoid arthritis, they showed that 1731 (17.1%) fulfilled the criteria for having fibromyalgia. The condition also has been found to occur in patients with back pain (Borenstein, 1995).

Some patients who are diagnosed with chronic Lyme disease may actually have fibromyalgia. Hsu, et al. (1993) discovered in a sample of 800 patients diagnosed with Lyme disease, that 70 of these patients actually had fibromyalgia.

Fibromyalgia, Work Disability, and Quality of Life

Fibromyalgia symptoms, including chronic pain, fatigue, weakness, hyperalgesia, and allodynia, can produce substantial work disability and disruption of quality of life, including impaired social and family functioning (Liedberg and Henriksson, 2002; Collado Cruz, et al., 2001). Despite the potential for major disability and impaired quality of life, many fibromyalgia patients are able to function normally and are able to continue working (Gordon, 1999).

Bernard, et al. (2000) evaluated quality-of-life issues for fibromyalgia patients using a sample of 270 fibromyalgia support group members from 3 states. Their results showed that the condition adversely affected patients' personal relationships, work experiences, and psychosocial functioning. Fibromyalgia patients ranked their current quality of life with the disease as 4. 8 out of a highest quality-of-life score of 10 and their future quality of life without the disease as 9.2.

The physical and emotional health and quality of life of persons with fibromyalgia have been compared to that of individuals with osteoarthritis. One investigation by Davis, et al. (2001) compared 50 women with fibromyalgia with 29 women with knee osteoarthritis who were scheduled for knee surgery and 22 women with osteoarthritis who were not scheduled for surgery. The findings revealed that both fibromyalgia and osteoarthritis surgery patients had similar levels of pain, and both groups had higher pain levels than the non-surgery group. However, the researchers showed that women with fibromyalgia had poorer emotional and physical health, reduced positive affect, and poorer social interactions than both groups of women with osteoarthritis.

Dr. Mark L. Goldstein offers the following case study to illustrate some of the difficulties patients go through in coping with fibromyalgia.

Case Study

Rachel is a 36-year-old Asian female, married, with three children. She has always been a homemaker, although she has two college degrees in business and accounting. She has always been actively involved with her three children, serving as room parent for each and volunteering in their classrooms at school. Rachel has always cooked gourmet meals, kept the house meticulously clean and has been very active in church. Approximately five years ago, Rachel noticed a decrease in her energy level, as well as muscle aches. Within one year of the initial symptoms, she experienced an increase in soft tissue pain, particularly in her shoulders, back of the neck and legs. Her lethargy increased, and she found that she felt tired even when she had slept for ten hours. In addition, she noticed that her thinking became fuzzy; she would lose her train of thought and forget words. Rachel had difficulty in being available to her children and husband. She felt "bad" on a daily basis and had no energy.

Eventually, she saw her physician, who diagnosed her as "stressed out" and recommended exercise. Rachel began to walk daily for 30–60 minutes, but noticed minimal improvement. Her condition deteriorated even further, as she was usually unable to help her children with their homework. In addition, she began to feel depressed. Finally, she went to see a new physician, who subsequently referred her to a neurologist who diagnosed her with fibromyalgia. The neurologist recommended massage therapy, vigorous daily exercise and antidepressant medication. The neurologist also had her complete a sleep study, which revealed that she was experiencing a sleep disorder, necessitating additional medication. She started to see a counselor, and her husband and three children attended some sessions with her where they learned more about fibromyalgia. At present, she continues to experience pain and has a lowered energy level, but her sleep is improved and she is able to do more with her children. Counseling continues to be a source of support and has helped her to accept herself and her limitations.

The high prevalence of fibromyalgia, the patients' perceptions of the severity of the disease, and poor functional status are factors that make fibromyalgia a common cause of work disability (White, et al., 1995). Even though the disease is a common and costly cause of work disability, it is a controversial diagnosis, and fibromyalgia patients experience obstacles in filing disability claims (Aronoff and Livengood, 2003; White, et al., 1995). The lack of diagnostic criteria, difficulties in quantifying the disability, the ineffectiveness of treatment, physician attitudes, and assessments from the insurance system are some of the reasons why patients face hurdles in filing disability claims for fibromyalgia (Aronoff and Livengood, 2003; White, et al., 1995).

A number of studies have investigated the prevalence of fibromyalgia-related disability and risk factors for this impairment. Based on a longitudinal survey of 1,604 fibromyalgia patients from 6 centers, Wolfe, et al. (1997) found that 26.5% of the patients reported obtaining at least one form of disability payment. More than 16% of the patients indicated that they were on Social Security disability. The authors discovered that pain symptoms, disability (as measured by the Health Assessment Questionnaire), and being single were risk factors for fibromyalgia-associated work disability. Payment awards and the prevalence of work-related disability varied among the 6 centers. The researchers suggest that these differences may be due to variations in referral patterns, physician attitudes, or patient socioeconomic status.

Using a sample of 100 fibromyalgia patients, 76 pain patients, and 135 control patients, White, et al. (1999) found that patients with the disease experienced significant impairment in functional status and disability. Their results showed that fibromyalgia patients reported more disability, were more likely to be receiving pensions, have lower functioning, spend more days in bed due to their disability, and lose more healthy years of life than the control group. In terms of risk factors, the researchers found middle age and prior heavy manual labor were related to work disability.

A survey of 176 women at a university pain or rheumatology clinic revealed that pain, sleep problems, excessive tiredness, muscle stiffness, and increased pain after muscle exertion were frequently reported symptoms of fibromyalgia (Henriksson and Liedberg, 2000). Twenty-three percent of the women surveyed indicated that fibromyalgia was the reason why they were not working. However, it is interesting to note that 50% of those surveyed reported that they were working, and 15% were employed full-time. These findings suggest that individuals with the symptoms of fibromyalgia vary in their ability to cope.

Another risk factor for fibromyalgia-related disability is an event, such as trauma, surgery, or a medical problem, that precedes the onset of the disease (Borenstein, 1995). Using a sample of 127 patients with the diagnosis of fibromyalgia, Greenfield, et al. (1992) found that that 29 of these patients had a precipitating event and were therefore classified as having reactive fibromyalgia. Patients with reactive fibromyalgia had a higher level of disability (70% had lost their jobs, 34% received disability payments, and 45% had reduced physical activity) when compared with those with primary or idiopathic fibromyalgia.

Stress, Coping, and Social Support for Persons with Fibromyalgia

Researchers are finding that some fibromyalgia patients are particularly vulnerable to stress. Psychosocial stress has been considered as one of the causes of the condition and as a factor that increases symptom severity (Dedert, et al., 2004).

How do fibromyalgia patients cope with their painful and disabling symptoms? Bernard, et al. (2000) showed that fibromyalgia patients make use of a variety of coping techniques. Coping strategies consisted of talking to their friends, praying, exercise, hobbies, relaxation techniques, professional consultations, and meditation.

Individuals with this disease may have less effective coping strategies than others with chronic pain. Davis, et al. (2001) compared coping techniques among women with fibromyalgia and those with osteoarthritis. Their findings showed that women with fibromyalgia employed less effective coping techniques and had weaker social networks than did the women with osteoarthritis.

These findings were noted for women who reported similar pain levels.

Other investigations have compared coping strategies and social support among fibromyalgia patients and patients with other chronic diseases. Da Costa, et al. (2000) compared the determinants of coping techniques and social support among 46 women with fibromyalgia and 59 women with systemic lupus erythematosus. The authors discovered some similarities and differences in the determinants of coping and social support among women in both groups. Among women with fibromyalgia, poorer psychosocial status was related to experiencing more generalized difficulties, more frequent use of emotion-focused coping techniques, and lower levels of satisfaction with social support. Among women with systemic lupus erythematosus, lower levels of mental health functioning was associated with lower income levels, more generalized problems, and higher levels of emotion-oriented coping.

Treatment and Rehabilitation Outcomes in Fibromyalgia Patients

Fibromyalgia is difficult to diagnose, lacks definitive etiology, and treatments are limited in their effectiveness (Horwitz, et al., 2003; Asbring and Narvanen, 2002; Noller and Sprott, 2003). It is thought that psychological and social issues affect the course of the disease and treatment outcomes (Blumenstiel and Eich, 2003). Attitudes toward this stigmatizing disease, self-management strategies, coping strategies, work, and interpersonal factors are some of the conditions that may influence the course and treatment of fibromyalgia (Jensen, et al., 2003; Blumenstiel and Eich, 2003; Raak, et al., 2003).

Treatment interventions for fibromyalgia patients consist of medications, exercise, cognitive behavioral therapy, meditation, physical therapy, occupational therapy, psychotherapy, patient education, and support (Blumenstiel and Eich, 2003; Astin, et al., 2003).

According to Cymet (2003), fibromyalgia patients frequently seek alternative medical treatments for their symptoms. These alternative medical therapies include nutritional treatment, acupuncture, and herbal treatments. Patients also rely on complementary treatments such as exercise, bed rest, vitamins, and the use of heat and or cold.

Based on a sample of 111 fibromyalgia patients, Nicassio, et al. (1997) measured the frequency and determinants of complementary treatment use. The investigators discovered that 98% of the sample had made use of at least one complementary treatment strategy during the previous 6 months. The following factors predicted the use of complementary treatment strategies: younger age, greater pain severity, and greater impairment. They also found that neither pain coping techniques nor the quality of social support was related to using complementary treatments.

Treatment interventions have various goals: increasing self-efficacy, reducing symptoms, increasing functioning, returning to work, improving the quality of life, and eliminating excessive health services utilization (Collado Cruz, et al., 2001; Burckhardt, 2002).

Studies have assessed both the short-term and long-term outcomes of treatment for fibromyalgia. Waylonis and Perkins (1994) conducted a follow-up study of 176 persons who received the diagnosis of post-traumatic fibromyalgia between 1980 and 1990. Patients were asked to compare their use of different therapies (biofeedback, medications, physical therapy, manipulation, massage therapy, and tenderpoint injections) for the first two years after onset of fibromyalgia as well as the year preceding the current evaluation. The investigators found that patients significantly reduced their use of physical treatments. Fifty-four percent continued to use over-the-counter medications, and 39% were taking antidepressants. Eighty-five percent of the patients continued to have major symptoms of fibromyalgia.

Using a sample of patients with chronic pain, including fibromyalgia, Collado Cruz, et al. (2001) evaluated the impact of multidisciplinary treatment of four weeks duration. Patients received medical treatment for pain control, physical therapy, occupational therapy, and participated in cognitive behavioral therapy. Based on an average follow-up of 10 months, the researchers discovered improvements in all outcome measures, including pain reduction, anxiety, depression, and improvement in functional status. Seventy-three percent of the patients went back to work at the time of discharge and 69% of the patients maintained their improvements and employment status at the end of the follow-up period.

Burkhardt (2002) suggests that non-pharmacologic management, including cognitive skill training, exercise, behavioral strategies, and progressive muscle relaxation, can help fibromyalgia patients if they are performed on a regular basis. In a review of the literature on treatment outcomes, he noted that there were no negative treatment outcomes, but a positive result was more likely when the patient obtained support from a therapist and maintained the intervention activities over the long term.

In a long-term, randomized, parallel clinical trial, Redondo, et al. (2004) compared the effectiveness of cognitive-behavioral therapy and physical exercise, both of which were of eight weeks duration. Both treatments were associated with improvements in some aspects of quality of life and strategies for coping with pain. All variables related to functional status improved among fibromyalgia patients in the physical exercise treatment, while among patients in the cognitive-behavioral therapy treatment, only physical activity of the vertebral column showed improvement. There were no improvements in psychosocial effects in either treatment group. Both groups returned to most of their baseline conditions one year after follow-up. However, functional capacity was still much better in the physical exercise treatment group than the cognitive-behavioral therapy group. The authors conclude that fibromyalgia patients sustain improvements in clinical conditions for only a short time and improvements in self-efficacy and physical capacity are not related to symptom reduction.

Another treatment approach to fibromyalgia is to focus on body awareness, including patients' body and self-image (Horwitz, et al., 2003). According to one treatment strategy, fibromyalgia patients view themselves on videotapes and afterwards were interviewed about their body and self-image. Horwitz, et al. (2003) found that the use of patient videotapes helped patients become more aware of their body and self-signals thus enabling therapists to customize treatment programs.

Researchers are beginning to investigate the role of religiousness in helping fibromyalgia patients cope with stress, which has been implicated as both a cause of fibromyalgia and symptom severity. Based on a sample of 91 women, Dedert, et al. (2004)

discovered that women with moderate or high levels of religious observance were likely to have high levels of cortisol in the morning and low levels in the evening. In contrast, women, who are not religious, tended to have flattened cortisol levels. The investigators believe that religiousness may protect against the physiological impact of stress among women with fibromyalgia.

Low Back Pain

Risk Factors for Low Back Pain

Low back pain can be acute (less than three months duration) or chronic. Approximately 90% of patients with acute low back problem recover spontaneously within one month (U.S. Agency for Health Care Policy and Research, 1994).

The risk factors for low back pain are complex and poorly understood. This complexity is due to the fact that the spine is made up of bones, joints, ligaments, fatty tissue, different layers of muscles and nerves (Tice, 2005). These structures are supplied by a complex arterial and venous system and lie close to the skin with its sensory receptors. It is assumed that spinal structures and tissues that contain either unmyelinated nerves or substance P or associated peptides have the ability to cause pain. These structures include the posterior facet joints, bones and periosteum, muscles, tendons, fascia, ligaments, nerve roots, dorsal root ganglia, dura mater, and the intervertebral disc (Haldeman, 1999). In less than 20% of cases can the specific tissue that is causing the pain be determined (Frymoyer, 1988).

There can be a variety of causes of back pain. Individuals who are obese are at greater risk for back pain, joint pain, and muscle strain than those who are not obese (Spine-health.com, 1999–2005, American Obesity Association, http://www.obesity.org). Being overweight or obese can help to cause symptoms related to osteoporosis, osteoarthritis, degenerative disc disease, spinal stenosis, and spondylolisthesis (http://www.spineuniverse.com). When a person carries excess weight, the spine is forced to take on the burden, which may bring about structural compromise and damage, such as injury and sciatica.

Lack of exercise and conditioning can lead to many types of back pain (Spine-health.com; http://www.spineuniverse.com). Lack of exercise and conditioning produces inadequate flexibility and weak muscles in the back, pelvis, and thighs, causing an increase in the curve of the lower back. As a result, the pelvis is caused to tilt too far forward. This process leads to poor posture, causing other regions of the spine (e.g., neck) to become painful.

Abnormalities in bones (e.g., fracture, osteoporosis, tumors, metabolic bone disease, infection, spondylolisthesis), muscles (e.g., sprain, strain, trigger points, fibromyalgia), discs (e.g., torsion injury, compression injury, degradation, herniation), zygapophyseal joint (e.g., osteoarthritis, capsular tear and or avulsion), ligaments (ligamentous pain in combination with annulus fibrosus pathology) and other conditions (e.g., duramater infection, inflammation) can cause back pain (Bhutra, 2001).

Acute low back pain can be due to potentially serious spinal conditions (e.g., tumor, infection, spinal fracture or a major neurologic condition, such as cauda equina syndrome), sciatica, and nonspecific back symptoms (U.S. Agency for Health Care Policy and Research, 1994).

As much as 40% of chronic low back pain has been reported to be due to problems with the intervertebral disc (Schwarzer, et al., 1995; Tice, 2005). However, the diagnosis and treatment of this problem has been controversial. Low back pain due to intervertebral disc abnormailities may be insidious or have a sudden onset. Individuals with this condition often suffer pain in the center of their backs and the pain may radiate to their buttocks or thighs. The pain can be increased by sitting and improved by lying down. Pain tends to get better within two weeks but a complete resolution may take up to 12 weeks.

Most back pain with a muscular origin is due to excessive effort or remaining in one position for too long. Work-related physical and psychosocial factors as well demographic characteristics, overweight and obesity, family factors, sports activities among sedentary workers, and smoking increase the risks of low back pain. In addition, risk factors may vary depending on whether the low back pain is acute (up to 3 or 4 weeks), sub-acute (from 3 or 4 weeks to 3 months), or chronic (3 to 6 months and longer) (Ozguler, et al., 2004).

Low Back Pain and Work-Related Physical Factors

A number of work-associated physical factors have been found related to low back pain. Based on a study of 3,042 Japanese workers with various job classifications in a manufacturing company, Matsui, et al. (1997) showed that low back pain can be job related. Van Nieuwenhuyse, et al. (2004) studied 278 young workers, who had no history of back pain and were employed in their first jobs. The researchers found that the young workers had an increased probability of developing their first experiences with back pain when their jobs involved the following actions: more than 12 flexion or rotation movements of the trunk per hour; long periods of seated work; and more than 3 years seniority in a job that involves lifting more than 25 kg at least once an hour. The authors suggest that when low back pain occurs in the first year of employment, it is probably due to the lack of work experience and/or training.

Based on a 3-year prospective, cohort study among workers in 34 companies in the Netherlands, Hoogendoorn, et al. (2000; 2002) discovered that flexion and rotation of the trunk and lifting at work were associated with low back pain. Employees who used their upper bodies in a minimum of 60 degrees of flexion for more than 5% of the time and/or those who worked in a minimum of 30 degrees of rotation for more than 10% of the time and/or workers who lifted a load of at least 25 kg more than 15 times a day, had an increased risk of developing low back pain.

Repetitive work that involves bending and the manual manipulation of heavy objects may increase the probability of low back pain. Using longitudinal data from the Hamburg Construction Worker Study, researchers discovered that workers who engaged in repetitive work involving bent positions and the manual manipulation of heavy stones resulted in an increased risk of future chronic low back pain (Latza, et al., 2002).

Certain types of sedentary work also may be related to a greater probability of low back pain. Using a sample of 94 crane operators, 95 straddle-carrier drivers, and 86 office workers, Burdorf, et al. (1993) discovered that workers who engaged in sustained sedentary work in a forced non-neutral trunk position were at increased risk of suffering low back pain.

Low Back Pain and Work-Associated Psychosocial Factors

Conditions, such as frequency of job stress, high job dissatisfaction, and low social support from supervisors or co-workers have been reported to be risk factors for low back pain among workers (Latza, et al., 2002; Nahit, et al., 2001). Latza, et al. (2002) examined a longitudinal study of 488 male construction workers, and reported that workers who had low satisfaction with their work achievements had a higher prevalence of chronic low back pain than those with high satisfaction.

A large population-based survey revealed that dissatisfaction with employment status doubled the chances of having a new low back pain episode among both employed and non-employed individuals (Papageorgiou, et al., 1988). Those persons who felt that their incomes were inadequate were three times more likely to have a new episode of low back pain regardless of their employment status.

Using the results of a cross-sectional study of 1,449 transit vehicle operators, Krause, et al. (1997) discovered that extended uninterrupted driving periods, frequent job problems, high psychosocial demands, significant job dissatisfaction and low support from supervisors increased the risk of back or neck pain. In another investigation, low supervisor support and low psychological job demands were risk factors for first-ever low back pain among workers (Van Nieuwenhuyse, et al., 2004).

Interactions between Physical and Psychosocial Risk Factors in Back Pain

Devereux, et al. (1999) used the results of a study of manual workers, delivery drivers, and office workers, to show that the highest risks for back disorders occurred among workers exposed to both high physical and psychosocial stress. The authors conclude that prevention strategies should emphasize not only ergonomic factors but also methods to reduce psychosocial stressors.

Sexual and Physical Abuse and Back Pain

Linton (1997) has found a possible link between physical and sexual abuse and back pain. The author compared three randomly selected groups of individuals, ages 35 to 45 years, from the general population (no pain group, n = 449; mild pain group, n = 229; pronounced pain group, n = 271) and 142 consecutive patients with chronic musculoskeletal pain as a clinical reference group. Sexual abuse was reported more frequently than physical abuse, and women reported more sexual abuse than men. Among women, the prevalence of physical abuse ranged from 2% in the no pain group to 8% in the pronounced pain group. The total amount of sexual abuse ranged from 23% in the no pain group to 46% in the pronounced pain group. The prevalence of abuse for the clinical reference group did not differ much from the pronounced pain group and was 35%. There was a clear association between abuse and back pain as physical abuse increased the risk of pronounced back pain by five-fold, and sexual abuse increased the risk of pronounced back pain by four-fold.

Demographic Factors and Low Back Pain

Certain demographic characteristics have been found to be related to an increased probability of low back pain. In a population-based, longitudinal study of 1,412 adults in northwest England, MacFarlane, et al. (1997) reported women had an increased chance of a first episode of back pain that necessitated seeing a physician.

Data from the Colorado Farm Family Health and Hazard Surveillance Survey was used to investigate back pain and risk factors in 759 farmers (Xiang, et al., 1999). The results showed that work activities were more likely to cause back pain in both men and women regardless of where the work was done.

Matsui, et al. (1997) showed that age, along with the physical demands of a job, increase risks for low back pain. However, as noted previously, young workers in their first employment also may be at increased risk of developing low back pain because of their lack of experience or training.

Family Factors and Low Back Pain

Using a sample of 3,042 Japanese workers, Matsui, et al. (1997) discovered that workers with a family history of low back pain had an increased chance of developing low back pain. Workers with a history of parental low back pain were significantly younger when they had their first episode of low back pain than those workers with low back pain who did not have a parental history of low back pain. The investigators recommend that a family history of low back pain should be taken into consideration when managing workers with low back pain.

Sports Activities among Sedentary Workers

Matsui, et al. (1997) found that sedentary workers who intermittently participated in sports activities had an increased chance of acquiring low back pain.

Estrogen Replacement Therapy and Back Pain

According to one cross-sectional and prospective investigation of a large cohort of elderly white women, the use of estrogen replacement therapy increased the risk of back pain and back dysfunction (Musgrave, et al., 2001).

Smoking and Increased Risk of Low Back Pain

Data on 562 individuals from a community-based prospective study revealed that among smokers, a job involving heavy lifting and substantial standing was related to low back pain. In contrast these two factors were not associated with low back pain among non-smokers. Smoking results in reduced perfusion and malnutrition of tissues in the spinal area, causing these tissues to react inefficiently to mechanical stress (Eriksen, et al., 1999).

Low Back Pain and Risk Factors for Work Disability

Overweight and obesity, poor general health, exercise or physical activity outside of work, smoking, bed rest, age, psychosocial, occupational, and Social Security system factors are some of the conditions that may influence disability outcomes and prevent a victim's return to work.

A review of the literature found that poor general health was a predictor of chronic low back pain and low rates of returning to work (Fayad, et al., 2004; Friedrich, et al., 2000). A study of 255 sewage workers showed that higher episodes of illness were positively associated with disability in the preceding 12 months (Friedrich, et al., 2000). Jacob, et al. (2004), in a longitudinal, community-based study in Israel, discovered that poor perceived general health was associated with recurring low back pain, pain symptoms, and poor functional status.

Using an observational, longitudinal study of 352 auto workers at two automotive plants, Oleske, et al. (2004) found that auto workers who exercised or participated in physical activity outside of work had better recovery rates from work-related low back disorders.

In their study of auto workers, Oleske, et al. (2004) reported that smoking predicted lower recovery rates among workers with work-related, low back disorders. They also discovered that workers in their study who reported bed rest following work-related low back disorders had poorer rates of recovery.

Friedrich, et al. (2000) revealed that age was one of the factors related to work disability in the prior 12 months.

Oleske, et al. (2004) showed that lower levels of stress predicted a good recovery from work-related, low back disorders among auto workers. Trief, et al. (2000) used a prospective study of 102 patients who underwent lumbar surgery to evaluate psychological predictors of surgical outcomes. The investigators found that failure to achieve improved functional capacity was related to pre-surgical somatic anxiety and depression.

Niemisto, et al. (2004) evaluated psychosocial problems and other risk factors for disability among persons with low back pain who received different types of treatment. In their investigation, patients were randomly selected to receive either a combined treatment consisting of spinal manipulation, exercise, and physician consultation or only a physician consultation. The authors showed that major emotional distress was associated with subsequent disability among patients who had received spinal manipulation therapy. Lack of control over one's life and generalized negative somatic symptoms predicted disability among the patients who were assigned only to the physician consultation group.

Watson, et al. (2004) revealed that feelings of anxiety and depression may reduce the rate of returning to work among sufferers of low back pain. Another longitudinal, community-based study revealed that experiencing a recent negative life event predicted recurring pain and poor functional status among low-back pain sufferers (Jacob, et al., 2004).

Various attitudes toward pain and control over one's environment among low back pain sufferers also may be related to disability rates (Woby, et al., 2004a; Woby, et al., 2004b; Niemisto, et al., 2004). Individuals who suffer low back pain may be less likely to recover and return to work if they fear that they will be re-injured. Using data from a randomized controlled study, Pfingsten, et al. (2001) reported that pain anticipation and fear-avoidance beliefs predict lower behavioral performance in patients with chronic low back pain. Woby, et al. (2004a and 2004b) also found empirical support for this association.

Injured persons who have a tendency to catastrophize the nature of their injuries also may be less likely to recover and go back to work, but Woby, et al. (2004b) did not find data to verify this relationship.

Occupational conditions, overweight and obesity, unemployment, Social Security, and health care delivery factors also may influence disability rates among patients with low back pain (Watson, et al., 2004; Jacob, et al., 2004; Poiraudeau, et al., 2004).

Using data from a study of sewage workers, Friedrich, et al. (2000) discovered that the weekly duration of stooping and lifting in the previous 5 years was positively related to disability.

In their longitudinal, community-based study in Israel, Jacob, et al. (2004) discovered that low satisfaction with work predicted recurring pain symptoms and poor functional status.

A review of return-to-work studies found that higher paid employees had a lower rate of recurring disability and higher rate of returning to work (Fayad, et al., 2004). In an evaluation of sickness absence due to back pain among office workers, Hemingway, et al. (1997) showed that workers in the lower-employment grades were more likely to have high rates of absences due to back pain than those in the higher-employment grades.

Poiraudeau, et al. (2004) reported that the highest rates of return to work are achieved by injured workers who attended functional restoration programs that provided them with appropriate modified job duties.

Obesity may increase the risk of back pain-related disability. According to a survey of 5,887 men and 7,018 women, aged 20 to 59 years, Lean, et al. (1999) found that obese women were 1.5 times more likely to suffer symptoms of intervertebral disk herniation than normal-weight women. In this sample, overweight women were more likely than women of normal weight to suffer problems related to low back pain, including impairment in daily activities, work absenteeism, and use of health care services.

In their review of disability rates associated with chronic low back pain, Fayad, et al. (2004) reported that worker compensation was moderately related to the rates of recurring low back pain and the workers' eventual return to work.

Providing prompt access to physiotherapy service for patients with new episodes of low back pain may reduce disability rates. Pinnington, et al. (2004) suggest that prompt access to physiotherapy is a cost-effective and feasible method for reducing disability among patients with new episodes of low back pain.

Stress, Coping Strategies, and Social Support for Persons with Low Back Pain

Low back pain sufferers can experience significant stress and psychosocial disorders. One study of back pain among farmers showed that being psychological depressed was significantly related to back pain (Xiang, et al., 1999).

Dr. Mark L. Goldstein provides a case study to illustrate the coping strategies of a patient with low back pain and sciatica, who also was later diagnosed with osteoarthritis of the spine.

Laura is a 67-year-old married Caucasian female, with two adult children. She had been a homemaker and was actively involved in her husband's church (he is a minister). Laura was the church organist for over twenty years and co-led the women's group at church as well. Approximately 15 years ago, she began to experience lower back pain as well as sciatica. She found it increasingly difficult to play the organ at church and at times, even had difficulty sitting in a pew during a church service. Laura's physician examined her, but did not perform any imaging tests. Instead, he recommended exercise and referred her for physical therapy. She began physical therapy, but had increased pain after treatment and soon discontinued the therapy. In addition, exercise also exacerbated her symptoms, resulting in the need for bed rest.

Over the next eighteen months, Laura's pain increased, particularly shooting pain in her buttocks and thighs. Eventually, Laura saw a rehabilitative medicine physician, who ordered an MRI. She was then diagnosed with osteoarthritis of the spine. Laura was placed on an anti-inflammatory drug, which helped reduce her pain somewhat. Over time, her pain increased and her physician utilized cortico-steroid injections, and recommended a weight loss diet, massage and heat treatments. Laura developed sleep problems due to the pain and was prescribed an antidepressant, Imipramine. This medication was helpful not only with sleep, but also with pain. She was also referred to a clinical psychologist specializing in hypnotherapy, which provided added relief. Although Laura can no longer play the organ at church, she is active in her church and community and enjoys travel, restaurants, theater and concerts. At times, Laura has exacerbations of pain, but is able to control severe pain through inflammatory and antidepressant medication and hypnotherapy.

Treatment and Rehabilitation Outcomes in Patients with Low Back Pain

Different multidisciplinary interventions have been employed to reduce low back pain and return the injured individuals back to work. These interventions include bedrest, medication, physical therapy, injections, surgery, spinal cord stimulation, cognitive-behavioral treatment, exercise, Back School, work hardening, work conditioning, and complementary and alternative therapies (Ozguler, et al. 2004; Childs, et al., 2004; Weiner and Ernst, 2004; Carter, 2004). It is important to note that pain always consists of both somatic and non-somatic processes, and therefore chronic pain will not be amenable to the best treatment if psychosocial problems and stressors are not taken consideration (Bhutra, 2001). In addition, although there is little scientific evidence to ascertain the optimal therapy for chronic low back pain, multidisciplinary specialists are developing practice guidelines to offer direction for clinicians (Rauck, et al., 1998).

Bedrest

Bedrest is the first treatment approach if the patient is suffering incapacitating back or leg pain (Bhutra, 2001). Bedrest is prescribed to reduce intradiscal pressure and impingement of the affected nerve root. However, bedrest for more than 4–7 days is rarely indicated and may lead to muscle loss, reduced cardiovascular conditioning, bone mineral loss, and reinforcement of the sick role.

Use of Pain Medications

Pain medications are frequently used in the treatment of both acute and chronic low back pain. A multiple dose, randomized controlled study by Dreiser, et al. (2003) tested the effectiveness and safety of Diclofenac-K in the treatment of acute low back pain. In this clinical trial, 124 patients treated with Diclofenac-K were compared with 122 patients who received Ibuprofen and 126 patients who were treated with a placebo. The results of the clinical trial revealed that Diclofenac-K (12.5 mg tablets) was superior to Ibuprofen and placebo. The authors conclude that the initial dose of 2 tablets followed by 1 to 2 tablets every four to six hours, with a maximum of 75 mg/day is effective and safe in treating acute low back pain.

Other research has evaluated the efficacy of Rofecoxib in the treatment of chronic low back pain (Katz, et al., 2004; Ju, et al., 2001). On the basis of a randomized clinical trial, Katz, et al. (2004) showed that about 2/3 of patients with chronic low back pain attained pain relief with Rofecoxib. Ju, et al. (2001) in another randomized clinical trial also showed that the daily administration of Rofecoxib reduced chronic low back pain and was tolerated well by the patients.

Injections in the Treatment of Back Pain

Four types of injections are used in the treatment of back pain: 1) Trigger point injections, 2) Epidural steroid injections, 3) Joint injections, and 4) Therapeutic spine injections (Bhutra, 2001).

Trigger point injection are the most common block. Local anesthetics with or without soluble or depot steroids, saline or neurolytic substances have been employed as injectate.

For about 40 years epidural steroid injections have been used for radiculopathy related to extrinsic disc conditions. It is thought that epidural steroid injections treat inflammatory changes in nerve root and inhibit transmission in normal nociceptive C fibers (Samanta and Samanta, 2004). Epidural steroid injections reach high concentration levels in the epidural space, and this procedure has been found to be safe for many patients. Injections in the zygapophyseal joint have both diagnostic and therapeutic benefits.

Permanent nerve blocks have been used in the management of chronic back pain. Three methods of nerve destruction are: 1) Injection of neurolytic substances, 2) Cryoanalgesia, and 3) Radiofrequency lesioning (Bhutra, 2001). Therapeutic spine injections of neurolytic agents, e.g., alcohol, phenol, and glycerole, have been employed for patients who suffer severe back pain related to metastasis (Bhutra, 2001).

Injection procedures, such as injection of trigger points in the back and injection of steroids, lidocaine, or opiods in the epidural space, have not been proven to be beneficial in treating acute low back pain (Banaszkiewicz, et al., 2003; Samanta and Samanta, 2004; U.S. Agency for Health Care Policy and Research, 1994).

Reviews of the effectiveness of epidural injections of steroids in clinical trials, have demonstrated mixed results (Samanta and Samanta, 2004). One review of 21 randomized clinical trials found that all types of spinal injections had some positive benefits, but the evidence was equivocal (Nelemans, et al., 2000). In a review by Koes, et al. (1996), 6 randomized clinical trials demonstrated the effectiveness of epidural steroids, whereas in 6 other clinical trials, patients did no better or worse than patients in comparison groups. Another review of 11 clinical trials revealed that patients receiving epidural steroids had a significant reduction of pain both in the short term and long term (Watts and Silagy, 1995). Banaszkiewicz, et al. (2003) suggest that epidural steroid injections may be beneficial in treating acute radiculopathy at intermediate follow-up periods, but these benefits seem to disappear over the long term.

Radiofrequency lesioning, which is based on the thermocoagulation of selected nerves using an electrode, can be effective for several reasons (Bhutra, 2001). Radiofrequency lesioning can accurately control the lesion size, recovery is quick, the nerve lesion heals without neuroma formation, and the procedure can be repeated when pain recurs. Yin, et al. (2003) found that sensory stimulation-guided sacroiliac joint radiofrequency neurotomy seems to have a major advantage over current treatments for chronic sacroiliac joint complex pain.

Spinal Cord Stimulation in Chronic Pain

Spinal cord stimulation is employed to treat low back pain and other types of chronic pain (Mailis-Gagnon, et al., 2004). The procedure involves an electrical generator that delivers pulses to a targeted spinal cord area. The leads can be implanted by laminectomy or percutaneously and the power source is provided by an implanted battery or by an external radio-frequency transmitter. The mechanism of action of the spinal cord stimulation is not well known. There is limited evidence to support using spinal cord stimulation for patients with the failed back surgery syndrome, and more trials are needed to assess the effectiveness of this treatment.

Physiotherapy

Physiotherapy is used to treat low back pain, but its effectiveness is unclear when compared to other modalities. Bronfort, et al. (2004), in their review of 69 randomized clinical trials, found moderate evidence that spinal manipulative therapy offers more short-term relief of pain than spinal mobilization and detuned diathermy for patients with acute low back pain. For patients with chronic low back pain, there was moderate evidence that spinal manipulative therapy has an effect similar to effective prescription non-steroidal anti-inflammatory medications. The investigators found that there is limited to moderate evidence that spinal manipulative therapy is superior to physical therapy and home back exercises in the long term.

Using a multi-center, randomized controlled trial, Frost, et al. (2004) compared the efficacy of regular physiotherapy to that of a patient receiving assessment and advice from a physiotherapist. The most common physiotherapy modalities were low velocity spinal joint mobilization and abdominal strengthening exercises. Based on a sample of 286 patients with low back pain from 7

National Health Service physiotherapy departments, the authors discovered that physiotherapy did not produce any long-term improvements in disability outcomes. The researchers concluded that physiotherapy was no more effective than one patient session with a physiotherapist.

Pinnington, et al. (2004) showed that prompt access to physiotherapy is a feasible and cost-effective treatment for adult patients with a new episode of low back pain.

Physical Exercise

Patients with low back pain have a reduced number of certain muscle fibers in the trunk which may explain why their physical endurance is less after their injury than before (Moffroid, 1997; Ozguler, et al., 2004). Inactivity may result in atrophy of these fibers. A variety of exercises can be effective in treating low back pain (Spine-health.com, 1999–2005). Stretching, strengthening/pain relief exercises, exercise ball therapy, and low impact aerobic conditioning are useful methods for reducing low back pain. Muscle strengthening exercises has been found to reverse the atrophy of muscle fibers in patients with chronic back pain (Rissanen, et al., 1995; Ozguler, et al., 2004). In patients who suffer either acute or chronic back pain, regular exercise, along with reducing excessive weight and changing activities, should be prescribed (Bhutra, 2001; Spine-health.com, 1999–2005)

A number of investigations have assessed the effects of physical exercise on patients with acute, sub-acute, and chronic low back pain patients (Ozguler, et al., 2004; Faas, 1996). For patients with acute low back pain, physical exercise has not been found to be effective in the reduction of pain, disability, or work absenteeism (Van Tulder, et al., 2000; Waddell, 1998).

Faas (1996) reported that physical exercise had a slight positive effect on improving the rate of return to work, absenteeism, physical mobility, and fitness, particularly among men.

Physical exercise, especially in combination with returning early to regular activities, has a positive effect on patients with chronic low back pain (Van Tulder and Koes, 2002; Faas, 1996). In a review of the literature, Faas (1996) and Waddell (1998) reported that physical exercise reduced pain intensity and disability and improved muscular strength.

Cognitive-Behavioral Treatment and Back Schools

The cognitive-behavioral treatment seeks to remove factors that reinforce pain-associated behavior and reinforce factors that promote physical reactivation, and resolve fears about the severity of the patient's back disorder (Woby, et al., 2004a; Ozguler, et al., 2004). This treatment involves identifying the patient's perception of pain and helping him/her to develop an understanding of pain and disability. Patients learn that their physical activities, exercise, or job activities will not cause their low back pain to recur. Patients are taught relaxation methods and learn how these methods can reduce stress and pain. Different books, brochures, and multimedia documents are used as part of this cognitive-behavioral treatment approach. One patient education brochure is the "Back book," and is a supplement to the "Clinical guidelines for the management of acute low back pain," which was published by the Royal College of General Practitioners in Great Britain in 1996 (Ozguler, et al., 2004).

A number of investigations have evaluated the effectiveness of cognitive-behavioral treatment in reducing low back pain and returning patients back to work. A study of the impact of the "Back book" in a population-based intervention found that it reduced the number of low back pain complaints, related health care costs, and absenteeism from work associated with low back pain (Ozguler, et al., 2004).

Hay, et al. (2005) compared a brief pain management program with physical therapy that incorporated manual therapy. In their study, patients with low back pain were randomly assigned to either a brief pain management program (n = 201) or physical treatments that included physical and manual therapies (n = 201). There were no differences in treatment outcomes (based on the Roland and Morris disability questionnaire), indicating that brief pain management methods are an alternative to physical treatments that incorporate manual therapy.

According to several studies, patients who received oral and written advice aimed at reducing fears about low back pain and encouragement about quickly returning to work had lower rates of absenteeism, less pain recurrence, and a more positive outlook on life at 6-month and 5-year-follow-ups (Woby, et al., 2004; Indahl, et al., 1998).

Woby, et al. (2004a) assessed the extent to which changes in cognitive factors were associated with changes in pain and disability in 54 patients with chronic low back pain. They found that there was no relationship between cognitive factors and changes in pain intensity. However, changes in fear-avoidance beliefs about work and physical activity and perceptions of control over pain were associated with reduced disability.

However, other investigations reported that patients with low back pain do not improve after receiving cognitive-behavioral treatment. Based on a sample of 486 employees, Hazard, et al. (2000) discovered that cognitive-behavioral treatment did not reduce the number of work-days lost due to low back pain. Giving employees a brochure that encouraged them to cope with their pain and quickly return to work had no impact at either the 6-month or 12 month follow-ups.

Cherkin, et al. (1996), in a study of nurses, also found that a similar kind of cognitive-behavioral treatment did not lead to improvements in knowledge and satisfaction after a 7-week follow-up. The researchers showed that patient knowledge and satisfaction had improved one week after the intervention, but these differences disappeared after seven weeks.

Using a sample of patients with acute or recurrent non-radiating low back pain, Burton, et al. (1999) compared patients who used the "Back Book" with a group who used another brochure that emphasized an explanation of the anatomy and biomechanics of the spine and gave recommendations about activity and ergonomics. Patients in the "Back Book" group had less negative attitudes toward the progression of their pain and reported being less disabled. However, no differences were found in pain intensity between patients in both groups.

Physical exercise for back patients is frequently combined with other treatments, including "back schools," work hardening, and work conditioning programs (Ozguler, et al., 2004). Back schools are group-oriented educational programs that give patients cognitive and sensorimotor information to help them reduce mechanic stress on their vertebral column and to attempt to change the participants' attitudes toward pain and medical care. There are various types of back schools, but all of them use interactions with participants to achieve these goals. The Swedish back school emphasizes ergonomics, while other back schools use psychology, education, and/or physical exercise. Back schools vary in their target population and their duration (from a 45-minute session to programs of several weeks duration) (Ozguler, et al., 2004).

Back schools reduce pain and disability in the short term (6 months), when compared to other modalities such as exercise, physiotherapy, anti-inflammatories, and manipulation (Van Tulder, et al., 2000; Ozguler, et al., 2004). However, after one year, these differences disappeared. Other research has shown that Swedish back schools that are used in work settings for over three weeks had the most significant positive changes (Koes, et al., 1994).

Work Hardening and Work Conditioning

Work hardening interventions are multidisciplinary programs that attempt to manage the physical and functional needs of patients with low back pain (Ozguler, et al., 2004). In work hardening programs experts develop simulations of a low back pain patient's work position and design psychosocial interventions to help the patient return to work. According to Weir and Nielson (2001), this approach has had mixed results. Work conditioning is another strategy that focuses on teaching the patient techniques for physical reconditioning and functional activities associated with job performance (Ozguler, et al., 2004).

In evaluating program effectiveness, Schonstein, et al. (2003) reported that combined work hardening and work conditioning programs produced better outcomes for patients with chronic low back pain than either program by itself. On the basis of 18 randomized studies, the authors found that physical conditioning programs, including those with cognitive-behavioral and intensive physical training components, resulted in fewer absences from work among patients with chronic low back pain, but the same was not true for those with acute low back pain.

Biopsychosocial Model

Biopsychosocial interventions are programs that integrate medical care with psychological, social, and professional support (Waddell, et al., 1993; Ozguler, et al., 2004). These multidisciplinary psychosocial programs frequently are initiated in pain treatment or rehabilitation centers and may also involve the workplace.

In a study in Canada, Loisel, et al. (1997) evaluated the effects of a multidisciplinary program that coordinated both medical care and an intervention program in the workplace. The intervention team consisted of an occupational therapist, an ergonomist, the employee, her or his supervisor, and management and union representatives. An analysis based on cost-benefit and cost-effectiveness, showed that this program was effective.

Lindstrom, et al. (1992) evaluated Volvo workers who had been absent from work for six weeks or longer due to low back pain. The experimenters measured the functional capacities of the experimental group, made visits to the work site, and used a back school and a behavioral-based, gradual physical reactivation program with the patients. The findings revealed that the study group participants returned to work more quickly and had greater functional capacity than did the workers in the control group.

Guzman, et al. (2001) evaluated intensive interventions using multidisciplinary and psychological programs which involved 100 hours of functional restoration therapy, versus shorter programs consisting of less than 30 hours. The results show that intensive programs are more effective than lighter programs in reducing low back pain and improving functional capacity.

In a review of 65 multidisciplinary interventions between 1960 and 1990, researchers discovered that that 68% of the experimental subjects had gone back to work after six months, while only 32% in the control groups (no intervention or single-approach intervention) had done so (Flor, et al., 1992; McCracken and Turk, 2002). Participants in the experimental groups had less pain and lower use of medications and felt less disabled than those in the control groups. Another analysis of by Cutler, et al. (1994) discovered that individuals in a multidisciplinary program had twice the rate of work return than did persons in the control group.

Manipulation (Adjustment)

Manipulation (also known as an adjustment) or the manual loading of the spine employing short or long leverage methods is fairly safe and can provide some benefit for patients in the first month of acute low back pain without radiculopathy (U.S. Agency for Health Care Policy and Research, 1994). Using a sample of 93 chiropractic patients and 45 family medicine patients, Nyiendo, et al. (2000) found that patients with chronic low back pain who were treated by chiropractors had greater improvement and satisfaction at a 1-month follow-up compared to those who were treated by family physicians. Some investigators suggest that patients with low back pain do achieve pain relief and enhanced functionality following spinal manipulation, although data to explain why this occurs are not available (Childs, et al., 2004).

A review of the literature has found that chiropractic treatment may offer some benefit. However, chiropractic and conventional therapies have been shown to be similar in efficacy (National Center for Complementary and Alternative Medicine, http:// nccam.nih.gov/health/chiropractic/; Assendelft, et al., 2003; Hurwitz, et al., 2002).

For example, an investigation comparing the effects of manual therapy, including spinal manipulations and exercise (including cycling, weight training, and stretching), showed that both treatments resulted in less low back pain, less disability, and better general health status among people with low back pain who were absent from work for 8 weeks to 6 months (Aure, et al., 2003). However, patients in the manual therapy treatment had more than twice the rate of returning to work and scored better on other criteria used in the study than those in the other group. While physical exercise has been shown to reduce pain and disability in patients with sub-acute and chronic low back pain, there is insufficient evidence to determine which types of exercise are the most effective (Ozguler, et al., 2004).

The risks of manipulation appear low, but there are few prospective studies on the prevalence of major complications (National Center for Complementary and Alternative Medicine, http://nccam.nih.gov/health/chiropractic/).

Surgery for the Treatment of Back Pain

The guidelines of the Agency for Health Care Policy recommend surgery for patients with major pathology or nerve root impairment associated with a herniated disc (Bhutra, 2001). In the

U.S., more than 300,000 laminectomies are performed each year and 15–45% of patients undergoing this procedure suffer persistent pain. Only 12% of patients with a herniated disc need surgery. Poor surgical outcomes are most commonly due to inadequate patient selection.

Researchers have evaluated the effectiveness of surgical interventions in improving low back pain. Despite the research, the scientific evidence of surgery for most surgical procedures is still mixed (Gibson, et al., 2000). For example, Fairbank, et al. (2005) conducted a multi-center randomized controlled trial to compare the effectiveness of surgical stabilization (spinal fusion) of the lumbar spine with an intensive rehabilitation program for patients with chronic low back pain. Drawing on a sample of 349 participants, aged 18 to 55 years, with chronic low back pain, they found that there were no significant outcome differences between the spinal fusion group and the intensive rehabilitation group. Both groups reported reductions in disability during the two years of follow-up. However, these improvements may not have been due to the interventions. The investigators concluded that spinal fusion surgery did not appear to be any more beneficial than intensive rehabilitation.

Fritzell, et al. (2004) evaluated the cost-effectiveness of lumbar fusion and non-surgical treatment for chronic low back pain. In their study, a total of 284 patients with chronic low back pain received either a lumbar fusion or non-surgical treatment. They discovered that all treatment effects (e.g., back pain, disability, and return to work) were significantly better after lumbar fusion. However, the 2-year costs for the surgery group were significantly higher compared to the non-surgical treatment group.

The Charite Artificial Disc was developed as an alternative to lumbar spinal fusion, the current surgical treatment for chronic low back pain due to degenerative disc disease (Tice, 2005). The device consists of two metallic endplates and a sliding plastic core which is designed to assist in aligning the spine and maintaining the spine's inherent flexibility. The Charite Artificial Disc is supposed to be superior to lumbar spinal fusion because it allows continued motion in the spinal segment. In contrast, lumbar spinal fusion limits range of motion, which may result in extra stress to discs above and below the fusion site.

A study of 105 French patients evaluated the effectiveness of the Charite Artificial Disc based on an average follow-up of 51 months (Lemaire, et al., 1997). The authors discovered that 79% of the patients had excellent outcomes and 87% went back to work. An investigation of 50 Dutch patients by Zeegers, et al. (1999) found that 70% of the patients had a satisfactory clinical outcome.

Physical Modalities

Physical modalities, such as massage, diathermy, ultrasound, cutaneous laser treatment, biofeedback, and transcutaneous electrical nerve stimulations (TENS), have been used to treat low back pain. However, scientific evidence regarding their efficacy has been mixed (Weiner and Ernst, 2004; U.S. Agency for Health Care Policy and Research, 1994). Weiner and Ernst (2004), in their review of clinical trials, discovered that percutaneous electrical nerve stimulation was effective for low back pain. However, the U.S. Agency for Health Care Policy and Research (1994) has not found physical modalities effective in treating low back pain.

Complementary and Alternative Approaches

There is increased use of complementary and alternative treatments for low back pain that include acupuncture, herbal therapies, and homeopathy (Weiner and Ernst, 2004; Guerreiro da Silva, et al., 2004; Ehrlich, 2003b). Acupuncture has not been found to be beneficial in treating acute low back pain (U.S. Agency for Health Care Policy and Research, 1994).

Weiner and Ernst (2004) did not find support for the use of traditional Chinese acupuncture and other complementary and alternative treatments for older adults suffering from musculoskeletal pain. Although the research findings did indicate that some herbals may have a modest analgesic benefit, there were insufficient data to support their use. In addition, some drug-herb interactions may make these herbals unsafe. The authors found that the risks of spinal manipulation of backs and necks outweighed the benefits that this treatment might bestow.

Other Therapies

The effectiveness of other treatments, such as the use of shoe lifts, shoe insoles, low back corsets, and back belts have been assessed. There is no evidence that shoe lifts are effective in treating acute low back pain, particularly when the lower limb length discrepancy is less than 2 centimeters. Shoe insoles are useful for persons with acute low back pain who have to stand for long periods. However, low back corsets and back belts have not been found to be useful in treating acute low back pain (U.S. Agency for Health Care Policy and Research, 1994).

Patient Education and Self-Management

Patient education and self-management programs have been developed in the United States and other countries to help patients with arthritis, osteoporosis, fibromyalgia, and low back pain (Damush, et al., 2003; Kralik, et al., 2004; Osborne, et al., 2004; Grainger and Cicuttini, 2004). These programs seek to increase patients' knowledge about their disease and prognosis, empower patients to cope with their condition, enhance their quality of life, increase their healthy activities, and strengthen their self-monitoring (Osborne, et al., 2004; Gold, et al., 1989).

Patient education programs should focus on improving outcomes associated with specific conditions. For example, Paier (1996) recommends that interventions with women who suffer postmenopausal vertebral fractures should help them regain or maintain their functioning, reduce pain, and help them develop strategies to cope with stress and isolation, and foster independent living skills.

Gold, et al. (1989) evaluated the impact of a 4-day osteoporosis patient education program that consisted of intensive education about the condition, education related to physical therapy, nutritional counseling, and medical evaluation and therapy. The results indicated that osteoporosis patients who had participated in the intervention had an improved outlook regarding their condition even though they continued to be concerned about pain and the chronic nature of their disease. Fewer participants reported depressive symptoms as their knowledge of their condition increased, and they felt that they had improved in their ability to manage their disease. The investigators recommend that patient education should be integrated in the management of osteoporosis and other chronic diseases.

There is some variability in how patients and health practitioners define self-management. According to Kralik, et al. (2004), clinicians may view self-management as formal patient education sessions, whereas as victims of arthritis may perceive self-management as the process of re-structuring their daily life. The researchers found that people living with arthritis deal with four issues in self-management: 1) identifying and evaluating their personal limitations, 2) accessing and using resources, 3) dealing with changes in their self-identity, and 4) re-organizing their daily activities in terms of planning, pacing, and setting priorities.

Investigators are assessing the role of the Internet in patient education interventions. Increasingly, patients are using the Internet to obtain health-related information. Shuyler and Knight (2003) used a content analysis of 793 free-text search queries they had submitted to a patient-education Web site to find out what patients are looking for when they access the Internet. The five most common reasons for accessing this website were: 1) to get information about the disease, 2) to learn more about treatment information, 3) to find out more information about symptoms, 4) to get advice about the symptoms, and 5) to receive treatment advice.

Prospective randomized trials have revealed that patient education activities had a variety of beneficial outcomes (Langer, et al., 2003). Arthritis patient education efforts have improved patient knowledge about their condition, enhanced their self-efficacy and self-help skills, reduced their helplessness and pain associated with arthritis, and lowered both their temporary and permanent disability.

Damush, et al. (2003) studied the effectiveness of a self-management program for low-income patients with acute low back pain from urban neighborhood health centers that demonstrated beneficial results. The program consisted of three group patient education sessions and a telephone follow-up that addressed such issues as understanding back pain, increasing physical activity, and coping with fears and frustration about acute low back pain. Compared to patients who received the usual care, patients who participated in the self-management program had lower disability levels, enhanced mental functioning, self-efficacy to manage their condition, more time involved in physical activity, and lower levels of fear about re-injury.

A randomized, controlled trial compared a patient education intervention consisting of a multidisciplinary information session 2 to 6 weeks before hip surgery with patients in a control group who did not participate in this session before surgery. The results showed that patients in the education intervention were less anxious and had less pain before surgery and were able to stand sooner after surgery than those in the control group (Giraudet-Le Quintrec, et al., 2003).

Patients may vary in their expectations and concerns concerning an upcoming surgery, so patient education efforts should take these factors into consideration. Using information obtained from a focus group of patients considering total knee replacement, Chang, et al. (2004) discovered some gender and racial differences in attitudes toward the surgical procedure. Whites had more concerns about anesthesia than other racial/ethnic groups. In addition, issues about recovery were more important for women than men.

Some research has shown that patient education programs have been inadequate in providing the necessary resources to help patients cope with their disease. A study of 194 persons with knee osteoarthritis discovered that individuals did not receive extensive information about their condition. Drawing upon patient interviews, patient diaries, and group teaching sessions, Victor, et al. (2004) found that 25% of the study participants had obtained support and advice about the disease itself, pain management, and the impact of the disease on their quality of life. Based on the results of a focus group of 112 persons with knee osteoarthritis, Tallon, et al. (2000) also found that patient education was not considered very effective.

6

Cardiovascular Disease

The spectrum of cardiovascular disease causes a huge medical, social and economic burden on society. Many of the risk factors for cardiovascular disease, also known as Syndrome X, are modifiable and are similar to the risk factors for type 2 diabetes (Gaillard, et al., 1997). Potentially modifiable risk factors for cardiovascular disease include smoking, hypertension, sedentary lifestyle, overweight and obesity, type 2 diabetes, high dietary fat intake, hypercholesterolemia, high-salt intake, dyslipidemia, significant alcohol consumption, and stress.

Below is a discussion of some of these risk factors.

Genetic Factors

The traditional cardiovascular risk factors explain about 50% of the variability in the risk for developing cardiovascular disease (Allen, 2000). Researchers have been analyzing the genetic component of cardiovascular disease to evaluate the additional unexplained variability and have determined that it is due to interactions between genetic and environmental factors (Corella and Ordovas, 2004; Allen, 2000; Amouyel, 1998).

Existing data show that plasma lipoproteins are major cardiovascular disease risk factors, and it is thought that gene-environment interactions influence plasma lipid concentrations and thus can enhance the potential risks for cardiovascular disease (Corella and Ordovas, 2004).

A family history of cardiovascular disease appears to be due to genetic and/or acquired factors (Acton, et al., 2004; Amouyel, 1998). Shared lifestyles, behaviors, and other common elements found among members of the same family may increase their predisposition to cardiovascular disease at a young age. Amouyel (1998) noted that this process may simulate a genetic risk factor. However, various twin studies have documented a genetic basis for cardiovascular risk.

Researchers have found that the Taq1B polymorphism of the CETP gene is a significant correlate of future cardiovascular disease events among patients with familial hypercholesterolemia who are treated with statins. Mohrschladt, et al. (2005) evaluated the influence of Taq1B polymorphism in the CETP gene on cardiovascular disease incidence. They used a sample of 300 familial hypercholesterolemia patients, of which 116 had cardiovascular disease at the study's baseline. Thirty-one percent of the Taq1B genotypes was B1B1, 49% B1B2, and 20% B2B2. At baseline, the only variation among the three genotypes was that the B1 allele was related to lower HDL-cholesterol levels. The results showed that the relative risk for cardiovascular disease events was higher for B2B2 carriers than for B1 allele carriers despite similar improvement of the lipoprotein status for both B2B2 and B1 allele carriers.

Several loci, e.g., APOA1, APOA4, APOE, and LIPC may lead to potential applications for cardiovascular disease risk prevention (Corella and Ordovas, 2004). They suggest that researchers need to go beyond simple approaches, such as relying on single nucleotide polymorphism, to emphasize models of multiple genes, dietary factors, and risks.

Age

Age is a known risk factor for hypertension and cardiovascular disease (Onal, et al., 2004). For example, Magro Lopez, et al. (2003) found that cardiovascular risk factors, including lack of physical activity, obesity, high blood pressure, glycemia, total cholesterol, triglycerides, and LDL-cholesterol increased with age. In another investigation of 629 patients, between 45 and 64 years, Devroey, et al. (2004) discovered that age above 50 years was associated with a low level of HDL-cholesterol, a major cardiovascular risk factor.

Based on a sample of 150 men, under the age of 55 years, with stable coronary artery disease (CAD), Skibinska, et al. (2004) discovered that the mean age of CAD patients was higher in patients with increased homocysteine levels, a known cardiac risk factor.

Fu and Fung (2004) in their study of 2,196 residents in selected metropolitan cities in China corroborated the fact that as people got older their cardiovascular health worsened. Azizi, et al. (2004) found that it is possible to identify predictors of cardiovascular risk factors in adolescents. They analyzed a sample of 290 adolescents in Tehran, Iran, and found that various dietary and life style factors predict cardiovascular risk factors. For example, they discovered an inverse relationship between calcium intake and systolic and diastolic blood pressure and serum triglycerides in female adolescents.

Gender

Some studies have documented that cardiovascular risk factors are more prevalent in males than in females. Devroey, et al. (2004) reported two cardiovascular risk factors: low HDL-cholesterol and high triglycerides were more prevalent in males than in females. Fu and Fung (2004) showed that, in general, females had better cardiovascular health than men.

Risk factors for cardiovascular diseases also vary among women. Postmenopausal status is linked to a twofold increase of risk for cardiovascular events. The loss of estradiol production at menopause increases the risk of coronary heart disease (Contreras and Parra, 2000). The risk for cardiovascular events also occurs in part because postmenopausal status is associated with adverse changes in plasma lipoproteins and endothelial function (McPherson, 2000). Because of these differences in risk factors between premenopausal and postmenopausal women, the use of hormone replacement therapy (HRT) in postmenopausal women is controversial. HRT has a beneficial impact on plasma lipids, flow-mediated vasodilation and fibrinolysis that could reduce the incidence cardiovascular events in many postmenopausal women. However, HRT also has procoagulant effects and increases the risk of venous thromboembolism.

For a majority of healthy women, these prothrombotic effects of oral estrogens may not be a major issue (McPherson, 2000). Epidemiologic studies indicate that among healthy women, long-term postmenopausal hormone therapy may reduce the risk for coronary artery disease (Hu and Grodstein, 2002). Adding progestin to the regimen does not weaken the benefit, and where estradiol is the prescribed form of estrogen, estrogen at lower doses may have the same benefit.

In their study of cardiovascular risk factors in middle-aged women, Shakir, et al. (2004) discovered that postmenopausal women who had ever used hormonal therapy had lower levels of serum total cholesterol, LDL-cholesterol, triglycerides and higher HDL-cholesterol than postmenopausal women who had not had hormone therapy. They also had lower rates of: systolic and diastolic blood pressures; lower rate of type 2 diabetes; of deep venous thrombosis and of coronary artery disease. The results showed that after controlling for other predictor variables, low-risk factors for cardiovascular disease and high educational attainment were related to use of hormonal therapy.

In contrast, analysis of the Nurses' Health Study has shown that among postmenopausal women with previous coronary disease, the risk for recurrent major coronary events appears to increase among short-term users of hormones (Grodstein, et al., 2001). With longer-term hormone use, the risk decreases.

In addition, the Heart and Estrogen/progestin Replacement Study (HERS) did not show a positive impact of oral HRT on cardiovascular events in older women with advanced coronary artery disease (Hulley, et al., 1998; McPherson, 2000). The acute prothrombotic impact of oral estrogen may outweigh the benefits of the long-term, anti-atherosclerotic impact of HRT in older women with advanced coronary artery disease. Therefore, HRT may not be advised for menopausal women with advanced cardiovascular disease.

Research is also underway to document possible gender differences in markers of inflammation, which increase the risk of cardiovascular disease. Godefroi, et al. (2005) found gender differences in the prevalence of one type of marker of inflammation, C-reactive protein (CRP). Their study showed that women had higher concentrations of CRP than men.

Other studies have focused on psychosocial factors that may promote coronary heart disease in women. Some of these may be: low socioeconomic status; the double loads of work and family; chronic emotional difficulties and lack of social support (Brezinka and Kittel, 1996).

Race/Ethnic Disparities

Like diabetes, there is a pattern of racial and ethnic disparities in the risk factors and morbidity related to cardiovascular disease. The results of the Third National Health and Nutrition Examination Survey revealed that among persons aged 25 to 99 years, non-Hispanic whites were more likely to have zero cardiovascular risk factors than Mexican-Americans and non-Hispanic blacks (Sharma, et al., 2004). Okosun, et al. (2001) reported that black men and women had a 1.58 and 1.39 elevated risk of hypertension compared to whites. Another investigation documented ethnic and racial disparities in stroke mortality, one of the outcomes of cardiovascular disease (McGruder, et al., 2004). Drawing on the results of the 1999–2001 National Health Interview Survey, they discovered that Hispanics and blacks stroke survivors were more likely than whites to report having diabetes and inadequate physical activity levels. Blacks were also more likely than whites to report having hypertension.

Morewitz (2005a), using the population-based 1998 National Health Interview Study, evaluated possible racial disparities in the hypertension history of pregnant women, and found that African-American women were more likely to have hypertension during pregnancy than white women, after controlling for income and other possible predictors.

There seems to be a pattern of racial and ethnic differences in accessing health care among patients with cardiovascular disease. Morewitz, (2005b) found that African-Americans who reported that hypertension impairs their daily activities were more likely than whites with similar levels of impairment to have had 2 to 3 emergency room visits in the prior 12 months, regardless of income. This study also found income differences; African-Americans and whites with self-reported hypertension impairment and incomes less than $20,000 were two to three times more likely to have used the emergency room in the previous 12 months than those with incomes of $20,000 or more.

In their study of black, Latino, and white patients seeking emergency care for chest pain symptoms, Haywood, et al. (1993) discovered that low-socioeconomic status patients were more likely to be black or Latino than middle-socioeconomic status patients.

It is unclear what accounts for the racial and ethnic disparities in the prevalence and risk factors for cardiovascular disease. Differences in socioeconomic status (e.g., education, occupation, and income), lifestyles, social environment, and access to preventive and clinical health services may influence ethnic and racial disparities (Kuller, 2004).

Socioeconomic Disparities and Cardiovascular Disease Risk Factors

In developed countries, cardiovascular disease risk factors and associated morbidity are shaped by socioeconomic disparities and problems in accessing preventive and clinical health services, with cardiovascular risk factors being more prevalent in disadvantaged minority groups (Sonmez, et al., 2004; Mcintyre and Mutrie, 2004; Kuller, 2004).

Haywood, et al. (1993) found that more low-socioeconomic status patients reported their health as fair or poor, had complained of frequent chest pain, suffered from other cardiovascular diseases, and were current smokers than middle socioeconomic status patients. In addition, few low-socioeconomic status patients knew their cholesterol levels, used estrogen, had a previous EKG or cardiac surgery, or had a stress test, and were less likely to have typical angina than middle-socioeconomic patients.

Sonmez, et al. (2004) showed that higher-income men had a worse cardiovascular disease risk factor profile than low-income men. Higher income in men was related to more cardiovascular risk factors: low HDL-cholesterol, high LDL-cholesterol, and central obesity. In contrast, among women, lower income and lower educational attainment were associated with central obesity.

Lee, et al. (2005) analyzed the link between low socioeconomic status and increased cardiovascular risk among women. Based on pooled data from 2,157 women with cardiovascular disease in 9 long-term cohort studies in the U.S., they showed that educational attainment was an age-dependent predictor of cardiovascular disease fatality. Non-high school graduates at age 60 years were more than two times likely to die from cardiovascular disease than high school graduates of the same age. However, by the age of 70, there was no longer any difference in the death rate.

Rutledge, et al. (2003) analyzed the link between socioeconomic status and risk factors for coronary artery disease in women. They used a sample of 743 women with chest pain who were referred for coronary angiography and then followed up for about two years. The researchers found that low socioeconomic status was related to various coronary artery disease risk factors such as higher body mass index and waist-to-hip ratios, cigarette smoking, sedentary behavior, and high risk of hypertension. Low income was linked to a higher probability of mortality from all causes after controlling for psychosocial and behavioral factors.

Sharma, et al. (2004) demonstrated that among non-Hispanic blacks, Mexican-Americans, and non-Hispanic whites the prevalence of having zero cardiovascular risk factors increased with educational level. Among all three ethnic and racial groups, the prevalence of zero risk factors increased from 6% to 14% among those with less than 12 years of education to 22–29% among those with 12 years or greater.

Morewitz (2002a) analyzed possible income disparities among individuals of Hispanic origin who suffer both stroke and heart attack using the population-based 1998 National Health Interview Survey. He found that the association between having a stroke and a heart attack was higher among persons of Hispanic origin who had incomes less than $20,000 than among persons of Hispanic origin with incomes at or above $20,000. These differences remained significant after controlling for possible predictor variables.

Based on a cohort of 3,410 patients with coronary artery disease, Horne, et al. (2004) discovered that patients from lower-socioeconomic neighborhoods had an increased risk of death or myocardial infarction. In addition, insurance type predicted risk of death or myocardial infarction. Self-pay, free care, and Medicaid, but not Medicare, predicted an increased risk of death or myocardial infarction, compared to private insurance.

Social Environment

The acculturation hypothesis describes the role of the social environment and changes in lifestyle in mediating ethnic and racial disparities in cardiovascular disease risk factors. The acculturation hypothesis suggests that immigrants who had low risk factors prior to immigrating to the United States will adopt high-risk lifestyles after they immigrate to the United States. Based on the results of the National Health Interview Survey, Singh and Siahpush (2002) showed that ethnic immigrant groups' risks of smoking, obesity, hypertension, and chronic disease increased with length of residence in the United States, although their risks remained significantly lower than for United States-born persons. Moreover other conditions in the social environment, such as employment opportunities, discrimination, prejudice, and access to preventive and clinical health services may alter the risk factors.

Hahn, et al. (1998) evaluated state and regional variations in cardiovascular risk factors based on the Behavioral Risk Factor Surveillance System, which is a survey of the 50 states and the District of Columbia. The study findings revealed that risk factors for cardiovascular disease were mostly lower in the western states and higher in the eastern states. The lack of physical activity and hypertension are major predictors of cardiovascular disease-related mortality rates. The results also showed that white women and white men were more similar in state risk factors than other race-sex combinations.

The residents of five southeastern states, (Alabama, Arkansas, Louisiana, Mississippi, and Tennessee) the so-called "Stroke Belt," bear an especially high stroke burden (Howard, et al., 2004). These five states have established the Delta States Stroke Consortium to help reduce the burden of this disease.

Psychosocial Stress, Social Isolation, and Social Support as Risk Factors

Psychosocial factors significantly influence the development of atherosclerotic heart disease, essential hypertension, and sudden cardiac death (Rozanski, et al., 2005; Horsten, et al., 2000; Frank and Smith, 1990). Psychosocial factors associated with these conditions include chronic stress, job strain, low socioeconomic status, negative emotions (e.g., depression, anxiety, and hostility), personality and character traits, social ties, lack of social support, and social isolation (Albus, et al., 2005; Strike and Steptoe, 2004; Rozanski, et al., 1999).

Stress, depression, anxiety, social isolation, inadequate social support, social conflict, and other psychosocial difficulties can have indirect effects in causing cardiovascular disease by fostering adverse health behaviors, such as smoking, poor nutrition, and inadequate use of health services (Albus, et al., 2005; Rozanski, et al., 1999). In addition, psychosocial factors can have a direct impact in producing cardiovascular disease by influencing neuroendocrine and platelet activation.

Both pre-existing vulnerability to cardiovascular disease, e.g., hypertension, obesity, and sedentary lifestyle, and major stressors can produce cardiac arrhythmias and/or plaque rupture, resulting in death (Ramachandruni, et al., 2004). However, more research is needed to clarify the link between psychosocial stress and the etiology of cardiovascular disease.

A number of pathophysiological mechanisms may explain the psychosocial effects on cardiovascular disease. The hypothalamic-pituitary-adrenal axis, hypertension and cardiovascular reactivity, inflammatory markers, platelets, coagulation factors, fibrinogen, lipids, and glucose metabolism may be involved in this process (Strike and Steptoe, 2004). Frank and Smith (1990) emphasize the interaction of the central nervous system's frontal cortex and hypothalamus with cardiovascular control functions in determining the effects of stress on the heart.

Research on animals has found a link between psychosocial stress and the worsening of coronary artery atherosclerosis, temporary endothelial dysfunction, and necrosis. These health effects may be triggered by an overworking of the sympathetic nervous system (Rozanski, et al., 1999).

Research on monkeys reveals that in premenopausal females, psychosocial stress produces ovarian dysfunction, hypercortisolemia and too much adrenergic activation (Rozanski, et al., 1999). These effects accelerate the process of atherosclerosis. Other studies indicate that acute psychosocial stress leads to myocardial ischemia, fosters arrhythmogenesis, triggers platelet dysfunction, and increases blood viscosity. In patients with existing coronary artery disease, acute stress produces coronary vasoconstriction. In addition sympathetic nervous system hyperresponsivity (reflected by exaggerated heart rate and blood pressure responses to psychological stimuli) may be related to the early development of carotid atherosclerosis (Rozanski, et al., 1999).

A variety of studies have assessed the link between psychosocial factors and adverse coronary events. For example, some research shows that low levels of social support have been found to be a predictor of mortality in coronary artery disease patients (Brummett, et al., 2005).

Other investigations focus on the role of depression in the development of coronary heart disease. According to epidemiologic reports, increased depressive symptoms in female and male patients are linked to an increased risk of myocardial infarction and a greater mortality rate after an acute cardiac event (Follath, 2003). However, in another study, researchers discovered that neither depression nor anxiety were associated with mortality 4 months after myocardial infarction (Lane, et al., 2000).

Patients who suffer depression after myocardial infarction may develop more complications, such as cardiac arrthythmias, compared to those who do not develop depression following a myocardial infarction. Follath (2003) demonstrated a link between depression in patients with coronary heart disease and subsequent negative outcomes, including diminished cardiac functional status, increased physical impairment, decreased quality of life, and increased dissatisfaction with treatment. Depressed cardiac patients are also less likely to adhere to their drug therapy.

The pathophysiological processes to explain the association between depression and subsequent adverse cardiac outcomes are not well-understood (Follath, 2003). Depression may lead to greater sympatho-adrenergic stimulation and increased platelet aggregation. Some anti-depressant medications may be responsible for cardiac symptoms and increase cardiac risks in coronary heart disease patients (Follath, 2003). For example, tricyclic antidepressant therapy has been linked to a higher risk of myocardial infarction, after controlling for other cardiovascular risk factors.

In some reports, both high psychological job demands and low decision latitude or high job strain has been linked to an increased risk of coronary events. Hammar, et al. (1998) evaluated psychosocial work aspects and the incidence of myocardial infarction using a case-control design. Their report, based on a sample of employed women and men in five Swedish counties, showed that men and women in jobs which had low decision latitude had an increased incidence of myocardial infarction.

Kuper and Marmot (2003) used the prospective cohort study, Whitehall II, which was based on a sample of 6,895 male and 3,413 female civil servants, aged 35 to 55 years. The study demonstrated that the highest risk for coronary heart disease occurred among workers with both low decision latitude and high job demands (job strain). The effect of job strain on the incidence of coronary heart disease was the strongest among younger employees.

In their occupational study, Hammar, et al. (1998) found that low social support at work and high psychological demands at work (high job strain) predicted an increased incidence of myocardial infarction primarily in men, ages 30 to 54 years. However, Kuper and Marmot (2003), in their study, found no association between social support in the workplace and increased risk of coronary heart disease.

Other reports found no association between job strain and an increased incidence of coronary events (De Bacquer, et al., 2005; Eaker, et al., 2004; Pelfrene, et al., 2003). One report, using the Belgian Job Stress Project cohort, concluded that job demands and decision latitude were not associated with an increased incidence of coronary events in a 3-year follow-up (De Bacquer, et al., 2005). The investigation revealed that low social support was a strong predictor of coronary events.

Analysis of data from the Framingham Offspring Study assessed the association between job strain and an increased risk of coronary heart disease or death in men and women (Eaker, et al., 2004). Using a sample of 1,711 men and 1,328 women, aged 18 to 77 years, the authors concluded that female and male workers under high job strain (high job demands-low control) did not have a significant risk for coronary heart disease or death. However men with higher education, income, and occupational prestige had a decreased risk for coronary heart disease or death.

Investigators in a large cohort study of female and male workers in Belgium analyzed the association between perceived job stress and coronary risk and also found no link between the psychosocial work environment and increased coronary risk among healthy worker (Pelfrene, et al., 2003).

Smoking

Incidence- and prevalence-based data show that smoking is a major cause of cardiovascular disease and related medical and social costs (Lightwood, 2003). One study of 1,398 adolescents and young adults showed that smoking, along with three other lifestyle habits, obesity, physical inactivity, and use of butter were related to a 5.5 times higher risk of three cardiovascular risk factors: high LDL-cholesterol, low HDL-cholesterol, and high diastolic blood pressure (Raitakari, et al., 1994).

In some research, smoking has been shown to be associated with homocysteine, which is considered a major cause of blood vessel damage and which has been linked to the incidence and progression of coronary artery disease (Skibinska, et al., 2004). Using the results of the ATTICA Study, a sample of 1,128 men and 1,154 women residing in Athens, Greece, area, one report discovered that the numbers of cigarettes smoked was related to plasma total homocysteine levels (Panagiotakos, et al., 2005).

Using a sample of 150 male patients, under the age of 55 years, with coronary artery disease (CAD), Skibinska, et al. (2004) evaluated conditions associated with homocysteine. Their results indicated that the proportion of CAD patients who smoked cigarettes was higher in those with high levels of homocysteine.

Another investigation, based on a sample of 292 men and 251 women, from the PILS II population study, did not report a link between smoking and homocysteine levels (Simon, et al., 1999). A study of an elderly population also did not reveal an association between smoking and homocysteine levels (Dankner, et al., 2004).

Smoking has also been linked to plasma fibrinogen, a protein involved in blood coagulation and a risk factor for cardiovascular disease (Sinha, et al., 2005). Increased levels of fibrinogen are thought to be a stronger risk factor for stroke than cholesterol because blood with higher levels of fibrinogen moves more slowly thus encouraging plaque formation (http://www.physicianschoicenews.com). Sinha, et al. (2005), based on a population-based study of 11,059 women and men, aged 45–74, discovered that average fibrinogen concentrations were higher in current smokers as compared to ex-smokers. They found that fibrinogen concentrations in men showed a reduction based on the number of years since the persons stopped smoking. In women, there was no association between fibrinogen concentrations and duration of quitting smoking.

High Normal Blood Pressure and Hypertension

Hypertension is one of the most important risk factors for cardiovascular disease, especially among whites (Li and Chen, 2005; Okosun, et al., 2001). Obesity has been found to cause or exacerbate hypertension (Redon, 2001; Okosun, et al., 2001). Redon (2001) states that the relationship between obesity and hypertension has been demonstrated in most racial, ethnic, and socioeconomic groups. However, he notes that the association between body mass index and blood pressure varies depending on age, gender, obesity type, and race. The hemodynamic profile of obese hypertensive patients differs from lean hypertensive patients. Moreover, obese hypertensive patients are more likely than lean hypertensive patients to develop left ventricular hypertrophy and kidney damage. In regard to treatment outcomes, obesity is one of the major causes of hypertension treatment failure. Several investigations have shown that obese patients need more antihypertensive drugs than lean hypertensives (Redon, 2001).

Inflammation and Prothrombotic Factors

Inflammatory and prothrombotic processes are known risk factors for both cardiovascular disease and diabetes (Grant, 2005; Erdmann, 2005; Balagopal, et al., 2005). Alterations in inflammatory mediators and coagulation/ thrombolytic factors increase the risk of cardiovascular disease, particularly among individuals with type 2 diabetes (Erdmann, 2005).

Li and Chen (2005) show that hypertension, by way of angiotensin and endothelin-1 and other vasoactive peptides, foster and speed up the atherosclerotic process by way of inflammatory mechanisms. They suggest that inflammation may be a bridge that links hypertension with atherosclerosis.

Inflammatory pathways also have been found to influence coronary plaque instability and subsequent rupture, leading to the onset of acute coronary syndrome. Elevated C-reactive protein (CRP), an inflammatory marker, is an independent risk factor for future cardiovascular events (Ostadal, et al., 2005).

Researchers have discovered that other inflammatory factors are associated with cardiovascular disease. They have found that the inflammatory factor, plasma fibrinogen, is a risk factor for cardiovascular disease (Sinha, et al., 2005). In addition, inflammatory factors, such as CRP, interleukin-6 (IL-6), and TNF-alpha, and fibrinogens, have been associated with obesity and sedentary lifestyles (Balagopal, et al., 2005; Grant, 2005).

Sedentary Lifestyle

Sedentary lifestyles foster obesity and low levels of aerobic fitness and are associated with increased cardiovascular disease risk factors (Borodulin, et al., 2005). Using data from the Finrisk 2002 Study in Finland, Borodulin, et al. (2005) found that aerobic fitness was associated with improved systolic and diastolic blood pressure, total cholesterol, triglycerides, and total cholesterol ratio. The results also indicated that aerobic fitness is related to enhanced cardiovascular risk factors, regardless of abdominal obesity levels in this Finnish sample.

Several investigations have revealed that sedentary life style habits are positively related to homocysteine levels, a major cause of blood vessel damage and a cardiovascular risk factor associated with the incidence and progression of coronary artery disease. In a study of 1,398 adolescents and young adults, Raitakari, et al. (1994) reported that physical inactivity was one of the lifestyle choices related to a 5.5 times higher risk of high LDL-cholesterol, low HDL-cholesterol, and high diastolic blood pressure.

Dankner, et al. (2004), using a sample of 423 men and women with a mean age of 69 years, showed that sedentary lifestyle was positively related to homocysteine levels. However, Simon, et al. (1999), in their study of 292 men and 251 women, did not find a link between physical activity and homocysteine levels.

Research is underway to evaluate the impact of different forms of physical activity on different social groups who have varying exposure to cardiovascular risk factors. Using the results of the Work, Lipids and Fibrinogen (WOLF) study, Fransson, et al. (2003) examined the association of leisure time, occupational, household, and total activity on four cardiovascular risk factors. Drawing on a sample of 10,413 employed individuals from two regions in Sweden, the researchers discovered that leisure time physical activity and total physical activity were related to decreased cardiovascular risk factors, especially HDL-cholesterol in both women and men. Overweight individuals involved in physical activity lowered their cardiovascular risk factors more than it did for lean persons. However, physical activity did not result in the same decrease in plasma fibrinogen among smokers as it did among non-smokers.

Another report, using the EPIC-Norfolk cohort in the United Kingdom, showed that television viewing and low participation in vigorous physical activity were independently related to obesity and other markers of cardiovascular disease (Jakes, et al., 2003).

Overweight and Obesity

As mentioned previously, overweight and obesity (including central obesity or adiposity), are major risk factors for cardiovascular disease and hypertension (Thomas, et al., 2004; Okosun, et al., 2001). Using data from the Third U.S. National Health and Nutrition Examination Survey, Okosun, et al. (2001) found that having a larger than expected waist girths was related to increased risks of hypertension in black men and black women.

Does central obesity contribute more to cardiovascular risks than general obesity? Thomas, et al. (2004) evaluated the relationships between general and central obesity and cardiovascular risk factors in 2,893 Hong Kong Chinese. Their results showed that general obesity predicted increased cardiovascular risks, but central obesity was a stronger predictor of adverse HDL-cholesterol, triglyceride, and insulin resistance levels.

Overweight and obesity factors predict cardiovascular risk among adolescents. Azizi, et al. (2004) assessed determinants of cardiovascular risk in Tehranian adolescents and showed that body mass index was positively related to both systolic and diastolic blood pressure in female and male adolescents. In addition, there were positive associations between body mass index and serum cholesterol in female and male adolescents. The researchers concluded that body mass index predict certain cardiovascular risk factors in adolescents.

Type 2 Diabetes

Individuals with type 2 diabetes have an increased risk of cardiovascular disease, coronary heart disease, and vascular disease (Lu, et al., 2004). The metabolic syndrome, which consists of a constellation of risk factors: genetic predisposition, central obesity, high triglyceride, low HDL-cholesterol, high blood glucose, high blood pressure, and insulin resistance, elevates the risk of cardiovascular disease. Investigators emphasize the need to manage the metabolic syndrome in order to prevent cardiovascular disease (Park, et al., 2004; Scuteri, et al., 2004). In addition to the metabolic syndrome, non-traditional risk factors, such as inflammation and atherosclerotic factors, increase diabetics' risks of developing cardiovascular disease.

Renal Endothelial Dysfunction

Impaired endothelial function is a risk factor for the development of hypertension. It is possible that reduced endothelial nitric oxide (NO) synthase activity, a lack or deficiency of L-arginine, increased endogenous NO synthase inhibitor, inactivation of NO by superoxide anions, and increased vasoconstrictors may lead to impaired endothelial function in persons with hypertension. However, the exact pathway is not known. In addition, it is not possible to ascertain whether endothelial dysfunction is a cause or consequence of hypertension (Higashi and Chayama, 2002).

Nutrition

Researchers have discovered that nutrition plays an important part of reducing hypertension and cardiovascular risk factors (Krousel-Wood, et al., 2004; Azizi, et al., 2004). Dietary factors influence coronary heart disease and stroke, since dietary factors can modulate blood lipids and their tendency for oxidation (Mera, 1994). A diet consisting of fruits, vegetables, and low-fat dairy products and low levels of sodium are recommended to prevent hypertension and related cardiovascular morbidity and mortality (Krousel-Wood, et al., 2004; Ketola, et al., 2000). Increased calcium intake is associated with decreased systolic and diastolic pressure and serum triglycerides in female adolescents (Azizi, et al., 2004). Dietary factors, especially fish oils, can influence the tendency for thrombosis (Mera, 1994).

Investigators have evaluated high dietary fat intake as a risk factor for stroke, which is a major manifestation of cardiovascular disease (Boden-Albala and Sacco, 2000). Although there is a debate over whether dietary fat determines excess body fat, it appears that the different types of fat are more important than the total amount of fat in the development of chronic disease (Khor, 2004). Ecological studies evaluating risks between populations have documented a relationship between saturated fat and total cholesterol and coronary heart disease mortality. However, within-populations studies have shown inconsistent results (Khor, 2004). High daily dietary fat intake is also related to obesity and may be an independent risk factor for stroke, or it may influence other stroke risk factors, including hypertension, diabetes, and hyperlipidemia.

There is growing concern because fat intake has increased significantly worldwide. For example, in East and Southeast Asia and China the fat intake rates have doubled and tripled, respectively, in the previous three decades (Khor, 2004). In developing countries, vegetable oils are a major dietary source, but animal fat intake has increased, from 8% of total calories in the 1960s to 13% in the 1990s.

A study based on a sample of 1,398 adolescents and young adults, aged 15–24 years, found that the use of butter over margarine was related to higher levels of low LDL-C in males and females (Raitakari, et al., 1994). The researchers showed that in male adolescents and young adults, the use of butter, along with obesity, smoking, and inactivity, was related to a 5.5 times higher risk of high LDL-cholesterol, low HDL-cholesterol, and high diastolic pressure, compared to those with a more positive lifestyle.

Glew, et al. (2004) studied the diet of men in Fulani, a rural area in northern Nigeria, and showed that the men abnormally high levels of homocysteine, a risk factor for cardiovascular disease. Based on a sample of 55 men, aged 20–70 years, they discovered that these men had low intakes of folate and vitamin B12 which may help to explain in part the abnormally high homocysteine levels in these men.

Diets high in flavonoids may reduce cardiovascular disease risk (Mennen, et al., 2004). Manios, et al. (2005) analyzed dietary intake and biochemical risk factors for cardiovascular disease among elderly women in two rural regions of Crete. The investigation used a sample of 37 elderly women from Avdou, an area with high consumption of wild greens, and 35 elderly women from Anogia, a region with low wild greens consumption. Wild greens have high amounts of vitamin C and E and flavonoids. The results indicated that the subjects from Avdou had higher total antioxidant capacity compared to those from Anogia.

Low levels of dietary vitamin E have been linked to hypertension. Using data from the 1946 British Birth Cohort study of 2,980 of persons, Mishra, et al. (2003) found that relatively low consumption of dietary vitamin E in childhood and adulthood predicted hypertension and high waist circumference in midlife.

The link between fish consumption and stroke risk has been inconsistent. Based on a sample of 4,775 adults, aged 65 years and older, Mozaffarian, et al. (2005) discovered that consumption of tuna or broiled or baked fish is related to a lower risk of ischemic stroke. In contrast, consumption of fried fish or fish sandwiches is linked to a higher risk of ischemic stroke. The authors conclude that the type of fish consumption may have an effect on the risk of ischemic stroke in the elderly, but the etiology needs further investigation.

Metabolic Disorders

A variety of metabolic disorders have been identified as risk factors for cardiovascular disease. In a person with damaged arteries, an excess of cholesterol, along with other fats, can build up at a lesion and create heart blockages. Cholesterol is a major risk factor for cardiovascular disease and associated morbidity and mortality (De Luca and Boccini, 2003; Ketola, et al., 2000). High levels of triglycerides, a type of fat in the blood stream, have been associated with excessive consumption of carbohydrates and alcohol. Triglycerides are risk factors for cardiovascular disease in that they are responsible for stroke and heart attacks. Triglycerides also affect blood clotting. Increased plasma total homocysteine is a known cardiovascular risk factor, and it is associated with several other established cardiovascular risk factors (Panagiotakos, et al., 2005; Dankner, et al., 2004). Total homocysteine blood levels are thought to be based on an interaction of genetic and lifestyle influences. Folates, vitamin B12, and pyridoxine intake are considered to be the main determinants of total homocysteine blood levels (Simon, et al., 1999).

Alcohol Consumption

Moderate alcohol consumption may protect against cardiovascular disease for it seems to have a beneficial effect on HDL/total cholesterol ratio, fibrinogogen, and homocysteine. (Burger, et al., 2004; de Gaetano, et al., 2003). Moderate consumption of alcohol is thought to produce anti-atherogenic changes in plasma lipoproteins, especially by increasing high-density lipoprotein (HDL) cholesterol. Another theory is that moderate alcohol use facilitates anti-thrombotic down control of blood platelet function and, coagulation and fibrinolysis balance.

Burger, et al. (2004) discovered the most favorable cardiovascular risk factor profile among women who drank a moderate amount of alcholol (10–20 grams) per day. In addition, the beneficial impact of moderate alcohol consumption appeared to be most evident among older men.

The association between alcohol use and incidence of ischemic stroke has been evaluated. Using a sample from 10 populations in northern and southern areas of China, Zhang, et al. (2004) discovered that the risk of ischemic stroke incidence was positively related to heavy alcohol intake among Chinese men. However, the investigators found that mild alcohol consumption was also linked to an increased risk of ischemic stroke.

However, high levels of alcohol consumption may increase the risk of cardiovascular disease, diabetes, liver disease, and accidental injuries (Waki, et al., 2005; Kurihara, et al., 2004). Kurihara, et al. (2004) assessed the association between heavy alcohol consumption and atherosclerotic cardiovascular risk in middle-aged male workers with normal blood pressure. Based on cross-sectional data, they discovered that heavy alcohol use (intake of more than 60 g of ethanol per day) was positively related to arterial stiffening, after controlling for traditional atherosclerotic cardiovascular risk factors.

Using 15 years of follow-up results from the Coronary Artery Risk Development in Young Adults Study, Pletcher, et al. (2005) evaluated the association between heavy alcohol consumption and coronary calcification, which is a marker for atherosclerosis. Their findings indicated that the prevalence of coronary calcification among 3,037 young adults, aged 33–45 years, increased with heavier alcohol intake. In addition, coronary calcification was more prevalent among binge drinkers. These results remained after controlling for confounding variables. The dose-response association was most clearly apparent for African-American men. Only heavier alcohol intake levels were related to coronary calcification in other race and sex sub-groups.

Alcohol use has been found to be positively associated with another cardiovascular risk factor, homocysteine levels. Based on a sample of Greek adults in the Athens area, Panagiotakos, et al. (2005) discovered that alcohol consumption was one of the lifestyle choices most strongly related to higher homocysteine levels.

Environmental Tobacco Smoke, Air Pollutants, and Cardiovascular Disease

There is emerging evidence that exposure to environmental tobacco smoke may be associated with increased cardiovascular risks (Zhang, et al., 2005). Using data from a population-based cohort study Zhang, et al. (2005) analyzed the link between husbands' smoking and prevalence of stroke among wives living in same household. They discovered that the prevalence of stroke among the wives increased with the intensity and duration of the husbands' smoking.

Kaur, et al. (2004) conducted a meta-analysis of 9 cohort studies to assess the association between environmental tobacco smoke exposure and the risk of cardiovascular disease mortality in women. They found that exposure to environmental tobacco smoke was related to a 15% increase in the risk of cardiovascular-disease related mortality among non-smoking women compared to non-smoking women who did not have environmental tobacco exposure. The investigators recommend warning women to reduce or avoid environmental tobacco smoke exposure as discussed in the American Heart Association guidelines for the prevention of cardiovascular disease.

Exposure to air pollution has also been identified as a possible cardiovascular disease risk factor and is also associated with total mortality (Lee, et al., 2003; Touloumi, et al., 2005). Epidemiological research has documented increases in the incidence of cardiovascular morbidity and myocardial infarction related to short-term and daily fine-particulate matter air pollution (Sullivan, et al., 2005). The elderly may be especially vulnerable to ischemic cardiovascular diseases related to cardiovascular diseases. In Seoul, Korea, Lee, et al. (2003) assessed the impact of ambient air pollution on hospital admissions for ischemic heart diseases and showed that hospital admissions for ischemic heart diseases were related to daily changes in ambient air pollution. During the summer months, for example, sulfur dioxide was associated with increased numbers of hospital admissions for ischemic heart diseases. The authors conclude that the elderly seem to be at risk from ambient air pollution.

Another report, however, did not find an association between fine-particulate matter air pollution and the onset of myocardial infarction. Using a case-crossover investigation of 5,793 patients with acute myocardial infarction, Sullivan, et al. (2005) showed no significant link between fine-particulate matter air pollution and the onset of myocardial infarction.

Disability, Quality of Life, and Cardiovascular Disease

A variety of demographic, socioeconomic, psychosocial, and disease-related factors influence disability and quality of life levels among persons with cardiovascular disease.

Age factors may affect disability and quality of life in individuals with cardiovascular disease. Froom, et al. (1999) found that older age was associated with a lower rate of work resumption following myocardial infarction. Other research has found that older patients experience more job strain and have lower return to work rates after myocardial infarction and coronary artery bypass surgery than younger patients (Karoff, et al., 2000). In an investigation of patients with peripheral arterial disease and claudication, age was also found to be one of the strongest predictors of lower extremity disability (Oka, et al., 2004).

Women with heart disease have poorer prognosis and higher levels of disability when compared with men with heart disease (Davidson, et al., 2003). In their review of research, Brezinka and Kittel (1996) found that women appear to have more difficulty in adjusting psychologically and socially after a myocardial infarction than men. However, gender differences in psychosocial adjustment following coronary artery bypass graft surgery are not conclusive.

Other research has shown that the rates of returning to work following myocardial infarction or coronary artery bypass graft (CABG) surgery are lower in women than in men (Brezinka and Kittel, 1996). There is a scarcity of data on women's sexual functioning after myocardial infarction or CABG surgery. In terms of cardiac rehabilitation outcomes, women have lower rates of participation, higher drop-out rates, and poorer compliance than for men. However, those women who complete cardiac rehabilitation have the same or better functioning as men who complete the program (Brezinka and Kittel, 1996).

Richardson (2003) assessed differences in physical functioning in older persons with angina. Using a sample of 624 older persons with angina pectoris, he discovered that older women who had suffered angina symptoms suffered more disability in lower extremity functioning than older men with angina symptoms. Disability was defined as requiring assistance in functional mobility or activities of daily living. The author concludes that angina symptoms may force older women to limit their more strenuous activities.

Kimble, et al. (2003) assessed a sample of 128 patients with coronary artery disease and chronic stable angina, and found that women reported greater physical impairment associated with anginal pain despite similarities in pain characteristics with those of men. The authors recommend that more research is warranted to analyze gender differences in functional disability related to anginal pain.

Racial and ethnic and socioeconomic disparities are increasingly recognized as predictors of disability in individuals with cardiovascular disease. Le, et al. (2002) examined possible African-American and white differences in hypertension and ankle pain, stiffness and aching in insulin-taking diabetics. The authors reported that hypertension was positively associated with ankle pain, stiffness, and aching among insulin-taking African-Americans, but not among insulin-taking whites. These findings remained significant after controlling for possible confounding variables.

Using data from the population-based 1998 National Health Interview Survey, Morewitz (2003b) evaluated possible African-American and white disparities in physical activity among persons with hypertension. According to the findings, African-Americans with hypertension were less likely to participate in vigorous activity than whites with hypertension. After controlling for income, both African-Americans and whites with hypertension who had incomes less than $20,000 were more likely to engage in vigorous physical activity than African-Americans and whites with incomes at or above $20,000.

Another investigation evaluated household income as a predictor of hypertension. This report found that after adjusting for possible confounding variables, men with a history of hypertension and incomes of less than $20,000 were about twice as likely those with hypertension history and incomes at or above $20,000 to report that hypertension impaired their daily activities. Similarly, women with a hypertension history and incomes of less than $20,000 were almost twice as likely as those with incomes at or above $20,000 to report hypertension impairment (Morewitz, 2004b).

Researchers have analyzed the impact of other aspects of socioeconomic status on disability. In one study, investigators evaluated the effects of education and other factors on physical function in 97 patients with peripheral arterial disease and claudication (Oka, et al., 2004). Their results indicated that education was a major predictor of lower extremity functioning.

Heart disease patients who do not have the money to buy their medications are at risk for exacerbating their problems. Morewitz (2004c) explored the possible association between coronary heart disease impairment and patients' ability to afford and access prescription drugs. He revealed that older coronary disease patients were more likely than younger coronary disease patients to report that at some time in the previous 12 months they were unable to purchase prescription drugs. The results persisted after adjusting for income and other possible confounding variables. These findings indicate that age is a possible predictor of inadequate access to medication, thus resulting in an exacerbation of their condition.

Overweight and obesity increase disease burden, disability, and impairment in quality of life among persons with chronic diseases. For example, one survey, based on the Third National Health and Nutrition Examination Survey, discovered the prevalence of having 2 or more co-morbid conditions was positively associated with increased weight in all racial and ethnic groups (Must, et al., 1999). Using a survey of 5,887 men and 7,018 women, aged to 59 years, Lean, et al. (1999) discovered that obese women and men were two times as likely to have problems in performing a range of regular daily activities when compared to women and men with normal weight.

The impact of overweight and obesity on disability may be especially evident among elderly persons. Based on a sample of 4,232 men, age 60–79 years, from 24 towns in the United Kingdom, Goya, et al. (2004) found that 25% of locomotor disability among the elderly men was related to overweight and obesity.

Smoking, excessive alcohol consumption, inadequate nutrition, and sedentary lifestyles are associated with low cardiorespiratory fitness, and an increased risk for cardiovascular disease-related disability and mortality. Using a sample of 25,714 adult men, Wei, et al. (1999) discovered that low cardiorespiratory fitness was an important determinant of cardiovascular disease risk and mortality.

Epidemiological studies indicate that patients who develop depression after myocardial infarction have more physical disability and impaired quality of life (Follath, 2003). In a 4-month follow-up study of 288 hospitalized myocardial infarction patients, Lane, et al. (2000) reported that both depression and anxiety were related to decreased quality of life.

Cardiovascular Disease, Stress, Coping Strategies and Social Support

Stress, social support, personality factors, and coping strategies may influence the extent to which individuals with cardiovascular disease become disabled. Dr. Mark L. Goldstein provides a case study of a patient whose whole outlook on life changed after his heart attack.

Case Study

Martin is a 65-year-old, single, Native-American Indian, who had owned a currency exchange for thirty years. He always had numerous friends and was considered "fun" by those who knew him. Martin was very active and enjoyed bowling, billiards, poker, movies and travel. His family, with whom he was not close, all lived in Canada. Approximately two years ago, Martin suffered a relatively minor heart attack. He was hospitalized briefly and counseled by a cardiologist to stop smoking cigarettes, change his high fat diet and begin exercising. Martin was 15 to 20 pounds overweight and had never exercised. He ignored the physician's suggestions and suffered a second, more significant heart attack less than one year later. Following the second heart attack, Martin had open-heart surgery. During his recovery in the hospital, he became withdrawn and severely depressed and was prescribed a number of antidepressants over the course of the next year. Despite medication, his depression remained. Martin adamantly refused to see a counselor. Although he was cleared to return to work, he chose not to and instead spent his days sleeping and watching television. Martin withdrew from friends and activities.

Within nine months, he suffered a third heart attack. Following hospitalization, he was referred to a skilled care facility for follow-up care. Martin was cantankerous to staff and vacillated between anger and depression. He expressed a desire to die. Martin's family arrived from Canada and offered to care for him, but he rejected their overtures. He died within four months.

Marital status and lack of social support have been implicated as possible predictors of disability among individuals with cardiovascular disease. Using the 1998 National Health Interview Survey, Morewitz (2004d) discovered that after adjusting for age, race, ethnicity, and income, widowed (12.8%), divorced (13.3%) or separated (14%) persons were more likely to report that hypertension impaired their daily activities than married persons (8.5%). These findings suggest that being married and living with someone may offer some protection against hypertension (Morewitz, 2004d).

In a population-based study of well-being among elderly Canadians after they had suffered a stroke, Clarke, et al. (2002) found that stroke survivors were more likely to have impairment in physical and cognitive functioning, co-morbidities, and worse mental health compared to seniors who had not suffered a stroke. Social support and educational resources, however, moderated the impact of disability.

Since female heart disease patients have a poorer prognosis and worse impairment compared to their male counterparts,

Davidson, et al. (2003) conclude from their literature review that women need more social support than do men.

Cardiovascular Disease Prevention, Treatment, and Rehabilitation Outcomes

Researchers have evaluated the effective of lifestyle interventions in reducing the risk factors for cardiovascular disease, stroke (Ketola, et al., 2000; Boden-Albala and Sacco, 2000). One of the basic questions is to what extent can a healthy-heart diet, exercise, weight loss, smoking cessation, and moderation in alcohol intake reduce cardiovascular disease and stroke risk factors and associated morbidity and mortality?

Aldana, et al. (2004) sought to replicate the original findings of the Ornish Program, an intensive lifestyle modification program for patients with cardiovascular disease. They used 50 patients, divided into six different cohorts from 8 independent medical centers located throughout the U.S. Baseline, 3-month, and 12-month follow-up data were obtained from them. Outcome data consisted of blood lipids, body fat, blood pressure, anginal pain, quality of life, and psychosocial conditions, such as stress, depression, and social support. The investigators' findings revealed that program participants experienced significant improvements in virtually all physiological and psychosocial outcomes. The authors conclude that patients with cardiovascular disease who participate in an intensive lifestyle modification program can significantly improve their physiological and psychosocial risk factors for cardiovascular disease.

Higashi and Chayama (2002) analyzed the effects of interventions on endothelial dysfunction. They found various approaches, such as the use of angiotensin-converting enzyme inhibitors and lifestyle interventions, e.g., exercise, weight loss, and sodium reduction, to be beneficial in essential hypertension patients with endothelial dysfunction of the forearm and renal circulation.

Lifestyle modification programs have also targeted health care providers. Lobo, et al. (2004) evaluated the effectiveness of a comprehensive intervention program for general practice staff on health-related quality of life of patients with cardiovascular disease and other chronic diseases. Outreach visitors provided a comprehensive intervention lasting 21 months for the staff of 62 general practices. The results indicated that while the health-related quality of life measures declined for all patients, the decline was greater in control patients. In cardiovascular disease patients, the differences between the intervention group and the control group were significant for physical functioning, vitality, and social functioning.

In a number of studies, investigators have assessed the impact of conventional treatment and cardiac rehabilitation. Conventional treatment for patients following acute myocardial infarction usually consists of general education on coronary heart disease and risk factor management by the patients' physicians (Boulay and Prud'homme, 2004). Cardiac rehabilitation after an acute myocardial infarction involves three components: 1) education, 2) exercise, and 3) encouraging resumption of work (Froom, et al., 1999).

Izawa, et al. (2004) evaluated the impact of an 8-week cardiac rehabilitation program on patients' physiologic measures, such as peak oxygen uptake, handgrip strength, and health-related quality of life using 82 cardiac rehabilitation patients and 42 control patients. Cardiac rehabilitation patients participated in supervised aerobic exercise and moderate resistance training from 1 month to 3 months after onset of an acute myocardial infarction. The researchers discovered that the cardiac rehabilitation patients had significantly greater improvements in physiologic measures than control patients. The cardiac rehabilitation patients also had greater improvements in 4 of the 8 health status measures (physical functioning, role-physical functioning, general health, and vitality) than control patients.

Boulay and Prud'homme (2004) compared the effectiveness of conventional treatment with short- and long-term cardiac rehabilitation. In this study, 54 control patients participated in a conventional treatment consisting of general education on coronary heart disease and risk factor management by their physician. Seventy-four experimental patients participated in a 2-phase, short-term cardiac rehabilitation program, and 37 of these patients participated for at least one year in a supervised third-phase, long-term cardiac rehabilitation program. The results showed a similar frequency of emergency room visits for chest pain or suspicion of cardiac-associated conditions at 1-year follow-up. However, the patients in the third-phase, long-term cardiac rehabilitation program had fewer hospital readmissions. Patients in the long-term cardiac program also had fewer emergency room visits and hospital readmissions between 3 and 12 months. The investigators found that control patients had a higher rate of recurrent myocardial infarction and fatal myocardial infarction compared to short- and long-term cardiac rehabilitation patients.

Froom, et al. (1999) evaluated resumption of full employment 24 months after acute myocardial infarction. Based on a sample of 216 acute myocardial infarction patients at an occupational medicine clinic, the authors discovered that 168 of these patients had attempted to return to work. Of these patients, 18 were unable to return to work. Of the remaining 150 patients, 54 obtained part-time employment and 96 were working full-time after 2 years. The findings revealed that for each month's delay in referral to the occupational medicine clinic there was a 30% reduction in the patient's chance for full-time employment. Delayed referral to the occupational clinic was related to work disability following an acute myocardial infarction. The researchers also noted that 6 (4%) of the 150 patients who returned to work had a recurrent acute myocardial infarction, two of them occurred in the workplace. The authors conclude that late referrals to occupational clinics should receive more intensive and long-term rehabilitation than patients referred early to the occupational clinics.

A variety of other factors may influence the rate at which cardiac patients return to work after myocardial infarction or coronary artery bypass graft. Keck (2000) emphasize the need to optimize the transition from inpatient cardiac rehabilitation phase to outpatient phase. This can be achieved by planning and implementing patient-focused approaches that involve the family physician, family members, workplaces, and local and community organizations, including health clubs, and therapeutic agencies.

Froom, et al. (1999) found that a number of risk factors were associated with failure to return to full-time work: diabetes, older age, Q wave acute myocardial infarction, angina before acute myocardial infarction, heavy work activities, and a late referral to the occupational medicine clinic.

Another study by Karoff, et al. (2000) reported that older patients after myocardial infarction and/or bypass operation were more likely to have job strain and lower rates of work resumption than younger patients. The investigators suggest that intensive after-care programs following cardiac rehabilitation can be helpful for older patients.

Kushnir and Luria (2002) note that the attitudes and behaviors of workplace supervisors play an important role in cardiac patients' resumption of work. This is one of a very few studies to investigate this process. The researchers surveyed 58 supervisors of employees who had resumed work after myocardial infarction or CABG. The supervisors felt that they play an important role in helping cardiac patients return to work, and they stressed the need to consult with occupational physicians on an on-going basis to ensure successful occupational rehabilitation. Many supervisors reported that myocardial infarction and CABG patients pose problems in the workplace because their initial work performance is impaired and they need special support on the job.

Another important determinant of return to work and other outcomes is the cardiac patient's psychosocial status. Cardiac patients frequently develop anxiety and depression, which impact their resumption of work, quality of life, and social and family functioning. In their study, Lane, et al. (2000) discovered that 4 months after hospitalization for an acute myocardial infarction, patients suffered both depression and anxiety that they associated with a lower quality of life. Cardiac patients who suffer anxiety and depression may have lower rates of return to work than those not suffering from these conditions despite their participation in cardiac rehabilitation.

Gender differences in prognosis and disability among heart disease patients may require changes in cardiac rehabilitation programs. Davidson, et al. (2003) suggest that cardiac rehabilitation programs be customized to meet the needs of women in heart disease who tend to have a poorer prognosis and higher levels of disability than men.

A growing policy issue in cardiac rehabilitation is improving access. One concern is that a large number of patients are not benefiting from cardiac rehabilitation due to the high costs of hospital-based programs. Home-based exercise training may be a better cost-effective alternative to hospital-based programs. In a randomized controlled trial, Arthur, et al. (2002) measured the exercise capacity, quality of life and social support of 120 CABG patients in a monitored home-based exercise program and 122 CABG patients in a hospital-based exercise program. They found that CABG patients in both groups experienced significant improvements in their exercise capacity as measured by peak oxygen consumption after 6 months of exercise. Patients in the monitored home-based program had greater social support and health-related quality of life by six months compared to those in the hospital-based cardiac rehabilitation program. The investigators suggest that home-based programs are comparable or better than hospital-based programs for low-risk CABG patients.

Another way of reducing the costs of cardiac rehabilitation is to reduce the duration of cardiac rehabilitation programs. To what extent can the duration of these programs be reduced without jeopardizing the effectiveness of these programs? Can the content of these programs be modified to produce similar results in less time?

Hevey, et al. (2003) compared exercise capacity and quality of life outcomes among myocardial infarction and CABG patients attending a 4-week multidisciplinary cardiac rehabilitation program with those participating in a standard 10-week program. The results of the study revealed no differences between the two groups. Six months after cardiac rehabilitation, patients in both groups experienced improvements in exercise time, metabolic measures, heart rate, energy, pain, emotional and social well-being, and general health. The researchers conclude from these preliminary findings that a shortened cardiac rehabilitation program may be effective and such programs may promote greater access to cardiac rehabilitation.

There has been concern about the high costs of CABG. Coronary catheter revascularization costs less than CABG because of lower direct costs (medical) and indirect costs (work loss). Pfund, et al. (2001) note that patients spend more time out of work following coronary procedures than necessary, and that this work loss increases the indirect costs to the extent that it exceeds the medical costs.

Another issue under investigation is the effectiveness of CABG compared to stent-assisted percutaneous coronary intervention (PCI) for patients with angina pectoris and multi-vessel coronary disease. The Stent or Surgery trial compared 206 women and 782 men with multi-vessel disease who were randomly assigned to either CABG or stent-assisted PCI (Zhang, et al., 2004). The study findings revealed that at three- and 6-month follow-ups, men, but not women, had greater improvement with CABG in physical limitations, angina frequency, and quality of life, compared with PCI. The authors conclude that CABG may be better than PCI in men, but in women, both procedures seem comparable.

Researchers have assessed the efficacy of enhanced external counterpulsation in treating angina and improving quality of life. Michaels, et al. (2004) demonstrated that at a 2-year follow-up, 73% of patients with chronic angina pectoris experienced a reduction by greater or equal to one angina class after undergoing enhanced external counterpulsation. Fifty percent of the patients also indicated that their quality of life had improved after having enhanced external counterpulsation.

Linnemeier, et al. (2003) evaluated one-year clinical outcomes among diabetic patients undergoing enhanced external counterpulsation for the relief of angina pectoris. They discovered that 69% of the diabetic patients who had the procedure had a reduction of angina by greater or equal to one angina class. Moreover, the diabetic patients after the treatment reported improvements in their quality of life.

Implantable devices for atrial defibrillation are likely to have an expanded future role. Tse and Lau (2004) have noted that implantable devices for atrial defibrillation are changing quickly. Currently employed technologies prevent and treat atrial defibrillation by combing pacing and cardioconversion treatments. Recent reports have demonstrated that these technologies are safe and can lower the incidence of atrial defibrillation as well as improve quality of life. In the future, implantable devices for atrial defibrillation should be increasingly used. Their expanded use is expected especially when they are employed with implantable cardioconverter defibrillator and cardiac resynchronization treatment for atrial defibrillation.

Studies have also been conducted to determine the effectiveness of clinical pathways in optimizing patient care for patients with cardiovascular disease. These pathways have the potential to promote high quality and cost-effective care that is based on the best available evidence and practice guidelines (Kwan and Sandercock, 2004).

Some investigations have shown that the implementation of a clinical or critical pathway has improved patient care outcomes for patients with a myocardial infarction. Pelliccia, et al. (2004) assessed the impact of a clinical pathway on patient care outcomes and processes for patients presenting to an emergency department of a large European hospital with acute chest pain and possible ST-elevation myocardial infarction. The sample consisted of 452 critical pathway patients, who were managed with pre-established criteria for diagnosis, thrombolysis, percutaneous coronary intervention, and admission to the coronary care unit in 2001 and 520 non-critical pathway patients, who were managed based on the emergency department cardiologists' decisions in 1997. The investigators discovered that critical pathway patients in 2001 were more likely to be sent to primary angioplasty compared to non-critical pathway patients, who were more likely to be given thrombolysis in 1997. Critical pathway patients also were more likely to be treated with aspirin and intravenous beta blockers soon after arriving at the emergency department compared to non-critical pathway patients. There were no differences between the two groups in their admission rates to the coronary care unit and cardiac wards. However, hospitalized critical pathway patients had a shorter length of stay and fewer major adverse coronary events and lower all-cause in-hospital mortality compared to non-critical pathway patients. It also took less time to initiate cardiac procedures for the critical pathway patients than for the non-critical pathway patients. The researchers conclude that a critical pathway increased the use of evidence-based practices and enhanced patient care outcomes for patients with acute chest pain and possible ST-elevation myocardial infarction.

Wolff, et al. (2004) evaluated whether the use of checklists and reminders in clinical pathways can enhance the quality of care for 116 patients with ST-elevation acute myocardial infarction and 123 patients with stroke. They found that after introducing the clinical pathway with checklists and reminders, treatment compliance for patients with ST-elevation acute myocardial infarction increased by 21.4% for patients being treated with aspirin in the emergency department, 42.7% for eligible patients being treated with beta-blockers within 24 hours of admission, 48.1% for eligible patients being prescribed beta-blockers on hospital discharge, and 41.2% for eligible patients receiving lipid therapy. After implementing the stroke clinical pathway with checklists and reminders, there was a 40.7% increase in treatment compliance for dysphagia screening within 24 hours of hospital admission, 55.4% for ischemic stroke patients beng treated with aspirin or Clopidogrel within 24 hours of admission, and 52.4% for patients having regular neurological observations during the first 48 hours after a stroke. The investigators conclude that the use of checklists and reminders in clinical pathways can significantly enhance patient care.

However, one study of Medicare patients with myocardial infraction at 32 non-federal hospitals in Connecticut did not find that critical pathways improve patient care outcomes (Holmboe, et al., 1999). The investigators compared 10 hospitals which had developed critical pathways for the care of Medicare patients with acute myocardial infarction with 22 non-pathway hospitals. They discovered that the hospitals that initiated critical pathways did not have increased use of evidence-based treatments, shorter lengths of hospital stays or reduced mortality compared to non-pathway hospitals.

Cardiovascular Disease Patient Education and Self-Management

Cardiovascular disease patient education and self-management interventions seek to improve the quality of life of patients, minimize symptoms, reduce the number of hospital admissions, and shorten the length of a hospital stay (Frattini, et al., 1998). These interventions determine the patients' needs, behaviors, an attitude, and then evaluate the impact of patient education and self-management activities on patient care outcomes.

Cardiovascular disease patients must have the requisite specialized knowledge to successfully engage in self-care practices, e.g., taking medications, monitoring their weight, exercising, and recognizing the signs of myocardial infarction, heart failure, and other health conditions. Various studies have documented low levels of knowledge among cardiovascular disease patients. Clinicians and patients need to work together to improve patient care outcomes in different areas of cardiovascular disease management include myocardial infarction and congestive heart failure. One report notes that improving patient knowledge and understanding of clinical practice guidelines can improve recovery from myocardial infarctions and ensure better compliance with recommended clinical guidelines (Dykes, et al., 2004). This report advocates the use of automated patient pathways, such as the Patient Education and Recovery Learning System to enhance patient adherence education and adherence to evidence-based, clinical practice guidelines.

Other reports have focused on the low levels of knowledge among heart failure patients. Based on a nurse questionnaire administered to 324 patients during their first visit to a new Heart Failure Unit in Spain, researchers found deficits in several knowledge areas. Only 30% of the patients understood the functioning of the heart and only 29% understood the nature of heart failure. Thirty-two percent of the patients in the study knew all of the names of their medications and only 23% understood the action of these drugs. On the positive side, 67% knew more than three signs of worsening symptoms (Gonzalez, et al., 2004).

Artinian, et al. (2002) found that the heart failure patients in their study had deficits in their knowledge about self-care practices. These patients did not know how to use their heart failure medications, monitor their weight, and they did not understand the definition of heart failure. The researchers found that older and more highly educated patients had higher levels of knowledge in these areas. Race and gender did not predict differences in knowledge about heart failure and self-care.

Gonzalez, et al. (2004) studied self-reported behaviors among heart failure patients and discovered both positive and negative self-care practices. In their investigation, 91% reported that they were taking all of their prescribed medications and 71% always carried their prescriptions. Eighty-five percent of the patients with ischemic heart disease knew how to use sublingual nitrogylcerine. Ninety-three percent of the patients surveyed indicated that they did not smoke and 83% reported that they rarely consumed alcohol. However, only 14% of the heart failure patients monitored their weight more than once a week, only 33% always followed a sodium restricted diet, and only 18% monitored their blood pressure more than once a week. Only 6% reported that they did some type of physical exercise, although 83% walked and engaged in daily activities.

Which factors predict whether cardiovascular disease patients will follow self-care practices? In Gonzalez, et al. (2004)'s study of heart failure patients, age and gender differences and referral patterns predicted self-care behaviors. The researchers discovered that younger patients, men, and patients referred from the Cardiology Outpatient Clinic participated in more physical activity than older patients, women, and patients referred from other departments. However, older patients were more likely to follow a sodium restricted diet than younger patients, and women were less likely to smoke and drink alcohol than men.

Psychosocial problems frequently occur after an acute myocardial infarction and are associated with other forms of cardiovascular morbidity (Lacey, et al., 2004). Heart disease patients who experience anxiety and depression may be less likely to learn the necessary information to follow self-care practices or lack the ability to follow these self-care procedures. Heart disease patients who are unemployed or who have limited financial resources may be especially at risk for developing psychosocial morbidity because they also have difficulty accessing health care providers. Researchers are investigating how interventions can be designed to help these patients better cope with the anxiety, depression, and other psychosocial problems associated with cardiovascular disease and financial distress.

Lacey, et al. (2004) measured the use of a home-based self-help package to reduce feelings of anxiety and depression among patients discharged from the hospital after an acute myocardial infarction. Patients in the experimental group received a home-based, self-help package plus usual after-care while those in the control group were given the usual after-care only. The results showed that patients in the experimental group improved significantly in terms of their feelings of anxiety and depression compared to the control group. In addition, patients who participated in hospital-based rehabilitation classes and those aged over 80 years showed improvements as a result of the intervention. These results indicate that a home-based, self-help package, along with hospital rehabilitation classes, are effective for improving the psychosocial status of patients of all ages.

7

Cancer

Cancer is a leading cause of death. Certain types of cancer share some of the same lifestyle and socioeconomic status risk factors as type 2 diabetes and cardiovascular disease. These findings suggest that lifestyle modification, including appropriate diet and nutrition, regular physical activity, weight control, and smoking cessation can help to prevent certain types of cancers.

Below is a summary of some of the risk factors for several prevalent types of cancer.

Lung Cancer

In 2000, there were 1.1 million lung cancer deaths worldwide (Whitrow, et al., 2003). Lung cancer incidence increased dramatically in the 20th century and continues to increase in the 21st century (Teixeira, et al., 2003; Bray, et al., 2004).

Smoking

Cigarette smoking is the leading cause of lung cancer, and the disease risks are proportional to the intensity and duration of smoking and individuals who quit smoking lower their risks of lung cancer compared to those who continue to smoke (Burns,

2003). In addition to smoking, a number of demographic, geographic, environmental, nutritional, genetic, hormonal, and lifestyle factors may be linked to an increased risk of lung cancer (Teixeira, et al., 2003). However, Whitrow, et al. (2003) note that there is limited evidence of causation other than for smoking.

Gender, age, racial/ethnic, and socioeconomic status differences in smoking habits have been reported (Teixeira, et al., 2003; Bray, et al., 2004; Patel, et al., 2004). With regard to gender, lung cancer is the leading cause of cancer-related deaths in U.S. women and accounts for as many deaths as breast cancer and all gynecological cancers combined (Patel, et al., 2004). In other developed countries, especially in Europe, there is an increased incidence of lung cancer in women (Teixeira, et al., 2003).

Despite all of the public health campaigns and interventions, 25% of women in the U.S. continue to smoke. Tobacco advertising targets women, and teenage girls face social pressures to smoke and engage in other risky behaviors (Patel, et al., 2004). Women begin to smoke earlier than men and have more difficulty trying to quit.

Moreover, women may be more susceptible to carcinogens than men, with women having a 1.5 times higher risk of developing lung cancer than men with the same smoking habits (Teixeira, et al., 2003). Research is showing that women have different risks for developing lung cancer when compared to men. Women's increased susceptibility to the negative effects of tobacco may occur because of their higher levels of DNA adducts, reduced DNA repair ability, increased frequency of mutations in tumor suppressor genes, and hormonal variations (Rivera and Stover, 2004).

There are a variety of gender differences in lung cancer presentation. Compared to men, there is a larger percentage of adenocarcinoma among women, a larger proportion of young women, and non-smoking women are more likely to be diagnosed with lung cancer (Rivera and Stover, 2004).

There are also age differences in the histological type of lung cancer, with young people having a higher prevalence of adenocarcinoma than older people (Teixeira, et al., 2003). Age differences may reflect differences in the type of cigarettes smoked and other factors (Marugame, et al., 2004).

With regard to racial/ethnic factors, smoking prevalence has been found to be higher among African-Americans compared to whites (Stellman, et al., 2003). African-Americans also have a higher risk for lung cancer compared to whites in the U.S. (Schwartz and Swanson, 1997). Among younger persons, this racial/ethnic disparity is greater.

African-American/white differences in lung cancer risks may be due to African- American/white differences in smoking habits. Stellman, et al. (2003), using a hospital-based case-control design, found that African-Americans and whites who had similar smoking habits had similar lung cancer risks, except for African-Americans who were very heavy smokers. The investigators suggest that modifying factors, such as cigarette type, diet, occupation, and the variations in the ability to metabolize smoke carcinogens may influence African-American/white differences in lung cancer risks.

Based on a survey of 5,588 cases of African-Americans and whites with lung cancer and 3,692 controls, Schwartz and Swanson (1997) analyzed the extent to which disparities in lung cancer risks are due to differences in smoking behaviors. The findings indicated that in the age range of 55 to 84 years, African-American/white differences in lung cancer were accounted for almost completely by differences in cigarette smoking behaviors. However, among men in the 40–54 year age group, African-Americans were 2 to 4 times more likely than whites to develop lung cancer even after controlling for smoking behaviors. The authors conclude that younger African-Americans may be especially susceptible to lung carcinogens or they may have unique exposures that remain unknown.

Socioeconomic status differences in smoking have been documented (Gulliford, et al., 2003; Lund and Lund, 2005). In a survey of persons with diabetes mellitus in a socioeconomically deprived area of London, Gulliford, et al. (2003) found that smokers were more likely than non-smokers to come from low-socioeconomic status backgrounds. Lund and Lund (2005), using a study of 5,125 persons, showed that smokers were more likely to have lower socioeconomic status than non-smokers. In lower socioeconomic status groups, larger number of people smoked and they were likely to smoke more dangerous cigarettes than those in the higher socioeconomic status groups. Young people begin smoking earlier and passive smoking is more accepted in the lower socioeconomic status groups.

Recently, there has been a relative increase of lung cancer of the adenocarcinoma type compared to the squamous cell carcinoma type, and this trend may be due to a shift from non-filter to filter cigarettes. Based on a case-control study of 356 patients with lung cancer and 162 control subjects, Marugame, et al. (2001) reported a decrease in both squamous cell carcinoma and adenocarcinoma among lifelong smokers of filter cigarettes. There was more of a reduction in cases of squamous cell carcinoma than for adenocarcinoma. However, among men, under 54 years of age, those who only smoked filter cigarettes had an increased risk of adenocarcinoma, but a risk reduction in squamous cell carcinoma. The researchers suggest that the change in histological type of lung cancer from squamous cell carcinoma to adenocarcinoma, especially among young smokers, may be associated with changes in the type of cigarettes smoked.

The tar yields of cigarettes also have been examined to determine if medium tar filter cigarettes are associated with a higher risk of lung cancer than low or very low tar cigarettes. Harris, et al. (2004) evaluated the relationship between the tar rating of the cigarette brand smoked in 1982 and lung cancer mortality in the following six years. The investigators discovered that regardless of the tar level of their current brand of cigarettes, all current smokers had a much higher risk of lung cancer than those who had stopped smoking or had never smoked. However, lung cancer risk was higher among female and male smokers of high-tar, non-filter brands compared to smokers of medium-tar, filter brands. In addition, the results showed no differences in lung cancer risks among male and female smokers of very low-tar or low-tar brands compared to smokers of medium-tar brands. The authors conclude that men and women who smoke high-tar, non-filter cigarette brands have an even higher risk of lung cancer than those who smoke medium-, low-, or very low- tar-filter brands.

Air Pollution

A number of studies have discovered a link between air pollution, including both outdoor and indoor air pollution, and lung cancer as well as ischemic heart disease and respiratory diseases in non-smokers (Whitrow, et al., 2003; Nafstad, et al., 2003; Boffetta and Nyberg, 2003). Nafstad, et al. (2003) found higher rates of lung cancer in urban areas, compared to rural areas, and the detection of known carcinogens in the urban atmosphere has led to the hypothesis that chronic air pollution increases lung cancer risk.

Investigators have discovered a causal relationship between exposure to environmental-tobacco smoke or second-hand smoke and lung cancer incidence. It is estimated that persons exposed to environmental tobacco smoke have a relative lung cancer risk of 1.2 (Boffetta and Nyberg, 2003).

However, exposure to environmental tobacco smoke is uneven in the population (Veglia, et al., 2003). Studies have evaluated determinants of exposure to environmental tobacco smoke to aid in the development of prevention programs. Veglia, et al. (2003) surveyed exposure to environmental tobacco smoke using a sample of 21,588 non-smokers in Italy. The researchers discovered that the most common exposure to environmental tobacco smoke comes from the workplace and individuals employed full-time were more exposed to environmental tobacco smoke than those employed part-time. The results also showed that white-collar employees had the highest exposures to environmental tobacco smoke.

Another known carcinogen, radon gas, can migrate from soils and rocks and accumulate in homes, underground mines, and other enclosed areas (Krewski, et al., 2005; Darby, et al., 2005; Boffetta and Nyberg, 2003). Research reveals that underground miners who are exposed to high levels of radon gas decay products (222Rn) have an elevated risk of developing lung cancer (Krewski, et al., 2005). Similar carcinogenic effects of exposure to radon decay products are demonstrated in experiments involving exposed laboratory animals (Field, et al., 2001).

Although high levels of radon produce an excess risk of lung cancer among underground miners, it is less clear if exposure to radon in homes results in a similar excess risk for lung cancer (Krewski, et al., 2005). Different factors may affect the association between residential-radon exposure and the risk of lung cancer. Levels of radon vary within residences. Blot, et al. (1990), in their study of indoor radon and lung cancer in Shenyang, People's Republic of China, found that radon levels were more likely to be higher on the first floor of multiple-story residences or in single-story houses. In their study, radon levels were also higher in residences which had coal-burning stoves that produced increased levels of indoor air pollution.

Several studies reveal a positive relationship between residential-radon exposure and increased lung cancer risk (Darby, et al., 2005; Krewski, et al., 2005; Lubin, et al., 1995). Lubin, et al. (1995) developed risk estimates based on pooling original data from 11 cohort studies of miners who were exposed to radon. The authors estimated that 10% of all lung cancer deaths may be a result of residential exposure to radon. In addition, 11% of lung cancer deaths among smokers and 30% of lung cancer deaths among persons who never smoked may be due to exposure to indoor radon.

Based on a combined analysis of 7 North American case-control studies, Krewski, et al. (2005) analyzed pooled data obtained from long-term alpha-track detectors to evaluate levels of residential radon. Using 3,662 cases and 4,966 controls, the investigation discovered that the risks for lung cancer increased with residential radon concentration.

Darby, et al. (2005) evaluated the risk of exposure to residential radon using data from 13 case-control studies of residential radon and lung cancer. The investigators discovered that for lifetime non-smokers, the absolute risks of lung cancer by age 75 years would be approximately 0.4%, 0.5%, and 0.7% at usual radon concentrations of 0, 100, and 400 Bq/m3 (becquerels or radon disintegrations per second per cubic meter), respectively. Cigarette smokers had about 25 time greater absolute risks of lung cancer at the usual radon concentrations.

In phase 1 of the Iowa Radon Lung Cancer Study, Field, et al. (2001) evaluated residential radon exposure using 413 incident lung cancer cases and 614 age-frequency matched controls. Their results indicated that cumulative exposure to radon in residences was positively related to increased lung cancer risk.

Other studies show that the precise effects of long-term radon exposure in residential settings are still not well known. A person's smoking history and other confounding factors need to be controlled to evaluate the link between radon exposure and lung cancer risk (Pearce and Boyle, 2005). Alavanja, et al. (1994) discovered that the magnitude of the risk for lung cancer from residential radon exposure in the U.S. seems low. An investigation in the People's Republic of China by Blot, et al. (1990) did not found a positive relationship between residential exposure to radon and lung cancer risks.

Research has documented that women in several Asian populations are at increased risk for developing lung cancer from cooking and heating (Boffetta and Nyberg, 2003). However, some investigations have yielded only modest evidence for causality (Whitrow, et al., 2003).

In one follow-up study of a cohort of 38,866 female and 6,824 male hairdressers, Czene, et al. (2003) showed that female hairdressers had an increased risk for lung cancer.

Arsenic

Studies have shown that consumption of water high in arsenic contamination increases the risk of lung cancer as well as the risk of bladder and skin cancer. Millions of people in Bangladesh, West Bengal India, and many other places around the world, are drinking ground water containing high concentrations of arsenic (Hossain, et al., 2005; West Bengal, India, and Bangladesh Arsenic Crisis Information Centre, 2003; Frisbie, et al., 2002). In Bangladesh, people had used to drink surface water, which often was contaminated with bacteria causing a range of diseases such as diarrhea, cholera, and typhoid (Frisbie, et al., 2002). Since independence in 1971, millions of tubewells were installed so that groundwater would be used for drinking instead of surface water. The use of groundwater reduced deaths from waterborne pathogens. However, it has been discovered that large areas of of Bangladesh now are exposed to arsenic and other toxic elements in the groundwater. Frisbie, et al. (2002) discovered that chronic arsenic poisoning may be the most important health risk from drinking Bangladesh's tubewell water. In their study, arsenic concentrations in the tubewell water samples were found to ranged from less than 0.007 to 0.64 mg/L, and 48% of the water samples had arsenic concentrations above 0.01 mg/L, which is the drinking water guideline established by World Health Organization. The survey also found that the groundwater contained unsafe levels of manganese, lead, nickel, and chromium, and four adjacent, populated states in India may have groundwater with unsafe levels of arsenic and other toxic elements.

Asbestos

Instances of asbestos contamination in public water supplies have triggered studies to evaluate the environmental health effects of asbestos contamination (Browne, et al., 2005; Andersen, 1993; Howe, et al., 1989). For example, very high concentrations of asbestos leachate in the drinking water in Woodstock, New York, were found in 1985. However, environmental health studies in the Woodstock, New York, area have not revealed a link between exposure to asbestos in drinking water and increased cancer incidence (Browne, et al., 2005). In fact, one study of the Woodstock, New York, area found the incidence of lung cancer was lower than expected for both women and men (Howe, et al., 1989).

Physical Activity

Several studies have shown that physical activity reduces lung cancer risk. For example, a population-based case-control study of 2,128 patients with lung cancer and 3,106 population controls in Canada found that recreational physical activity reduced the risk of lung cancer (Mao, et al., 2003). Both men and women who participated in physical activity had a reduced risk for lung cancer. A greater reduction in risks occurred for women with squamous cell carcinoma, while there was a greater reduction in risks among men for small cell carcinoma. Furthermore, smokers and those with low and moderate body mass indexes exhibited a greater risk reduction for lung cancer. The researchers recommend that more research is needed to substantiate the link between physical activity and histologic sub-types of lung cancer and gender as well as the biologic etiology (Varo Cenarruzabeitia, et al., 2003).

Nutrition and Lung Cancer

Some investigations show that the consumption of certain foods, such of fruit and vegetables, dietary supplements, and vitamins may protect against lung cancer (Miller, et al., 2004; Mannisto, et al., 2004). For example, foods high in beta-cryptoxanthin, such as citrus fruit, may lower the risk of lung cancer. However, other investigations using cohort and case-control study designs have reported no protective effects. Intervention studies have demonstrated that supplemental beta-carotene has either no beneficial effect or a harmful impact on risk of lung cancer (Mannisto, et al., 2004). However, until recently research has been limited by the lack of databases for specific types of carotenoids.

Using data from 478,021 persons who participated in the European Prospective Investigation into Cancer and Nutrition, Miller, et al. (2004) discovered that fruit consumption was associated with a reduced risk of lung cancer. This relationship was significant after controlling for age, smoking, height, weight, and gender. The association between fruit consumption and lower lung cancer risk was strongest among persons from the Northern Europe centers, among current smokers, and was enhanced when 293 persons with lung cancer diagnosed in the first two years of follow-up were not used in the analysis. The researchers reported no relationship between consumption of vegetables or subtypes of vegetables and risk of lung cancer. However, the impact of fruit consumption on lung cancer risk is probably small compared to the effect of smoking cessation.

Breast Cancer

There are multiple risk factors for breast cancer and premalignant breast cancer (Tyrer, et al., 2004). Some of these factors are genetic and are associated with family history, while others are personal, lifestyle or environmental/occupational factors (Tyrer, et al., 2004). Various studies focus on the interactions between genetic susceptibility and environmental exposure in the etiology of breast cancer (Bernstein, et al., 2004; Millikan, et al., 2004).

Genetic Factors and Family History of Breast Cancer

Genetic factors increase a woman's risk of developing breast cancer (Tyrer, et al., 2004; Colditz, et al., 2004). Mutations in the BRCA1 or BRCA2 genes are possible precursors of breast cancer. In southern Sweden, Loman, et al. (2001) evaluated the nature and prevalence of two germline mutations in a population-based series of early-onset breast cancer. Their results indicated that 48% of the women in the study with early-onset breast cancer have had some positive history of breast or ovarian cancer. BRCA1 or BRCA2 germline mutations were found in 9% of the women with early-onset breast cancer. Mutation carriers were more prevalent among young women with at least one or more first- or second-degree relatives with breast or ovarian cancer, and among women with bilateral breast cancer.

BRCA1 and BRCA2 mutations do not account for all of the familial aggregation of breast cancer (Tyrer, et al., 2004). The RPS6KB1 gene is enhanced and over expressed in about 10% of breast cancers and has been related to a poor prognosis of the disease (van der Hage, et al., 2004).

Han, et al. (2004) found that a human sulfotransferase (SULT1A1), which activates the sulfation of different phenolic and estrogenic compounds, predicted increased breast cancer risk in Chinese women. Zheng, et al. (2004) suggest that CYP11A gene polymorphism may increase susceptibility to breast cancer risk.

Other research focuses on the gene-environment interaction in influencing the risk of breast cancer. For example, the manganese superoxide dismutase (MnSOD) gene may increase breast cancer risk if specific environmental exposures, such as smoking, radiation to the chest, and occupational exposure to ionizing radiation, are present (Millikan, et al., 2004).

Benign Breast Disease

Research has revealed that a history of benign breast disease is related to an elevated risk of breast cancer (Wang, et al., 2004; Altaf, et al., 2004; Colditz, et al., 2004). More research is needed to clarify this relationship, especially the ways in which the type of benign breast disease and other risk factors may mediate this relationship. Using a sample of 11,307 women with no history of atypical hyperplasia or in situ breast cancer, Wang, et al. (2004) discovered that women with benign breast cancer had an elevated risk of breast cancer. As noted previously, this relationship was especially pronounced among women in the 50 and older age group. These findings were independent of other major epidemiologic breast cancer risk factors.

Reproductive and Hormonal Factors

A number of reproductive and hormonal factors have been linked to increased risk of breast cancer. Studies have found that risk factors for breast cancer include: early menarche; late age at birth of first child; low parity; years of menstruation and menopausal status (Walker, et al., 2004; Colditz, et al., 2004; Zheng, et al., 2004). A women's first pregnancy has been found to have an adverse effect on breast cancer risk (Colditz, et al., 2004).

Early age at first full-term pregnancy and increasing parity are related to a lower breast cancer risk. However, the effect of pregnancy on BRCA1 and BRCA2 germline mutation carriers is unknown. Jernstrom, et al. (1999) conducted a matched case-control study that evaluated the relationship between pregnancy and the risk of early breast cancer in carriers of BRCA1 and BRCA2. Cases consisted of carriers who had acquired breast cancer by age 40, and controls were carriers of the same age who had not developed breast cancer. The findings revealed that cancer cases were more likely than controls to have had a full term pregnancy. The cancer cases had a higher number of childbirths than controls. Breast cancer risks increased with the number of births. Cases and controls were of similar ages at their first and last births. The authors concluded that BRCA1 and BRCA2 mutation carriers who have children have a greater chance of developing breast cancer by age 40 than carriers who are nulliparous. They also noted that each succeeding pregnancy is linked to an increased risk of breast cancer and an early first pregnancy is not protective for them.

Jernstrom, et al. (2004) found, in general, that breast cancer risk decreases with increasing duration of breast-feeding. In order to find out if the same is true for women who carry the BRCA1 and BRCA2 mutations, the researchers analyzed breast-feeding and the risk of breast cancer in 965 cases of women who had been diagnosed with breast cancer and 965 matched controls who had no history of breast or ovarian cancer. Women carrying BRCA1 mutations who breast-fed for more than 1 year had a lower probability of developing breast cancer than those who had never breast-fed. This association was not found among women carrying BRCA2 mutations. The authors conclude that women carrying the BRCA1 mutations who breast-fed for more than one year had a lower risk for acquiring breast cancer.

Menopausal status has been related to breast cancer risk and other risk factors for breast cancer. For example, body mass index after menopause was associated with positive progesterone receptor tumors but not with negative progesterone receptor tumors. Differences in the incidence of estrogen-positive and estrogen-negative tumors were associated with past use of post-menopausal hormones (Colditz, et al., 2004).

Estrogen plays a major role in breast cancer risk (Boyapati, et al., 2004). One report notes that women who undergo more than five years of estrogen treatment have a 30% increase in breast cancer (Martin-Du, 2003). One hypothesis is that various known risk factors for breast cancer are influenced by endogenous sex hormones. Boyapati, et al. (2004) studied 420 post-menopausal healthy women, and discovered that body size was strongly associated with endogenous sex hormones. Specifically, weight, waist circumference, and hip circumference were positively related to levels of testosterone, estradiol, and estrone. These results indicate that the risk of breast cancer related to body size may be partially influenced by endogenous sex hormone levels.

There has been concern about the safety of hormonal contraceptives ever since their introduction in the 1960s (Burkman, et al., 2004; Narod, et al., 2002). Research has found an association between use of oral contraceptives and elevated breast cancer risk (Burkman, et al., 2004; Braaten, et al., 2004). Burkman, et al. (2004) note that based on a recent meta-analyses, there may be a small increase in the risks of breast and cervical cancer associated with using hormonal contraceptives.

Researchers have investigated whether oral contraceptives use is related to increased breast cancer risk in women who carry one of the adverse BRCA1 and BRCA2 mutations. Narod, et al. (2002) used a matched case-control study of women with adverse BRCA1 and BRCA2 mutations, recruited from 52 centers in 11 countries, to evaluate oral contraceptives and breast cancer risk. Their findings revealed that among BRCA1 but not among BRCA2 carrier, long term use of oral contraceptives was modestly related to increased breast cancer risk. Those BRCA1 carriers who used oral contraceptives for at least five years had a greater chance of developing breast cancer compared with BRCA1 carriers who had never used oral contraceptives. Those BRCA1 carriers who were on oral contraceptives before the age of 30 years, those who were diagnosed with breast cancer before the age of 40 and those who initially went on oral contraceptives before 1975 had a greater probability of acquiring breast cancer than BRCA1 carriers who never had used oral contraceptives. The investigators found the oral contraceptive use does not seem to be related to increased breast cancer risk, but more data are needed to assess this association.

Leptin, a hormone which helps regulate body weight and sexual maturation, may be related to breast cancer risk. Tessitore, et al. (2004) analyzed the link between leptin and tumor, hormonal, and cachexia markers among patients with breast and gynecological cancer. The authors reported that among patients with breast cancer, increased leptin levels were related to elevated levels of progesterone and estradiol and increased tissue levels of estrogen receptor and progesterone receptor. These findings suggest that leptin levels are associated with hormonal status but not cachexia. The authors propose that leptin triggers the production of sexual hormones, which are risk factors for breast and gynecological cancers. They conclude that leptin is an important prognostic marker for these cancers.

Obesity, Insulin Resistance, and Breast Cancer Risk

Obesity and insulin resistance have been implicated as risk factors for breast cancer (Mantzoros, et al., 2004; Boyapati, et al., 2004; Kaaks and Lukanova, 2002). Breast cancer risks related to obesity may be impacted by endogenous sex hormones. For example, in a case control study of post-menopausal Chinese women, Boyapati, et al. (2004) discovered that measures of body size, including weight, waist circumference, and hip circumference were positively correlated with testerone, estradiol, and estrone.

Adiponectin, an adipocyte-secreted hormone, is inversely related to insulin resistance. Studies suggest that adiponectin is inversely correlated with endometrial cancer and may be inversely associated with breast cancer as well. Mantzoros, et al. (2004) believed that decreased adiponectin levels may influence the relationship between obesity/insulin resistance and breast cancer. In a case-control study consisting of 174 women with breast cancer and 167 controls, they found that a lower level of adiponectin was related to an increased risk of breast cancer among postmenopausal women. However, no association was discovered among premenopausal women.

Insulin-like Growth Factor (IGF)

The IGF family, consisting of ligands, receptors, binding proteins and proteases is essential for the development and maintenance of normal tissue homeostasis (Perks and Holly, 2003). Two substances that are thought to influence tumor development are insulin-like growth factor (IGF-I) and its primary binding protein (IGFBP-3) (Renehan, et al., 2004). Some studies have shown that high concentrations of circulating IGF-I and low concentrations of IGFB-3 are related to an elevated risk of breast, colorectal, and prostate cancers (DeLellis, et al., 2004; Allen, et al., 2005).

The link between circulating IGF-I and risk of breast cancer may vary by menopausal status (Schernhammer, et al., 2005). Using a case-control study of 117 cases and 350 matched controls Allen, et al. (2005) discovered that high levels of circulating IGF-I and low levels of IGFB-3 were related to an increased risk of breast cancer in premenopausal women, while among postmenopausal women, neither IGF-I nor IGFB-3 was related to breast cancer risk. Schernhammer, et al. (2005) also found that circulating IGF-I appeared to be modestly associated with breast cancer risk among premenopaual women but not among postmenopausal women. In contrast, free IGF did not predict breast cancer risk among either premenopausal or postmenopausal women.

Jernstrom, et al. (2004) analyzed the associations between IGF1 genotype, early-onset breast cancer, breast volume, circulating IGF-I, and use of oral contraceptives. Using a prospective cohort of 258 healthy women, 40 years or younger, from high-risk breast cancer families, they discovered that lack of the 19-repeat allele was related to high levels of IGF-I in nulliparous users of oral contraceptives. The absence of the 19-repeat allele was also associated with larger breast volumes in parous women and users of oral contraceptives. In addition, breast cancer was more prevalent in women without the 19-repeat allele. The investigators conclude that the absence of the 19-repeat allele influences levels of IGF-I, breast volume, and possibly the risk of breast cancer after exposure to hormones in young women from high risk-families

Nutritional Factors

Given the association between obesity/insulin resistance and elevated breast cancer risk, it is not surprising that researchers, such as Mattison, et al. (2004) have implicated nutritional factors as risk factors or protective factors for breast cancer. Based on a sample of postmenopausal women, they reported that high-fat intake was related to elevated breast cancer risk.

Some studies indicate that an increased dietary (n-3) fatty acid intake and/or increased (n-3)/(n-6) polyunsaturated fatty acid (PUFA) ratio are related to lower risk of breast cancer. Goodstine, et al., (2003) assessed these associations by combining two related case-control studies in Connecticut. The results revealed that when the data were limited to one population-based study site, a higher (n-3)/(n-6) PUFA ratio predicted a lower breast cancer risk.

There have been inconclusive findings regarding the impact of fruits, vegetables, and antioxidant micronutrients on the risk of breast cancer (Gaudet, et al., 2004; Nkondjock and Ghadirian, 2004; Zhang, et al., 1999). Using the cohort of 83,234 women, aged 33–60 years, from the Nurses' Health Study, Zhang, et al. (1999) showed that there were weak negative associations between intakes of beta-carotene from food and nutritional supplements, lutein/zeaxanthin, and vitamin A from foods and breast cancer risks among premenopausal women. However, among premenopausal women with a positive family history of breast cancer, there were strong inverse relationships between intakes of alpha-carotene, beta-carotene, lutein/zeaxanthin, total vitamin C from foods, and total vitamin A and breast cancer risk. Premenopausal women with a positive family history of breast cancer had a much lower breast cancer risk if they consumed five or more servings of fruits and vegetables per day compared to those who had less than two servings. They suggest that consumption of fruits and vegetables high in specific carotenoids and vitamins may reduce the risk of breast cancer in premenopausal women.

Based on a sample of 414 women with breast cancer and 429 controls, one report found that consumption of high amounts of both total carotenoids and decosahexaenoic acid may lower lower breast cancer risk (Nkondjock and Ghadirian, 2004).

Gaudet, et al. (2004) evaluated whether the association between consumption of fruits and vegetables and breast cancer risk is affected by menopausal status or with clinical aspects of breast cancer. Using 1,463 cases and 1,500 controls, the authors found that among postmenopausal but not premenopausal women, there was a decreased risk of breast cancer risk with the increased use of fruits and vegetables. This inverse association was shown to be stronger for postmenopausal women with estrogen receptor (ER) + tumors.

Alcohol Use

Epidemiologic reports have linked alcohol use to increased breast cancer risk (Laufer, et al., 2004; Mattisson, et al., 2004). However, a causal association has not been ascertained. In addition, the mechanisms underlying this association have not been established. One hypothesis is that alcohol affects the development of breast cancer by way of altered folate and vitamin B (12). These two vitamins are necessary for DNA methylation and nucleotide synthesis, and therefore are essential for cell integrity. Further research is needed to clarify the quantity of alcohol associated with increased breast cancer risk and the extent to which other breast cancer risk factors, e.g., high fat intake and menopausal status, influence the relationship between alcohol intake and breast cancer.

Mattison, et al. (2004) addressed some of these issues by evaluating the associations between alcohol and high fat intake and breast cancer in post-menopausal women. Based on data from the Malmo Diet and Cancer cohort study, they reported that high wine use, but not high alcohol use, was related to an elevated risk of breast cancer. High-fat intake was associated with breast cancer risk.

Laufer, et al. (2004) also evaluated the effects of moderate alcohol intake on folate and vitamin B (12) status using a sample of 53 post-menopausal women. They discovered that moderate consumption of alcohol was associated with reduced vitamin B (12) status, but had no effect on folate status. These results suggest that among healthy, well-nourished post-menopausal women, moderate alcohol use may increase breast cancer risk by diminishing vitamin B (12) status.

Physical Activity and Breast Cancer

Physical activity has been identified as a possible protective factor in reducing the risk of breast cancer (Varo Cenarruzabeitia, et al., 2003; Walker, et al., 2004; Kaaks and Lukanova, 2002). Regular physical activity helps individuals control their weight and may reduce the breast cancer risks associated with obesity and associated insulin resistance. Some investigations have shown a protective effect of physical activity on breast cancer risk. According to a meta-analysis by Thune and Furberg (2001), 48 studies showed that high levels of physical activity were associated with a reduced chance of breast cancer. Likewise, other research has revealed that low levels of physical activity have been associated with an increased risk of breast cancer (Varo Cenarruzabeitia, et al., 2003).

The menopausal status of women may mediate the association between physical activity and breast cancer risk. A case-control study of 1,233 women with breast cancer and 1,237 controls analyzed the possible association of lifetime physical activity and risk of breast cancer in premenopausal and post-menopausal women

(Friedenreich, et al., 2001). The researchers discovered no relationship between lifetime physical activity and breast cancer risk in premenopausal women. However, among postmenopausal women, total lifetime physical activity was associated with reduced breast cancer risk. Household and occupational activity had the greatest risk reduction, while recreational activity was not related to any reduction in risks. Among those with the highest total lifetime physical activity, non-smokers, non-alcohol drinkers, and nulliparous women had stronger risk reductions.

Cigarette Smoking and Breast Cancer Risk

Research evidence indicates that cigarette smoking is associated with an elevated risk of breast cancer. More research is needed to quantify this relationship among current and former smokers. Based on cohort study of 604,412 women who were cancer-free at the start of the study, one report found that the number of cigarettes smoked per day and the total number of years smoked were positively associated with breast cancer risk among current smokers (Calle, et al., 1994). Current smokers of 40 or more cigarettes per day had a high risk of breast cancer.

Aspirin Use and Breast Cancer Risk

It is thought that aspirin and other NSAIDs may inhibit estrogen biosynthesis by reducing prostaglandin synthesis. Using a study of 1,442 women with breast cancer and 1,420 controls, Terry, et al. (2004) assessed the frequency and duration of the use of aspirin and other NSAIDs and risk of breast cancer. They discovered that frequent use of aspirin and other NSAIDs (greater or equal to 7 tablets per week) was related to a decreased risk of breast cancer. The reduction in breast cancer risk with aspirin use occurred among women with hormone receptor-positive tumors but not among those with hormone receptor-negative tumors. These findings are consistent with other investigations that show reduced breast cancer risk with regular use of aspirin and other NSAIDs.

Breast Cancer and Environmental and Occupational Exposures

Research studies have shown a possible association between environmental and occupational exposures and elevated breast cancer risk. Passive smoking may be linked to increased breast cancer risk. One investigation found that prolonged passive smoking exposure in the workplace may be related to increased breast cancer risk (Shrubsole, et al., 2004). However, this study did not find an association between exposure to a husband's smoke and increased breast cancer risk.

Ionizing radiation is a well known risk factor for breast cancer (Adjadj, et al., 2003; Bernstein, et al., 2004). Both radiation and genetic susceptibility influence the development of bilateral breast cancer (Bernstein, et al., 2004).

Exposure to cosmic radiation at high altitude has been suggested as a possible risk factor for breast cancer among airline cabin attendants. Rafnsson, et al. (2003) found that airline cabin attendants who had been employed for five or more years before 1971 had a higher risk of breast cancer compared with those who had less than five years of employment before 1971. These results were based on 35 breast cancer cases and 140 matched controls selected from a cohort of 1,532 female cabin attendants, and these results were adjusted for reproductive factors. Since 35 cases do not make a definitive study, more research is necessary to clarify any association between occupational factors and increased breast cancer risk among airline cabin attendants.

There has been some concern that residential and occupational exposure to magnetic fields increases the risk of breast cancer among women (Feychting, et al., 2005; Johansen, 2004; Ahlbom, et al., 2001). One issue concerns the frequency of magnetic fields. To what extent does occupational exposure to extremely low frequency magnetic fields increase breast cancer risk? Another problem is clarifying the impact of residential and occupational exposure to magnetic fields from high-voltage power lines. Also of interest is whether a woman's estrogen receptor status and menopausal status influence their risk of breast cancer that may result from their exposure to magnetic fields.

One study of 608 postmenopausal women with breast cancer and 667 controls discovered a small increased risk for breast cancer associated with lifetime occupational exposure to extremely low frequency magnetic fields at medium or high intensities (Labreche, et al., 2003). Women workers who were exposed before age 35 had elevated risks. In addition, women workers with progesterone receptor positive tumors had increased risks of breast cancer.

An investigation by Kliukiene, et al. (2004) examined whether residential and occupational exposure to high-voltage power lines were linked to increased breast cancer risk among women. The authors discovered that women with residential exposure to high-voltage power lines had an increased risk of breast cancer compared to unexposed women. Women workers with the highest occupational exposure had an increased risk of breast cancer compared to women who were not exposed at work.

In contrast, Feychting et al., in their review of the literature, conclude that there is probably not an association between extremely low-frequency electric and magnetic fields (EMF) and increased risk of breast cancer. Forssen, et al. (2005), using Swedish population registers and job exposure data, did not find a link between occupational magnetic fields and breast cancer.

In a study of occupational exposure to EMF in the Danish utility industry, Johansen (2004) also did not show that EMF exposure was linked to an increased risk of breast cancer. However, research has indicated that there is an increased risk for childhood leukemia linked to EMF exposure. Ahlbom, et al. (2001) noted that the association between EMF exposure and breast cancer remains unresolved.

Some organochlorine pesticides have been linked to breast cancer in post-menopausal women (Garcia, 2003). The possible association between occupational exposure to ethylene oxide and breast cancer has been assessed. In a mortality follow-up of 18,235 men and women exposed to ethylene oxide at work, Steenland, et al. (2004) reported no overall excess in breast cancer mortality in the sample. However, there was an excess of breast cancer mortality among those workers with the highest cumulative exposure to ethylene oxide.

Experimental research has shown a link between melatonin and tumor growth, and indirect data from observational studies suggest that decreased melatonin production resulting from night work may increase the risk of breast cancer among women night shift workers (Pauley, 2004; Davis, et al., 2001; Schernhammer and Schulmeister, 2004; Blask, et al., 2002). Environmental lighting suppresses the physiologic release of melatonin which typically peaks in the middle of the night (Schernhammer and Schulmeister, 2004). Suppression of normal night-time production of melatonin could increase the risk of breast cancer by increasing the release of estrogen by the ovaries (Davis, et al., 2001).

In a study of 813 cases and 793 controls, Davis, et al. (2001) discovered that the risk of breast cancer increased among subjects who often did not sleep during the period of the night when melatonin levels peak. Subjects with the brightest bedrooms had an increased risk of breast cancer. In addition, working on the graveyard shift was linked to an increased risk of breast cancer. The investigators conclude that exposure to light at night may be related to the risk of developing breast cancer.

Age and Breast Cancer

Age factors in relationship to reproductive and hormonal factors have been associated with breast cancer risk. For example, age at menarche, age at a woman's first child birth and age at menopause have been related to breast cancer risk (Walker, et al., 2004; Oestreicher, et al., 2004). Protective factors for breast cancer in developed countries have included early age at the birth of a first child (Walker, et al., 2004). Other research has found that differences in the incidence of estrogen-receptor positive and estrogen-receptor negative tumors were found with a woman's age, both before and after menopause (Colditz, et al., 2004).

Wang, et al. (2004) used the National Surgical Adjuvant Breast and Bowel Project to discover that women, aged 50 years and older, with lower-category benign breast disease, had an elevated increase in breast cancer risk.

Age also is related to breast tumor proliferation. Using a sample of 484 women, aged 40 years and older, Oestreicher, et al. (2004) showed that breast tumor cell proliferation decreased with increasing age. Their findings were similar to those of other investigations.

In addition to breast cancer incidence and tumor proliferation, age has been associated with educational differences in mortality rates among women with breast cancer. In one study of socioeconomic differences in mortality rates in Korea, Khang, et al. (2004) discovered that higher educational levels were associated with increased mortality rates among older women with breast cancer. The authors propose that this association reflects the changing social distribution of risk factors that have occurred due to Korea's rapid economic development.

Socioeconomic Factors and Breast Cancer

Some studies have discovered that women with breast cancer are more likely to come from higher socioeconomic status backgrounds (Reynolds, et al., 2002). One report, using data from the San Francisco Bay Area, showed that high socioeconomic status was related to increased breast cancer risk only among Hispanic women (Krieger, et al., 1999).

Using the findings from a cohort study of 102,860 women from Norway and Sweden, Braaten, et al. (2004) discovered that women with more than 16 years of education had a greater chance of developing breast cancer than those with 7 to 9 years of education. Among postmenopausal women, this association was slightly stronger than among premenopausal women. However, among both groups, the relationship between educational attainment and risk of breast cancer was no longer significant after adjusting for breast cancer risk factors such as reproductive and hormonal factors.

Colorectal Cancer

Colon cancer is a major public health problem in Western countries. The incidence rates of colorectal cancer differ widely between the high rates in Western countries and the low rates in developing countries. It is estimated that there is a 20-fold difference between the rates of colorectal cancer in Western countries compared to developing countries (Kaleta Stasiolek, et al., 2003). In

Western countries, colorectal adenocarcinoma is the second cause of death due to cancer (Pasetto, et al., 2005).

In the United States, colon cancer incidence is higher in African-Americans than in other racial and ethnic groups (Satia-Abouta, et al., 2003). More research is needed to clarify the underlying mechanisms for these ethnic and racial differences in colorectal cancer incidence.

Socioeconomic disparities also may be linked to the prevalence of colon cancer among African-Americans. Using the population-based 1998 National Health Interview Survey, Morewitz (2002b) reported that among adult males with incomes below $20,000, being African-American was positively related to having colon cancer. In contrast, among adult males with incomes at or above $20,000, there was no association between being African-American and having colon cancer. Persons in low-income groups may be especially at risk for developing colon cancer.

Although many mechanisms remain unclear, colorectal cancer may be associated with dietary, sedentary lifestyle, or environmental factors as well as genetic factors (Giovannucci, 2002). Increased colorectal cancer risks have been attributed to: family history and genetic susceptibility, cigarette smoking and exposure to cigarette smoke, physical inactivity, poor diet and nutrition, obesity, increased insulin production (hyperinsulinemia), chronic ulcerative colitis, and genetic susceptibility (Pan, et al., 2004; Slattery, et al., 2003; Slattery, et al., 2003).

Family History and Genetic Susceptibility

Slattery, et al. (2003) evaluated the association of family history of colorectal cancer in first-degree relatives and the risk of developing colorectal cancers using two population-based case-control studies of colorectal cancer. The findings showed that a positive family history in any first-degree relatives was slightly increased the risk of rectal cancer. Family history of colorectal cancer was related to the greatest risk among persons diagnosed at age 50 years or younger for rectal tumors, distal colon tumors, and proximal colon tumors. Among those with a family history of colorectal cancer, factors related to increased colorectal cancer risk included not having a sigmoidoscopy, a non-prudent diet (e.g., low in fruits, vegetables, whole grain, and poultry), a western diet (e.g., high in red meat, fat, refined grains, processed, and fast foods), and smoking cigarettes. Physical inactivity was not related to increased risk of colorectal cancer in this group.

Slattery, et al. (2002) identified specific genetic factors related to the development of colon cancer. For example, the inactivation of the p53 tumor suppressor gene has been linked to the initiation of colon cancer. In a case control study of 1,458 incident cases and 2,410 controls, they found that p53 mutations were identified in tumors of 47.1% of the cases and 81.9% of the individuals with p53 mutations had a missense mutation. The results indicate that persons with a p53 mutation were more likely to follow a Western-style diet compared to controls. Specifically, western-style diets with a high glycemic load, high in red meat, fast food, and trans-fatty acid had the greatest association with the p53 mutation compared to controls. Diets with a high glycemic load, high intake of red meat, fast food, and trans-fatty acid were related to missense mutations. These findings suggest that diets that are high in red meat and that increase the glycemic load are related to a p53 disease pathway.

Cigarette Smoking and Colorectal Cancer Risk

Cigarette smoking is a risk for colon cancer (Slattery, et al., 2003). Both active and passive cigarette smoking have been found to increase the risk of colon cancer.

However, less is known about the association between cigarette smoking and rectal cancer. Using a case-control study of 952 persons with rectal cancer and 1,205 controls, Slattery, et al. (2003) evaluated the possible association between active and passive smoking and risks for rectal cancer. The researchers also studied whether two genotypes, GSTM-1 and NAT2, change these relationships. The results showed that male smokers, especially those who smoked more than 20 pack-years, had an increased risk of rectal cancer. This relationship may be increased by the GSTM-1 genotype. In addition, the researchers reported that passive cigarette smoking may increase rectal cancer risk among men who do not smoke.

Low Physical Activity and Colorectal Cancer Risk

Physical inactivity, along with high energy intake and obesity, are consistently linked with an increased risk of colorectal cancer (Mao, et al., 2003; Giovannucci, 2002). Using on a population-based, case-control study, Mao, et al. (2003) reported that low recreational physical activity was related to an increased risk of rectal cancer. Other research has found that high physical activity is related to lower risks of colon cancer (Varo Cenarruzabeitia, et al., 2003).

Nutrition and Colorectal Cancer Risk

Micronutrients commonly found in fruits and vegetables, especially folate and calcium, may be protective factors in colorectal cancer (Satia-Abouta, et al., 2004; Giovannucci, 2003; Fung, et al., 2003). In their study of African-Americans and whites, Satia-Abouta, et al. (2004) discovered that high and frequent consumption of vegetables, especially dark green vegetables, was related to a 20 to 50% reduction in the risks of colon cancer, regardless of ethnic/racial group.

In a study of 76,402 women, Fung, et al. (2003) compared the effects of a prudent diet consisting of higher intakes of fruits, vegetables, legumes, fish, poultry, and whole grains with the western-style diet comprising higher consumption of red and processed meats, sweets and desserts, French fries, and refined grains. In a 12-year follow-up, the authors showed that there was a non-significant negative association between the prudent dietary pattern and colon cancer risk. In contrast, the western-style diet was related to an increased risk of colon cancer. With regard to rectal cancers, there was no link between dietary patterns and colon cancer risk. In their population-based study, Slattery, et al. (1998) also showed that the prudent diet was protective, especially among persons diagnosed before the age of 67 years and among individuals with proximal colon tumors.

Using data from the Swedish Mammography Cohort of 61,433 women, aged 40 to 75 years, Larsson, et al. (2005) discovered that there was a weak negative association between poultry consumption and colorectal cancer risk. The results showed no link between fish consumption and colorectal cancer risk at any anatomical site.

Goldbohm, et al. (1994), in their prospective cohort study of 120,852 men and women, aged 55 to 69 years, in the Netherlands, discovered that chicken and fish consumption were not related to increased colon cancer risk.

However, high daily intakes of total energy (caloric input) and low levels of dietary fiber in diets have been associated with increased colon cancer risk (Satia-Abouta, et al., 2003). High consumption of the Western-style diet, e.g., red meat, fast food, sweets, desserts, trans-fatty acid is associated with p53 mutations, a common event in the etiology of colon cancer (Slattery, et al., 2002).

A number of epidemiological investigations have found a positive link between the Western-style dietary pattern and increased risk of colon cancer (Fung, et al., 2003). Chao, et al. (2005) note that many but not all investigations have found a positive relationship between high consumption of red and processed meat and increased colorectal cancer risk. The authors evaluated possible risk of colon cancer associated with long-term meat intake. Using a cohort of 148,610 adults, aged 50 to 74 years, they discovered that higher consumption of red and processed meats was related to a higher colon cancer risk after controlling for age and caloric energy intake but after additional adjustment for body mass index, cigarette smoking, and other predictor variables. Among individuals who had the highest consumption of meat during the study periods, consumption of processed meat predicted a higher risk of distal colon cancer. In contrast, long-term consumption of poultry and fish was negatively associated with the risk of both proximal and distal colon cancer. Prolonged high consumption of red and processed may increase the risk of cancer in the distal portion of the large intestine.

A prospective cohort study of 120,852 men and women, aged 55 to 69 years, in the Netherlands evaluated the link between consumption of processed meat and other dietary habits and colorectal cancer risk (Goldbohm, et al., 1994). The investigators found that consumption of processed meat was related to an increased colon cancer risk, while total fresh meat, beef, pork, and minced meat consumption was not linked to an increased risk of colon cancer.

One population-based study, using data from Northern California, Utah, and Minnesota, also found that consumption of the western-style diet predicted a higher risk of colon cancer in both women and men (Slattery, et al., 1998). The association was strongest among individuals who were diagnosed before the age of 67 years and among men with distal colon tumors.

Likewise, analysis of data from the Swedish Mammography Cohort of 61,433 women, aged 40 to 75 years, revealed that high red meat consumption may increase the risk of distal colon tumors (Larsson, et al., 2005).

As previously noted, there is a higher colon cancer incidence in African-Americans compared to other racial and ethnic groups, and ethnic and racial differences in diet and nutrition may help to explain some of these differences. Based on a sample of 613 persons with colon cancer and 996 matched controls in North Carolina, Satia Abouta, et al. (2003) found that a higher average daily caloric intake was associated with increased colon cancer risk in both African-Americans and whites. Among African-Americans, large consumption of dietary fiber was related to a statistically significant 50–60% reduction of colon cancer risk. In contrast, among whites, a high level of dietary fiber was associated with only a 30% decrease in colon cancer risk.

Based on a pooled analysis of 8 cohort studies, Cho, et al. (2004) discovered that having more than 2 alcoholic drinks a day predicted an increased risk of colorectal cancer. This relationship was significant for cancer at three anatomical sites: proximal colon, distal colon, and rectum. There were no differences in the relative risks of colorectal cancer associated with consuming different types of alcohol.

Folate levels may be especially significant for alcohol users since alcohol use increases the risk of colorectal cancer, especially when intake of folate is low (Giovannucci, 2003). Methylation of DNA, which may help to regulate gene expression, is dependent on dietary folate and methionine. It is believed that abnormal DNA methylation may help to trigger the start or growth of colon cancer. One theory is that inadequate consumption of folate or methionine and high intake of alcohol, an antagonist of methyl-group metabolism, increases the risk of colon cancer (Giovannucci, et al., 1995).

Su and Arab (2001) used the First National Health and Nutrition Examination Survey to evaluate folate intake and colon cancer risk. Their results indicated that a high folate intake was linked to lower risks for colon cancer among men and non-alcohol drinkers. Men who had low intake of both folate and methionine and high alcohol intake had an elevated risk of colon cancer, compared to male non-drinkers who had high intake of both folate and methionine. There was no association found between folate intake and colon cancer risk among women. The authors suggest that there may be a synergistic interaction between intake of folate, methionine, and alcohol and risk of colon cancer.

Frequent coffee consumption has been linked to a reduced risk of colorectal cancer. It is possible that this inverse relationship is due to coffee-related reductions of cholesterol, bile acids and neutral sterol secretion in the colon, anti-mutagenic properties of coffee, and increased colonic motility (Tavani and La Vecchia, 2004).

Michels, et al. (2005) analyzed the consumption of coffee and tea and colorectal cancer incidence using data from two large prospective cohorts of men and women. Based on the results of the Nurses' Health Study and the Health Professionals' Follow-up Study, the authors discovered that consumption of caffeinated coffee or tea with caffeine or intake of caffeine was not related to colorectal cancer incidence in either cohort. However, consumption of decaffeinated coffee was linked to a reduced incidence of rectal cancer.

Tavani, et al. (1997) evaluated coffee and tea intake and colorectal cancer risk by combining data from two case-control studies in Italy. The authors showed that drinkers of 4 or more cups of coffee per day had a reduced colon cancer risk, compared to coffee non-drinkers. There was no relationship between coffee consumption and rectal cancer risk. In the study, drinkers consumed low amounts of decaffeinated coffee and there was also an inverse association between decaffeinated coffee intake and colorectal cancer risk. Tea intake was low (one cup a day or occasional consumption) and did not influence colorectal cancer risk. The investigators also found that the protective effects of coffee were stronger in persons having 3 or more meals per day. The authors conclude that coffee consumption has a protective effect on risk of colon cancer.

Another report analyzed coffee and tea consumption and colorectal cancer risk based on a population-based case-control study in Stockholm, Sweden. Baron, et al. (1994) found that high coffee consumption, e.g., drinking 6 cups or more per day was protective of colon cancer, compared to drinking one or fewer cups per day. No link was found between coffee intake and rectal cancer. The researchers discovered no relationship between tea consumption and colon cancer. For rectal cancer, however, tea intake of two or more cups per day was protective of rectal cancer, compared to non-tea drinkers.

Obesity

Obesity, along with low physical inactivity and poor nutrition are related to increased colorectal cancer risk (Giovannucci, 2003; Kaaks and Lukanova, 2002). Excessive adiposity, particularly if it is distributed around the waist, is associated with greater colorectal cancer risk (Giovannucci, 2003). Obesity triggers insulin resistance that elevates the risk of colorectal cancer.

In a case-control study of 21,022 persons with 19 types of cancer and 5,039 controls, Pan, et al. (2004) discovered that obese men and women (body mass index greater or equal to 30kg/m^2) had an elevated risk for cancers and an increased risk of colon cancer.

Insulin, Hyperglycemia, Insulin-Like Growth Factors

Colorectal cancer and type 2 diabetes share many of the same risk factors, such as physical inactivity, poor dietary habits, and obesity. Both hyperinsulinemia (excessive production of insulin in the body) and hyperglycemia (excessive presence of sugar in the blood) appear to increase the colorectal cancer risk (Wei, et al., 2005; Ma, et al., 2004). More research is needed to assess whether elevated insulin production and hyperglycemia are independent predictors of colorectal cancer risks. One study by Ma, et al. (2004) used plasma C-peptide, an indicator of insulin production, to evaluate whether high levels of insulin production are linked to increased colorectal cancer risk. Based on a sample of 176 patients with colorectal cancer and 294 age- and smoking status-matched controls, the investigators discovered that elevated insulin production may predict colorectal cancer risk, independent of vigorous exercise, body mass index, factors associated with insulin resistance, and the insulin-like growth factor I (IGF-I) and its binding protein 3 (IGFBP-3).

The insulin-like growth factor system, which includes IGF-I and IGF-II, IGF receptors (IGF-IR and IGF-IIR) and IGFBPs affect the epithelial growth, anti-apoptosis, and mitogenesis (Durai, et al., 2005). IGFs influence the growth and proliferation of several types of cancer. As previously noted, high levels of insulin-like growth factor 1 (IGF-1) and low levels of IGF binding protein-3 (IGFBP-3) have been related to an elevated risk of colorectal, breast, and prostate cancers (Durai, et al., 2005; DeLellis, et al., 2004; Wei, et al., 2005) For example, DeLellis, et al. (2004) used a random sample of 1,000 participants from the Multiethnic Cohort Study, and evaluated the association between IGF-I and colon cancer incidence. The findings revealed that IGF-I levels were positively related to the incidence of colon cancer by race/ethnicity for both women and men.

Chronic Ulcerative Colitis and Colorectal Cancer Risk

Chronic inflammation predisposes to cancer, and chronic ulcerative colitis and Crohn's colitis have long been associated with an increased risk for developing colorectal cancer (Ullman, 2005; Ullman, et al., 2003; Chen, et al., 2005). The continuous process of DNA mutations, clonal expansion via crypt fission and clonal succession may trigger inflammatory-related colon cancer (Chen, et al., 2005). Crypt cell turn-over and cell death may moderate this mutational process. The authors suggest that this model may apply to other inflammatory-associated cancers.

Various risk factors have been identified for colorectal cancer among patients with ulcerative colitis and Crohn's colitis (Ullman, 2005). Among ulcerative colitis patients, those with more extensive colitis, longer disease duration, concomitant primary sclerosing cholangitis, and a family history of colorectal cancer have the highest risk. Two other risk factors, young age at disease onset and greater disease disability, have been proposed as possible risk factors for colorectal cancer in this group.

Colorectal cancer surveillance has not been found to reduce colorectal cancer morbidity or mortality, although it is recommended in practice guidelines. Various factors, such as the low levels of agreement among pathologists interpreting surveillance specimens, patients lost to follow-up, and the physicians' failure to recommend colectomy once dysplasia has been identified, limit the effectiveness of surveillance activities (Ullman, 2005).

There is no universal agreement about the most effective management of ulcerative colitis patients with low-grade dysplasia in flat mucosa (Ullman, et al., 2003). Some experts recommend prompt colectomy, while others favor continued surveillance. Ullman, et al. (2003) evaluated the frequency in which flat low-grade dysplasia in ulcerative colitis progressed to cancer. Based on a sample of 46 ulcerative colitis patients with flat low-grade dysplasia, they found no clinical features that predicted progression to cancer. Despite frequent follow-up surveillance, cancers developed. The investigators conclude that during ulcerative colitis surveillance, the finding of flat low-grade dysplasia is a major predictor of progression to advanced neoplasia. They recommend early colectomy for these patients.

Colorectal Cancer and Exposure to Light at Night

Research has found a link between exposure to light at night and increased risk of colorectal cancers in night shift works (Pauley, 2004). Suppression of melatonin, because of exposure to light at night, may increase the risk of colorectal cancers in night shift workers.

Skin Cancer

An estimated 1.3 million Americans were diagnosed with skin cancer in 2002. Fifty-three thousand of these individuals were diagnosed with melanoma, which is the most prevalent fatal type of skin cancer, and more than 7,000 persons died of melanoma (Geller and Annas, 2003). The increase in the rate of cutaneous melanoma is larger than all other preventable cancers.

Malignant melanoma is mainly a disease of the skin but may rarely occur at other sites, including the mucous membranes, such as the vulva, vagina, lip, and in the eye. Melanomas develop from melanocytes, which are cells that are responsible for producing pigment. Most melanomas are dark in color but some do not contain pigment and are hard to diagnose.

Non-melanoma skin cancers (primarily basal cell carcinoma and squamous cell carcinoma) have the highest incidences of all cancers. Each year there are more than one million persons diagnosed with basal cell and squamous cell carcinoma in the United States (Vargo, 2003).

On a world-wide basis, the incidence of basal cell carcinomas differs depending on the region. Australia has the highest annual rate of 1% to 2%. The incidence of basal cell carcinoma increases by 5% per year. Mortality from non-melanoma skin cancers is low, and these diseases are highly curable if detected and treated early (Vargo, 2003). However, non-melanoma skin cancer is a major public health problem because approximately 50% of the cancers will recur in 5 years, and the local invasiveness of these types of skin cancers lead to high medical costs (Corona, 1996). In the United States, the rising incidence of non-melanoma skin cancer in the aging population will result in increased health care costs, morbidity, and mortality (Strom and Yamamura, 1997).

Genetics and Skin Cancer

Risk factors for skin cancer include a number of genetic conditions, including: family history of skin cancer, phenotypic risk factors, such as fair complexion, hair and eye colors, and nevus

counts, as well as xeroderma pigmentosum, vitiligo, senile and seborrheic keratitis, Bowen's disease, and hereditary basal cell nevus
syndrome (Almahroos and Kurban, 2004; Bataille, et al., 2004;
Masini, et al., 2003).

Different factors cause non-melanoma skin cancer and
researchers are evaluating the interaction among environmental,
lifestyle and genetic factors. It is believed that the interaction of
these three factors predict the development and progression of
non-melanoma skin cancer (Strom and Yamamura, 1997).

One report evaluated risk factors for cutaneous squamous cell
carcinoma using a hospital-based case-control study in Italy
(Masini, et al., 2003). The study findings indicated that family
history of skin cancer and light eye color were related to an
increased occurrence of cutaneous squamous cell carcinoma.

Ultraviolet exposure may contribute to the risk of skin cancer
in these genetically vulnerable individuals. Kraemer, et al. (1994)
evaluated xeroderma pigmentosum (XP), an inherited cancer-
prone, DNA-deficient disorder, with significant clinical and laboratory ultraviolet hypersensitivity. Based on a sample of 132 white
patients with XP, the authors reported that malignant skin cancers
were present in 70% of the sample at a median age of 8 years, which
is 50 years earlier than the incidence in the rest of the white population in the United States. The researchers concluded that DNA
repair helps to prevent skin cutaneous cancers in the general population, and ultraviolet exposure may be responsible for the induction of skin cancers in persons with XP.

Racial/Ethnic, Demographic, Socioeconomic, and Sociocultural Factors

Racial/ethnic, demographic, socioeconomic, and sociocultural
differences may be associated with different risks for skin cancer
(Reynolds, et al., 2002; Strom and Yamamura, 1997; Suarez-Varela,
et al., 1996). In the United States, whites have a much higher
absolute risk of developing cancer compared to African-Americans
(Pennello, et al., 2000). In whites, non-melanoma skin cancers are
the most prevalent malignancies (Zak-Prelich, et al., 2004; Corona,

1996). Ultraviolet B radiation exposure increases the risk of melanoma and non-melanoma skin cancers in Whites (Pennello, et al., 2000).

Reduced immunity, possibly related to aging, is also associated with an elevated risk of skin cancers (Strom and Yamamura, 1997). Skin cancer has become a major public health concern with the increasing average life-span in western countries. The results of epidemiological, biological, and molecular studies indicate that skin cancer is mainly a disease of older persons (Syrigos, et al., 2005). About 53% of skin cancer-associated deaths occur in individuals over 65 years.

Gender differences in non- melanoma skin cancer were noted by Suarez-Varela, et al. (1996) in a case-control study of 276 cases and 552 matched control subjects in Valencia, Spain, between 1990 and 1992. The results showed a statistically significant elevated risk in men with high non-occupational exposure, i.e., participation in open-air activities in the sun and sun bathing. In women, there were no statistically significant associations between high non-occupational exposure and increased risk of non-melanoma skin cancer. The investigators suggest that gender differences in non-melanoma skin cancer risk may be sociocultural, for women's work is usually different than men's, and their work and leisure activities differ.

Investigations have shown that persons with melanoma are more likely to have higher socioeconomic status (Reynolds, et al., 2002).

Exposure to Ultraviolet Radiation

Studies show that each of the three main types of skin cancer, basal cell carcinoma, squamous cell carcinoma, and melanoma, is caused by sun exposure (solar ultraviolet radiation) (Armstrong and Kricker, 2001; Bataille, et al., 2004). In addition to the sun, ultra violet radiation exposure can come from artificial sources which are widely used in industry as well as in hospitals, laboratories, and other settings (Ohnaka, 1993).

Ultraviolet radiation can be classified into three regions based on its wavelength: UVA (320–400 nm), UVB (320–280 nm), and UVC

(280–200 nm). Of the three regions, the UVC has the most detrimental health effects (Ohnaka, 1993). There are many harmful effects of ultraviolet radiation, including erythema, sunburn, photodamage (photoaging), photocarcinogenesis, eye damage, changes in the immune system of the skin, and chemical hypersensitivity (Guenel, et al., 2001; Ohnaka, 1993). There is major concern that stratospheric ozone depletion is allowing more ultra violet radiation to reach the earth and thus contribute to the rising incidence and mortality rates of sun exposure-related skin cancer (Marks, 1995).

The relationship between ultraviolet exposure and the development of skin cancer is complex for melanoma and basal cell carcinoma (Armstrong, et al., 1997; English, et al., 1997; Kricker, et al., 1995). The incidence rate of each type of skin cancer is based on phenotypic features, including skin tone, eye and hair color, and number of nevi present (Armstrong and Kricker, 2001; Berwick, et al., 2004). For example, the skin cancer rate is higher in fairer skinned, sun-sensitive persons than in dark skinned, less sun-sensitive persons. Armstrong and Kricker (2001) note that increasing ambient solar radiation exposure also increases skin cancer risk and the highest densities of skin cancers are on the most sun-exposed parts of the body. Elevated risks are related to total sun exposure (mainly squamous cell carcinoma), occupational sun exposure (mainly squamous cell carcinoma), and recreational or non-occupational sun exposure (primarily melanoma and basal cell carcinoma). Higher skin cancer risks are also associated with a history of sunburn and benign sun-damaged skin.

Sun Exposure in Childhood

Sun exposure in childhood may be one of the risk factors for all common skin cancers (Marks, 1995). However, more research is needed to assess the association between sun exposure levels during childhood and the development of skin cancer. Stanton, et al. (2003) assessed solar ultraviolet radiation exposure among 49 children aged 3 to 5 years in Australia. Solar ultraviolet radiation exposure was investigated under 4 conditions (e.g., teacher's instruction to use sunscreen and stay in the shade) using a repeated measures design. The results showed that the potential amount of solar ultraviolet radiation exposure for young children who were outside on a sunny day from 9–10 A.M. was 1.45 Minimum Erythemal Dose. Yet, on average they only received 0.35 Minimum Erythemal Dose, which is not sufficient to produce an erythemal response on light skin even without sunscreen use.

Solar and Seborrheic Keratoses

Solar keratoses are risk factors for non-melanoma skin cancer and are precursors of squamous cell carcinoma (Masini, et al., 2003; Marks, 1995). Using data from a hospital-based case-control study in Italy, one report found that a large number of solar keratoses and seborrheic keratoses on the body surface are factors that predict an increased occurrence of cutaneous squamous cell carcinoma (Masini, et al., 2003).

Solar keratoses seem to be more sensitive indicators of carcinogenic sunlight exposure than invasive tumors. Solar keratoses are labile and change in appearance over time. The routine use of sunscreens can prevent the development of new solar ketoses and increase the likelihood of remission in existing ones (Marks, 1997).

Occupational Exposure and Skin Cancer

Workers in certain occupations and industries may be at increased risk for skin cancer due to their occupational exposure to natural and artificial sources of ultraviolet radiation, ionizing radiation, cosmic radiation, arsenic, and carcinogens (Ohnaka, 1993). More research is needed to evaluate the radiation doses of individual workers and the confounding effects of certain phenotypic characteristics, sun exposure in other settings, sun burn history, and other risk factors for skin cancer (Freedman, et al., 2003). Below is a description of some of the skin cancer risk factors associated with several types of industries and occupations.

Outdoor Work and Exposure to Natural Sources of
Ultraviolet Radiation

The risk of solar ultraviolet radiation exposure to outdoor workers has been knowned for some time. This risk is especially prevalent among building and construction industry workers who frequently do little to protect themselves against solar ultraviolet radiation. In Australia, where ultraviolet radiation levels in the spring and summer are very high, there have been governmental efforts to implement and encourage ultraviolet radiation protection measures by outdoor workers (Gies and Wright, 2003).

In Australia, Gies and Wright (2003) quantified ultraviolet radiation exposure in the building and construction industry using ultraviolet radiation-sensitive polysulphone film badges. Their findings revealed that the individual doses of radiation were frequently in excess of exposure limits. In addition, many of the workers had high-risk skin types, did not use appropriate sun protection measures, and exhibited signs of sunburn.

Another study in a high occupational risk country, Israel, estimated risk of skin cancer using a national sample of 450 employers involved in outdoor work and 5,000 of their workers (Azizi, et al., 1990). Outdoor workers were given one of five total risk levels based on combinations of skin sensitivity to ultraviolet radiation, total weekly outdoor occupational sun-exposure, and percent of skin surface exposed during outdoor work in the summer. The findings revealed that of the 379,000 workers in outdoor occupations, 44% are at elevated risk for skin cancer due to their occupational exposure to solar ultraviolet radiation. The researchers estimated that their lifetime skin cancer risk is 1.5 to 20 times higher than workers who have low or minimal risk levels.

A case-control study of 276 cases of non-melanoma skin cancer and matched control subjects in Spain revealed an increase in the risk of cancer proportional to an increase in the hours of occupational exposure to the sun (Suarez-Varela, et al., 1996).

Occupational Exposure to Artificial Sources of Ultraviolet Radiation

Artificial sources of ultraviolet radiation are used widely in industry, especially in industries that involve welding (Perez-Gomez, et al., 2004; Gies and Wright, 2003; Tenkate, 1999). Dentists, physiotherapists, and lithographers are exposed to artificial sources of ultraviolet radiation (Perez-Gomez, et al., 2004). Workers in hospitals and laboratories use artificial sources of ultraviolet radiation for germicidal purposes, and artificial ultraviolet radiation is also used for cosmetic purposes (Ohnaka, 1993).

An occupational cohort study of risks of cutaneous melanoma among Swedish male workers found that workers exposed to ultraviolet radiation sources had elevated occupational risk ratios for different body locations (Perez-Gomez, et al., 2004).

Occupational Exposure to Ionizing Radiation

Workers, who have protracted and fractionated exposure to ionizing radiation, may be at increased risk of skin cancer, leukemia and other cancers (Freedman, et al., 2003; Wang, et al., 2002). Friedman, et al. (2003) analyzed the risk of melanoma among medical radiation workers based on a sample of 68,588 white radiological technologists. According to the results, melanoma was significantly related to phenotypic characteristics (skin tone, eye and hair color), personal history of non-melanoma skin cancer, family history of melanoma, and residential sun exposure. Risk of melanoma was elevated among individuals who had worked prior to 1950, especially among those radiological technologists who worked five or more years before 1950, when radiation exposures were likely to be highest. Melanoma risk was modestly higher among radiological technologists who did not routinely use a lead apron or shield when they first began working.

In China, Wang, et al. (2002) studied cancer incidence among 27,011 medical x-ray workers in China, during the period, 1950 to 1995. They used reconstructed dosimetry methods to show that medical x-ray workers had significantly elevated risk for cancers of the skin, along with leukemia, female breast cancer, and other cancers. They believe that the high risks of these cancers, and possibly thyroid cancer may be related to occupational exposure to x-rays.

Gallagher, et al. (1996) found that x-ray treatment for skin conditions may increase the risk of squamous cell and basal cell carcinoma of the skin. In a case control study of males in Alberta, Canada, using 406 cases (180 squamous cell carcinoma and 226 basal cell carcinoma) and 406 randomly selected male controls, the researchers found that non-diagnostic x-ray treatment for skin diseases increased the risk of both types of skin cancer.

Occupational Exposure to Cosmic Radiation

Pilots and cabin attendants may have prolong exposure to cosmic radiation along with electric and magnetic fields and chemicals, and research is underway to determine if they are at risk for developing skin cancer and other cancers (Zeeb, et al., 2003; Reynolds, et al., 2002; Rafnsson, et al., 2003; Pukkala, et al., 2002). Some studies have revealed a higher than expected rate of skin cancer and other cancers. However, the link between cosmic radiation and skin cancer has not been established. One investigation of cancer incidence among 10,211 commercial airline pilots in Denmark, Finland, Iceland, Norway, and Sweden, found an increased incidence in skin cancer among airline pilots (Pukkala, et al., 2003). The investigators obtained elevated cancer risks for melanoma, squamous cell carcinoma, and basal cell carcinoma. However, the study did not suggest that the marked increase is due to cosmic radiation, although some influence of cosmic radiation on skin cancer cannot be completely excluded.

Reynolds, et al. (2002) investigated California flight attendants and reported that compared to the general population, flight attendants had a malignant melanoma rate that was about twice than expected, and female breast cancer incidence was over 30% higher than expected.

Exposure to Carcinogens and Skin Cancer

A link between prolonged or multiple exposure to carcinogens and increased risk of developing skin cancer and other cancers has been found (Czene, et al., 2003; Richter, et al., 2003; Yu, et al., 2001).

Based on a case-control study of males in Alberta, Canada, Gallagher, et al. (1996) evaluated the risks for squamous and basal cell carcinoma associated with exposure to various chemicals. According to the study findings, males exposed at the highest tertiles to insecticides, herbicides, fungicides and seed treatments and petroleum products, grease and several other products had increased risks for squamous cell carcinoma. With regard to basal cell carcinoma, males exposed to dry cleaning agents had an elevated risk for basal cell carcinoma.

Research has shown that workers exposed to polychlorinated biphenyls (PCBs) have an excess mortality from malignant melanoma (Ward, et al., 1997). A study of 138,905 men employed at five electrical power plants discovered that mortality from malignant melanoma increased with exposure to PCBs (Loomis, et al., 1997). The investigators indicate that the link between PCBs exposure and malignant melanoma is a concern for workers in this industry.

In a study of cancer risks among hairdressers, Czene, et al. (2003) conducted a follow-up study of a cohort of 38,866 female and 6,824 male hairdressers. In their study, female hairdressers had an increased risk for in situ skin cancer, and cancers of the pancreas, lung, and cervix. In terms of in situ skin cancer, the increased risks were related to the scalp and neck of the hairdressers, the sites of contact for hair dyes.

Research also has linked chronic occupational exposure to arsenic and increased risk of skin cancer and other skin diseases (Yu, et al., 2001). In Taiwan, chronic arsenic exposure resulted in an endemic of hyperpigmentation, keratosis, and skin cancer. The arsenical skin cancers presented as multiple lesions at different disease stages. Arsenical skin cancers were often found in body areas not exposed to the sun. The fact that this type of cancer is inhibited by Ultraviolet radiation B may explain why they occur in body areas not covered by clothing.

Moran (1992) investigated the epidemiological factors of cancer in California and found a possible link between occupational exposures to dusty environments and an increased incidence of skin cancer, gastric cancer, and lymphoma. In their case-control study of males in Alberta, Canada, Gallagher, et al. (1996) discovered that exposure to fiberglass dust was related to an increased risk of basal cell carcinoma.

Individuals employed as divers in polluted waters may be at increased risk of skin cancer. Richter, et al. (2003) studied cancer risks in five successive cohorts of 682 naval divers with multiple exposures to carcinogens from Israel's most polluted waterway and showed an increased incidence of skin cancer and other cancers. Cohorts first diving after 1960 had increased risks of cancer compared to those diving before 1960. The researchers also found short induction periods for the cancers. These results suggest that direct contact with and absorption of various toxic compounds is associated with an increased risk for cancer and short induction periods.

Sunscreens

The effectiveness of those sunscreens, which block only ultraviolet B, in reducing the risk of skin cancer has been debated by scientists, and their use has been implicated as a major risk factor for skin cancer (Uhoda, et al., 2002; Garland, et al., 1993). Melanoma incidence and mortality rates have increased since the 1970s and 1980s despite the fact that sunscreens with high sun protection factors became widely used beginning in that period (Garland, et al., 1993). In the past, widely used chemical sunscreens blocked ultraviolet B radiation but were ineffective in blocking ultraviolet A radiation, which constitutes up to 90 to 95% of ultraviolet energy in the solar spectrum. Sunscreens that blocked only ultraviolet B, by preventing erythema, sunburn, and accommodation of the skin to sunlight, may have facilitated excessive exposure of the skin to other types of solar radiation that cause skin cancer. These results are suggested by laboratory studies, which show that ultraviolet B sunscreens may be ineffective in preventing these cancers, and their use may actually increase sun cancer risks (Garland, et al., 1993).

New sunscreens now block both ultraviolet B and ultraviolet A, and these sunscreens will presumably decrease the risk of skin cancer.

Sunbeds

Bataille, et al. (2004) evaluated the cancer risk of using sunbeds based on a case-control study of melanoma (413 cases and 416 control subjects) in the United Kingdom. The results indicated that the risk of melanoma increased only for fair skinned, young persons, after adjusting for sun exposure characteristics, such as a history of more than 10 severe sunburns and having sunburns before the age of 15 years. The investigators suggest that use of sunbeds may moderately affect persons with sun-sensitive skin types. However, they note that the magnitude of the melanoma risk in relationship to natural and artificial solar exposure is small compared to skin type, nevus counts, and other phenotypic risk factors.

Smoking

Ultraviolet radiation exposure in relationship to smoking and other risk factors may be linked to an elevated risk of a sclerosing form of basal cell carcinoma known as morpheaform basal cell carcinoma (Erbagci and Erkilic, 2002; Zak-Prelich, et al., 2004). Morpheaform basal cell carcinoma contains more mast cells than other forms of basal cell carcinoma. As yet, the causes and clinical significance of high levels of mast cells are not known. It has been noted that smoking and exposure to ultraviolet radiation may be associated with the creation of morpheaform basal cell carcinoma. Erbagci and Erkilic (2002), using a retrospective study of occupational ultraviolet exposure using 34 patients with morpheaform basal cell carcinoma and 50 patients with solid basal cell carcinoma, showed that morpheaform basal cell carcinoma was significantly more prevalent in smokers compared to patients with solid tumor basal cell carcinoma. In patients with morpheaform basal cell carcinoma, smokers had a higher average number of mast cells than non-smokers. In addition, the average number of mast cells among smokers with morpheaform basal cell carcinoma was significantly higher than that of smokers with solid basal cell carcinoma. Exposure to ultraviolet radiation alone did not predict either the frequency of mast cells or morpheaform basal cell carcinoma. The researchers note that smoking can play an important part in the development of morpheaform basal cell carcinoma by increasing the number of peritumoral mast cells.

Immunosuppression

Immunosuppressive therapy has been related to an elevated risk of basal cell carcinoma and non-Hogkin lymphoma (Sorensen, et al., 2004; Zak-Prelich, et al., 2004). One study found that patients treated with glucocorticoids, a common immunosuppressive therapy, have an increased risk of developing squamous cell carcinomas and non-Hodgkin lymphoma (Sorensen, et al., 2004). Organ transplant recipients also frequently develop skin cancers, especially cutaneous squamous cell carcinoma (Lindelof, et al., 2003). Excessive sun exposure and other risk factors may increase the risk of skin cancer in these patients, but these associations are unclear. Based on a case-control study with 95 kidney transplant recipients who had developed cutaneous squamous cell carcinoma, Lindelof, et al. (2003) discovered that poor tanning ability, rather than level of sun exposure, was related to the development of cutaneous squamous cell carcinoma in kidney transplant recipients. Bordea, et al. (2004) discovered that renal-transplant recipients have an increased risk of developing skin cancers, particularly squamous cell carcinoma. The investigators recommend that renal transplant patients be advised about possible skin complications, obtain regular dermatological follow-ups, and their immunosuppressive therapy should consist of minimum effective doses with good graft function.

Human Papillomavirus Infection

In their hospital-based study in Italy, Masini, et al. (2003) discovered that human papillomavirus type 8 predicted an increase occurrence of cutaneous squamous cell carcinoma, while human papillomavirus type 15 was negatively related to cutaneous squamous cell carcinoma. According to the investigators, viral infection could serve as a co-factor in the development of cutaneous squamous cell carcinoma.

Disability, Quality of Life, and Cancer

Innovations in cancer detection, treatment, and rehabilitation have led to the increased survival of cancer patients. As cancer survivors live longer, they may face increased work disability and quality of life problems.

Research has been conducted to determine the prevalence of work disability among cancer survivors. Hewitt, et al. (2003) used data from the population-based 1998–2000 National Health Interview Survey to analyze disability and health status of cancer survivors and individuals with other chronic diseases. The researchers discovered that cancer survivors without other chronic diseases had a higher probability of reporting fair or poor health, work disability under the age of 65 years, psychological disability, and impaired activities of daily living than individuals without a history of cancer or other chronic condition. Cancer survivors who had co-morbid chronic conditions were more likely to report poor health and disability compared to those who did not have co-morbid chronic diseases (Hewitt, et al., 2003).

A variety of factors influence disability and quality of life among cancer survivors (Al-Otaibi, 2004). Work disability and impaired quality of life are caused by major side effects, which can be due to different types of cancer, cancer therapies, and therapeutic doses (Spelten, et al., 2003; Schneider, et al., 2002; Delbruck, 1997).

Sometimes combined cancer therapies result in adverse outcomes for cancer survivors. One report showed that heart and lung injury caused by irradiation and chemotherapy in the treatment of Hodgkin's disease can produce shortness of breath or difficulty breathing and reduced maximal exercise heart rate (Lund, et al., 1996). In addition, patients may be at risk for the late effects of chemotherapy and radiotherapy. Side effects can lead to work disability, increased levels of fatigue, and disabling muscular weakness.

Fatigue is a major side effect of the disease itself as well as the treatment and has been identified as a major predictor of work disability and reduced quality of life (Spelten, et al., 2003; Winningham, 2001; Lucia, et al., 2003). Spelten, et al. (2003) assessed cancer-related fatigue symptoms and rates of return to work using a prospective cohort study of 235 cancer patients who went through curative treatment. In their study, 64% of the cancer survivors went back to work within 18 months. Fatigue predicted return to work independent of cancer diagnosis and treatment, but not cancer-associated symptoms. The investigators suggest that enhanced management of cancer-associated symptoms will help cancer survivors return to work.

Other related cancer-related effects include cognitive impairment, decreased sexual relations, pain, nausea, and dyspnea, and these problems can be disabling for cancer survivors. The loss of physical functioning, diminished quality of life, work-related discrimination, insurance loss, and reduced life expectancy can produce severe psychological problems in this population. In addition, depression, anxiety, hostility, and sleeping problems, are all factors which can lead to diminished health outcomes, impaired quality of life, and increased disability (Collins, et al., 2004; Spelten, et al., 2003; Davies, et al., 2003).

Axillary lymph-nodal dissection produces upper limb edema, pain at the thoracic wall, and lower limb function, leading to impaired work disability, reduced quality of life, and emotional distress (Collins, et al., 2004; Boccardo and Capisi, 2002).

Based on qualitative data from interviews with 24 women with breast cancer, Collins, et al. (2004) discovered that returning to normal functioning took longer than expected for both the women and their physicians. Many women indicated that they had difficulty performing upper-body tasks, which led to impaired functioning, reduced employability at work, and discomfort while driving, doing housework, or sleeping. The adverse physical effects resulted in psychological strain for the women were reminded of the trauma of their illness and the fact that they might never regain normal functioning.

Based on a survey of 378 breast cancer survivors, Stewart, et al. (2001) explored the impact of breast cancer on women's employment, insurance coverage, and their disclosure of the disease to family, friends, and work supervisors. They found that over 50% had disclosed their condition to their work colleagues and supervisors. Forty percent of the women reported that breast cancer had changed their priorities or progress at work, and 5% were afraid to change their jobs in case they became ill again. A significant percentage of the cancer survivors stated that they had been refused insurance or had their premiums increased due to their past diagnosis of breast cancer.

Aspects of the work environment may increase a cancer survivors' risk of disability. Drawing on a sample of 235 cancer patients in the Netherlands, one investigation showed that the type of workload was related to return to work (Spelten, et al., 2003).

Older age, co-morbidity and other factors increase the risk of disability and impair the quality of life among cancer survivors. Older persons with co-morbid chronic conditions, such as cancer, stroke, and hip fracture may be at increased risk for severe mobility disability (Guralnik, et al., 2001).

Gender disparities in disability among cancer survivors have been found (Lund, et al., 1996; Spelten, et al., 2003). Based on a national cohort study of 116 Hodgkin's disease patients, one investigation found that being female gender a significant risk factor for cardiac and pulmonary sequelae following mediastinal irradiation with or without chemotherapy.

Gruber, et al. (2003) evaluated the long-term impact of hematopoetic stem cell transplantation on a sample of 163 patients who had undergone the procedure during a preceding 16-year period. The authors discovered that unemployed patients had a greater risk of pain and psychosocial impairment, including sleep disorders, anxiety, depression, and disruption in intimate and family relations.

Lifestyle behaviors, such as sedentary lifestyles, smoking, alcohol use, being overweight, and obesity may influence disability rates in cancer survivors. Sedentary behaviors can promote muscle catabolism and worsen functional capacity in persons with cancer (Lucia, et al., 2003).

Stress, Coping Strategies, and Social Support

How do cancer survivors cope with the stresses of their condition, the potential disruption of family, social, and occupational functioning, and the possible shortened life expectancy? Are certain coping strategies more effective than others in helping cancer survivors deal with these obstacles and uncertainties?

Dr. Mark L. Goldstein offers a case study of a patient with non-Hodgkins lymphoma to describe some of the problems that cancer patients experience in their social, occupational, and family functioning.

Case Study

James is a 52-year-old married Caucasian male, who has no children. He had owned his own successful business for the past twenty years and was actively involved in his local Rotary club and school board. James always had a problem with obesity, but his weight never slowed him down. Then he began to feel generally ill, with concomitant weight loss, sweating at night, and a low-grade fever. Despite these symptoms, he did not see a doctor for several months. Ultimately, he was diagnosed with non-Hodgkins Lymphoma. He then began chemotherapy on an outpatient basis, which he tolerated poorly. James was unable to work, withdrew from friends and family and became chronically anxious. He began to develop panic attacks and was constantly in fear of dying, debilitating him. In turn, his wife became angry and began an affair.

While receiving chemotherapy in the hospital, he began psychotherapy with a clinical psychologist, who specialized in hypnotherapy (a technique that assists patients in tolerating the chemotherapy). When James' anxiety worsened, he began to see the same psychologist, who provided him with individual counseling and later provided marital counseling to James and his wife. The therapist utilized primarily cognitive-behavioral strategies, including hypnotherapy, imagery, Jacobsonian muscle relaxation, biofeedback and breathing exercises as well as thought-stopping techniques to assist James with his anxiety. His physician also placed him on an anxiolytic, specifically Alprazolam (Xanax) to help reduce his anxiety.

At present, James is in remission, has returned to work and reconciled with his wife. He continues to have periodic anxiety and panic attacks and continues in counseling. However, he only utilizes anti-anxiety medication as needed.

The above case study and other research show that psychosocial distress and anxiety are major psychosocial problems associated with cancer and can lead to maladaptive coping strategies (Grassi, et al., 2004; Hammerlid, et al., 1999). An investigation of 105 women with breast cancer revealed that higher levels of health anxiety were associated with greater maladjustment based on the Mini-Mental Adjustment to Cancer scale (Grassi, et al., 2004).

Based on a sample of 87 cancer patients undergoing radiotherapy, Fritzsche, et al. (2004) discovered that mental and behavioral disorders, most of which were adjustment disorders, were diagnosed in 51% of the patients. The need for psychotherapy was assessed by patients and by a professional. The professional determined that 32.2% of the patients were actually in need of psychotherapy, compared to 43% of the patients who accepted the offer of psychotherapy. There was a significant difference in the viewpoint of the patients and the professional towards anxiety as a justification for psychotherapy, while the professional considered it an important indicator for psychotherapy, the patient did not.

Depression and anxiety are prevalent psychosocial disorders among cancer patients and is related to pain, suicide risk, diminished quality of life, impairment, and maladaptive coping strategies (Grassi, et al., 2004a; Grassi, et al., 2004b; Grassi, et al., 2004c). Using findings from the Southern European Psycho-Oncology Study, Grassi, et al. (2004c) reported that 34% of 277 cancer patients had pathological scores on the anxiety component of the Hospital Anxiety-Depression Scale and 24.9% on the depression component.

An investigation of 148 randomly selected postoperative ambulatory breast cancer patients revealed that 23% of the patients exhibited psychiatric morbidity using the Hospital Anxiety-Depression Scale (Akechi, et al., 2001). Various factors were found to be associated with the patients' psychiatric morbidity, including pain, dyspnea, having children with health difficulties, and poor coping strategies such as feelings of helplessness and hopelessness.

A prospective multi-center investigation of head and neck cancer patients in Sweden and Norway by Hammerlid, et al. (1999) showed that about one third of the patients were classified as having a possible or probable mood disorder six times during a one-year study period. The investigators also discovered that anxiety levels were highest at the time of diagnosis, while depression was most prevalent during treatment. Females had higher anxiety levels than males at the time of diagnosis, and patients under the age of 65 years had higher levels of anxiety than head and neck cancer patients who were 65 years and older.

Dr. Mark L. Golstein's case study of James illustrates that cancer patients may engage in a variety of positive and negative coping and harm appraisal strategies. Researchers constructed the Mental Adjustment to Cancer Scale to measure the different ways in which cancer patients cope with cancer (Osborne, et al., 1999). The Mental Adjustment to Cancer Scale measures such constructs as fighting spirit, anxious preoccupation, feelings of helplessness and hopelessness, fatalism, and loss of control.

Haase and Phillips (2004) suggest that hope-fostering coping techniques and use of spirituality may be especially effective in helping adolescents and young adults adjust to cancer.

Researchers have found that cancer patients use emotion-focused and adaptive-problem-focused strategies (Burker, et al., 2004; Bishop and Warr, 2003). Some of these passive or emotion-focused strategies, such as disengagement, avoidance, ruminating and venting emotions, and failing to request emotional support, are dysfunctional, and have been associated with psychosocial distress and impairment (Burker, et al., 2004; Bishop and Warr, 2003).

Using a sample of 68 breast cancer patients with chronic pain, Bishop and Warr (2003) evaluated the possible relationship between coping styles and disability, and found that active coping strategies predicted less disability, while passive coping techniques predicted higher disability levels.

Other researchers have shown that emotional approach coping is actually adaptive in chronic pain patients. Based on a sample of 80 patients suffering from chronic myofacial pain, Smith, et al. (2002) discovered that emotional approach coping, such as the use of emotional processing and emotional expression, were related to lower pain levels and less depression. These findings contrasted with the patients' use of passive pain-coping strategies, which were related to poor adjustment and higher pain levels.

Austenfeld and Stanton (2004) indicate that measures of emotion-focused strategies are confounded with psychosocial distress and self-deprecation. They suggest that aspects of the environment, stressful experience, and individual characteristics moderate the association between emotion-focused coping and health outcomes. According to the authors, longitudinal and experimental data support the finding that emotion-focused strategies are adaptive in patients with breast cancer, chronic pain and infertility.

Cognitive processes underlying emotional reactions may alter the ways in which patients cope with their disease. Based on a survey of 148 women with possible breast disease, Lowe, et al. (2003) discovered that acceptance/resignation coping was related to self-accountability and pessimistic appraisals of both the future and emotion-focused coping potential.

In a study of peritoneal disease patients, Pucheu, et al. (2004) found that patients had higher physical quality of life if they felt that their behavior could influence their health status. Patients who believed that their health condition was less controllable were more likely to report low psychological quality of life and more maladaptive, emotion-focused coping strategies, e.g., avoidance coping strategies.

Pain catastrophizing is another response used by some cancer patients. Pain catastrophizing involves characterizing pain as awful, horrible or unbearable, and it is considered an important aspect in the experience of pain (Gracely, et al., 2004; Bishop and Warr, 2003).

The level of physical distresses may influence coping strategies in cancer patients. Chen and Ma (2004) evaluated the possible association between symptom and coping techniques in breast cancer patients who had undergone a mastectomy in the past two years. In their study, the degree of biopsychosocial distress among mastectomy patients ranged from none to mild. The mastectomy patients who had high levels of physical discomfort and pain were likely to also have a high degree of psychological distress and functional impairment. Patients who suffered symptom distresses were more likely to use problem-focused coping techniques, and these strategies were helpful in reducing symptom distresses.

A variety of other factors may influence the effect of coping strategies among cancer patients. In a study of patients with large tumors of the mouth, Kollbrunner, et al. (2001) discovered that patients with higher self-esteem were able to develop better coping techniques than those with low self-esteem. They also found that psychosocial burden in early childhood were associated maladaptive coping strategies. The authors reported that higher psychosocial burden was related to defensive coping strategies, including distrust, cognitive avoidance, and distraction.

Stress and coping strategies for cancer patients may differ from those used by their caregivers. Based on a convenience sample of 257 cancer patients and 196 of their caregivers from 2 hospitals in Seoul, South Korea, Kim (2003) compared stress and coping techniques of cancer patients and their caregivers. Cancer patients had higher stress levels than their caregivers, and were more likely to use emotion-focused coping methods than problem-focused coping techniques. In contrast, caregivers used problem-focused coping techniques more than emotion-focused coping methods and they frequently used positive coping and information seeking strategies. When caregivers used emotion-focused methods, they used the "wish" strategy more than patients did. Patients were more likely to use two coping emotion-focused techniques, "blame" and "emotion expression" more than caregivers.

Ben-Zur, et al. (2001) compared coping strategies between breast cancer patients and their spouses based on a sample of 73 breast cancer patients and their spouses. Their results showed that the patients had higher psychosocial distress than their spouses but a similar degree of psychosocial adjustment. The patients in this study relied more on problem-focused coping techniques than their spouses. Emotion-focused coping strategies included ventilation and avoidance techniques and were significantly related to the patient's distress and maladjustment. The findings of the study also revealed that the spouses' emotion-focused coping techniques were significantly related to the patients' distress and poor psychosocial adjustment.

Barrera, et al. (2004) compared psychosocial adjustment of mothers of children newly diagnosed with cancer with mothers of children with acute illnesses. Based on a sample of 69 mothers of children with cancer and 22 mothers of children with acute illnesses, the researchers found that the mothers of children with cancer had more psychosocial adjustment that were associated with their child's behavior.

Social support can have a major impact on the daily lives of cancer patients and it can take many forms. Family members and friends can offer affection, provide health-related information about cancer, promote self-care behaviors, and provide assistance in household chores (Biffi and Mamede, 2004). Cancer survivors frequently obtain social support and health-related information from other cancer survivors (Skalla, Bakitas, and Furstenberg, et al., 2004). The Internet has provided an important setting for cancer survivors to receive social support and education from other cancer survivors. Health care providers also can offer social support by providing patients with information and encouragement.

Studies have documented the impact of social support on cancer patients' quality of life. Based on a sample of 636 veterans with colorectal cancer, Sultan, et al. (2004) found that regardless of the social network size, the availability of emotional and instrumental support had an impact on health-related quality of life.

Using a convenience sample of 146 newly diagnosed gastrointestinal cancer patients, Yan and Sellick (2004) studied symptoms, psychological distress, social support, and quality of life issues. Their findings indicated that depression, symptom distress, and social support explained 44% of the total variability in health-related quality of life measure.

Difficulties can develop in providing social support to cancer survivors (Haley, 2003; Biffi and Mamede, 2004). Partners, family members, and others who provide social support are vulnerable to significant stressors as they try to care for cancer survivors (Haley, 2003; Cliff and MacDonagh, 2000).

Biffi and Mamede (2004), based on qualitative interviews with 9 breast cancer survivors, found that problems can occur in sexual relations between breast cancer survivors and their partners. Women with mastectomies and their partners may be reluctant to

engage in sexual relations. In addition, the authors discovered communication problems between breast cancer survivors and their
partners and family members. Breast cancer survivors also are con-
fronted with feelings of impotence and insecurity over their cancer
diagnosis and ability to adjust to family chores.

How effective is social support in influencing health-related
quality of life outcomes for cancer survivors? One report in Japan
analyzed the impact of social support on mental health status
among 176 patients with early stage uterine cervical cancer (Ohara-
Hirano, et al., 2004). The study employed the Center for Epidemiologic Studies Depression Scale to measure mental health
problems. Their results showed that the absence of a husband or a
partner was related to increased pain and worse mental health outcomes in uterine cervical cancer patients. The authors conclude that
the presence of a husband or partner played an important social
support function for these patients by reducing their level of
depression.

Health care providers may also affect the impact of social
support on cancer survivors' adaptation to their condition.
Drawing on a sample of 325 women with recently diagnosed breast
cancer, Han, et al. (2004) reported that breast cancer patients who
had perceived problems in their interactions with physicians and
nurses had higher levels of cancer-associated traumatic stress, less
emotional self-efficacy in dealing with cancer, and less satisfaction
with social and family support. Women who were less satisfied
with emotional support from family and friends were less likely to
be satisfied with their physicians.

Cancer Treatment and Rehabilitation Outcomes

Various factors influence the outcomes of cancer treatment.
Cellular targets and activating enzymes limit the anti-tumor activity of most anti-cancer agents. Constitutive genetic polymorphisms
may curtail drug bioavailability and affect either the effective of
anti-tumor activity or toxicity (Peters, et al., 2004).

Below is a review of cancer treatment outcomes for lung,
breast, colorectal, and skin.

Lung Cancer

Lung cancer is still the leading cause of cancer-associated deaths in the world (Rigas and Dragnev, 2005). In the United States, non-small cell lung cancer is the leading cause of deaths related to cancer (Budde and Hanna, 2005). Enhanced treatments are needed to reduce these high mortality rates.

For patients with operable non-small cell lung cancer, surgery alone has been the standard therapy. Unfortunately, despite complete resection, 5-year survival rates have not been good. Approximately 50% of patients eventually relapse and die from the disease. In the last 10 years, thousands of patients have participated in randomized trials, resulting in findings that show that post-operative platin-based adjuvant therapy has a definite survival benefit (Pisters and Le Chevalier, 2005).

In patients with non-small cell lung cancer, Platinum-based combination treatments containing Gemcitabine, Vinorelbine, or Taxanes resulted in response rates of 30–40%, median survival time of 8 to 10 months and 1-year survival rates of about 35% in advanced non-small cell lung cancer patients. Some clinical trial data show that Gemcitabine-Platinum-based therapies produce beneficial overall and progression-free survival compared to other Platinum combinations. Gemcitabine-Platinum 2-agent combinations may produce the best benefit-risk ratio in treating patients with advanced non-small cell lung cancer (Langer, et al., 2005).

Winton, et al. (2005) evaluated whether adjuvant Vinorelbine plus Cisplatin increases overall survival among patients with completely resected early-stage non-small cell lung cancer. They randomized a total of 482 patients to receive Vinorelbine plus Cisplatin or observation only. The results showed that patients who were treated with Vinorelbine plus Cisplatin had sigificantly higher overall survival than patients in the observation group (69% vs. 54% five-year survival). The adjuvant chemotherapy also had an acceptable level of toxicity.

An increasing number of non-small cell lung cancer patients are feeling better after front-line chemotherapy, are in good status and are willing to undergo additional treatment (Ardizzoni and Tiseo, 2004). Unfortunately, second-line treatment options have been limited in the management of non-small cell lung cancer. A multi-targeted antifolate Pemetrexate has therapeutic activity as a single agent and as part of combined chemotherapy against non-small cell lung cancer (Budde and Hanna, 2005). A recent phase III clinical trial found similar survival outcomes for patients treated with Pemetrexed or Docetaxel in second-line treatments. However, Pemetrexed with vitamin B (12) and folate supplementation has less toxicity than Docetaxel (Budde and Hanna, 2005; Ardizzoni and Tiseo, 2004). Pemetrexed has been produced fewer episodes of neutropenia, neutropenic fever, and infections, and with Pemetrexed, there has been less use of granulocyte colony-stimulating factor support (Ardizzoni and Tiseo, 2004). Pemetrexed has the potential to be used in the treatment of metastatic disease, as adjuvant therapy, and for locally advanced breast cancer (Budde and Hanna, 2005).

Researchers have analyzed the effects of Getfitinib and Erlotnib, which are small molecules that selectively inhibit epidermal growth factor receptor (EGFR)-tyrosine kinase activity (Pao and Miller, 2005). Gefitinib and Erlotinib are being assessed in second- and third-line settings for patients with non-small cell lung cancer. Both drugs have shown favorable response rates and toxicity. For example, in a recent phase III trial, Erlotinib demonstrated a survival advantage of two months compared to the placebo group (Ardizzoni and Tiseo, 2004).

Retinoids help to regulate cell division, growth, differentiation, and proliferation, and show promise for targeted lung cancer treatments. Investigators are studying the effectiveness of several synthetic retinoids that bind to retinoic acid receptors. Rexinoids are synthetic agents that bind specifically to retinoid X receptors. Adverse effects of rexinoids include cheilitis, skin reactions, severe headaches, and hypertriglyceridemia. One multi-targeted synthetic rexinoid under investigation for use in the treatment of non-small cell lung cancer is Bexarotene. Bexarotene, combined with chemotherapeutic agents, have produced favorable median survival for advanced non-small cell lung cancer patients compared to combination chemotherapy by itself. In progress are two phase III trials to further investigate the effects of Bexarotene in treating non-small cell lung cancer (Rigas and Dragnev, 2005).

Overexpression of cyclooxygenase-2 (COX-2) is often present in lung cancer and may influence carcinogenesis, invasion, and metastasis. Overexpression of COX-2 has been found to be related to decreased survival in patients who have a resected early-stage lung adenocarcinoma (Gore, 2004). Cox-2 inhibition has been shown to reduce tumor cell proliferation in vivo and improve tumor radiosensitivity. In addition, COX-2 inhibition may protect normal pulmonary tissue from radiation-related fibrosis. Studies are in progress to evaluate the risks and benefits of COX-2 inhibition in lung cancer therapy.

Breast Cancer

In 2004, more than 215,000 women in the United States were diagnosed with breast cancer and over 40,000 died. Fortunately, breast cancer mortality has gone down despite an increase in the incidence of breast cancer. This decline in breast cancer mortality may be due to enhanced screening for better detection of tumors and innovations in early disease treatment (Eneman, et al., 2004).

The goals of neoadjuvant treatment for locally advanced breast cancer include reducing the size tumors to permit breast conservation and possibly enhance survival rates (Freedman, et al., 2005). Neoadjuvant treatment initially was dominated by chemotherapy. Chemotherapy produced increased rates of breast conserving surgery, but has not brought about increased survival rates compared to standard adjuvant chemotherapy.

Endocrine therapy came to the fore in breast cancer treatment because of its ability to rapidly and routinely assess the predictive factors of responses including estrogen (ER), progesterone (PR), and human epidermal growth factor receptor 2 (HER2) nu receptor status (Freedman, et al., 2005). Endocrine therapy has proved effective for women with estrogen receptor-positive and/or progesterone receptor (PR) positive breast tumors (Eneman, et al., 2004). For breast cancer, the selective estrogen-receptor modulator (SERM) Tamoxifen for many years has been the "gold standard" among anti-estrogen therapies (Robertson, et al., 2005). Tamoxifen has been proven to be safe and efficacious in the adjuvant treatment of both pre- and postmenopausal women with hormone-receptor-positive early disease. However, endocrine therapy is not effective for breast tumors which lack ERs and PRs. Ovarian suppression is an important option for premenopausal women (Eneman, et al., 2004).

SERMs, such as Toremifene, Droloxifene, Idoxifene, Raloxifene, and Arzoxifene, have minimal activity in fighting Tamoxifen-resistant disease and have not been found to be better than Tamoxifen as first-line therapies for advanced disease. For advanced disease, the selective aromatase inhibitors (AIs), Anastrozole, Letrozole, and Exemestane have had advantages over Tamoxifen as first-line therapies for patients with early, operable breast cancer (Robertson, et al., 2005). Recently, the AIs have been shown to be efficacious in postmenopausal women.

AIs are increasingly being employed in the adjuvant setting and have been shown to be effective in the metastatic and adjuvant settings. In addition, AIs have been shown to be effective in the neoadjuvant setting. Neoadjuvant endocrine therapy with AIs has grown from being an experimental palliative therapy for women with locally advanced breast cancer who were unsuitable for surgery or chemotherapy to become an effective and possibly preferred alternative for postmenopausal women with hormone receptor positive large tumors or locally advanced breast cancer. Neoadjuvant trials have also facilitated research on predictive biomarkers of breast cancer in order to clarify the nature of treatment resistance and sensitivity and help to identify new systemic therapies (Freedman, et al., 2005).

Research is underway to investigate the best sequencing of therapy with Tamoxifen or an AI (Eneman, et al., 2004). Women with breast cancer have the benefit of various treatment options, including the steroidal AI, Exemestane, and the ER antagonist, Fulvestrant (Harwood, 2004). The steroidal estrogen receptor (ER) antagonist, Fulvestrant (Faslodex), downregulates the cellular levels of the estrogen receptor (ER) and progesterone receptor (PR) and has no agonist activity (Robertson, et al., 2005). Fulvestrant may have a potential role as one of the endocrine therapies for advanced disease.

Gemcitabine (Gemzar) has been effective in fighting breast cancer because of its positive outcomes (e.g., favorable time to disease progression and survival outcomes) and low toxicity. Combining Gemcitabine with other cyotoxic agents has the potential for non-overlapping toxicities, a novel mechanism of action, and a potential lack of cross-resistance. Response rates, time to disease progression, and survival rates have been enhanced by adding Gemcitabine to Paclitaxel as a first-line therapy. Gemcitabine is being studied for the treatment of early breast cancer (Yardley, 2004).

Researchers have analyzed the efficacy, safety, and pharmaco-kinetics of Trastuzumab (Herceptin) monotherapy as a first-line therapy for women with HER2-positive metastatic breast cancer. A phase II study, based on a sample of 105 patients with HER2-positive metastatic beast cancer, showed that administering higher doses of Trastuzumab once every three weeks did not adversely affect efficacy or safety of the therapy (Baselga, et al., 2005).

There is a risk of Trastuzumab-induced cardiotoxicity when combined with Anthracyclines or other potentially cardiotoxic agents after Anthracyclines treatment. The combination of Gemcitabine and Cisplatin or Carboplatin (Paraplatin) might reduce these cardiotoxic risks. Clinical evidence suggests that Trastuzumab plus Gemcitabine and Trastuzumab plus Gemcitabine plus Cisplatin or Carboplatin should be analyzed in clinical trials (Konecny and Pegram, 2004).

Phase I clinical trials have suggested that the combination of Gemcitabine and Paclitaxel is safe in metastatic breast cancer patients. One hundred and fourteen of 221 patients (52%) responded to the combination of Gemcitabine and Paclitaxel. Among patients who had undergone previous chemotherapy, the response rates were lower (45% second-line treatment and 70% first line treatment). For the Gemcitabine-Paclitaxel therapy, toxicity has been low. Compared to Paclitaxel alone, the phase III registration trial found that the Gemcitabine-Paclitaxel treatment is superior in terms of time to disease progression, response rate, and survival (Colomer, 2004).

For the adjuvant treatment of patients with node-negative breast cancer, clinical trials have evaluated the efficacy of Uracil and Tegafur (UFT). Based on a review of pooled analysis of six randomized trials, Noguchi, et al (2005) concluded that the survival of women with node-negative breast cancer improved with adjuvant UFT. Because UFT had milder adverse effects, it can be an effective alternative to Doxorubicin and Cyclophosphamide, or Cyclophosphamide, Methotrexate, and Fluorouracil in the adjuvant therapy for women with node-negative breast tumors.

Other therapeutic alternatives for advanced breast cancer include high-dose estrogens and progestins. High-dose estrogens and Tamoxifen have similar response rates, but the toxicity of estrogens limits their use. Therefore, there is a need for new endocrine therapies, especially for disease that is resistant to Tamoxifen or AIs (Robertson, et al., 2005).

Breast cancer treatment also may be enhanced through the use of clinical pathways. For example, clinicians at the National University Hospital, Singapore, have developed a mastectomy clinical pathway to improve the quality and cost-effectiveness of breast cancer treatment (Santoso, et al., 2002). In their prospective study, Santoso, et al. (2002) compared two groups of mastectomy patients, 83 clinical pathway patients and 69 non-pathway patients. They discovered that patients in the clinical pathway group had a significant reduction in their average length of hospital stay and average cost per patient compared to patients in the non-pathway group. There were no differences in the rates of complications and hospital readmissions between the clinical pathway and non-clinical pathway patients. The researchers conclude that the use of a mastectomy clinical pathway enhanced the consistency in therapy, the quality of patient care, and lowered the costs of health care and hospital length of stay. In addition, the investigators conclude that the analysis of the mastectomy pathway helps clinicians identify problems in order to enhance patient outcomes.

Investigators are evaluating the impact of a new diagnostic procedure, sentinel lymph node biopsy, on patients with breast cancer. Sentinel lymph node biopsy is used to determine whether breast cancer has mestastized to axillary lymph nodes. Breast cancer cells begin to escape from the primary tumor site in the breast and they travel to the lymph nodes under the arm. The first lymph nodes that they reach are known as the sentinel lymph nodes. A sentinel lymph node biopsy necessitates the removal of only one to three lymph nodes for review by a pathologist. If the sentinel lymph nodes do not consist of cancer cells, it may not be necessary to remove additional lymph nodes in the axillary region. As a result, patients who have the sentinel lymph node biopsy may have less pain and fewer complications, such as lymphedema, than patients who have the standard axillary dissection.

Purushotham, et al. (2005) evaluated 298 patients with early breast cancer (tumors 3 centimeters or less on ultrasound examination) and clinically node negative. These patients were randomly assigned to either a sentinel lymph node biopsy followed by an axillary lymph node node dissection if they were subsequently found to be lymph node positive or a control group who received an axillary lymph node dissection. The investigators discovered that patients who received the sentinel lymph node biopsy had a significant reduction in post-operative arm swelling, rate of seroma formation, numbness, and loss of sensitivity to light touch and pinprick compared to patients in the control group.

However, some patients who receive a sentinel lymph node biopsy report having pain, nerve damage, or lymphedema after the procedure. These problems occur more often when other lymph nodes are removd along with the sentinel lymph nodes. A majority of patients who receive the sentinel node biopsy stay one day or less in the hospital, and sometimes the procedure can be performed on an outpatient basis (http://www.cancer.org; http://www.imaginis.com)

Many surgeons believe that breast cancer may be staged accurately without having to take out any lymph nodes besides the sentinel lymph nodes. However, investigators have discovered that a low percentage of sentinel node biopsies produce false negative results. These false negative findings can occur because of several factors, including: the timing of the dye injections, the type of dye/tracers employed, the presence of more than one sentinel node, and the way in which the initial node was sectioned or stained (http://www.cancer.org; http://www.imaginis.com).

Colorectal Cancer

The primary treatment for lymph-node-positive colon cancer (stage III) is surgical resection, which cures 50 to 60% of patients with this condition. Chemotherapy after surgical resection (adjuvant chemotherapy) has produced a 4-year survival rate of almost 80% (Allegra and Sargent, 2005).

Over the years, the treatment of patients with metastatic colorectal cancer has changed significantly. For the last 40 years, 5-Fluorouracil (5-FU)-based treatment regimens have been employed in the treatment of colorectal cancer. Clinicians have a number of therapeutic options for treating patients relapsing after surgical excision of their primary tumor. These options include 5-FU used with FA, Irinotecan and Oxalipatin and the oral Fluoropyrimidines: Capecitabine and Uracil/Tegafur (UFT). In the first-line treatment of metastatic colorectal cancer, clinical trials have found that combination treatment with 5-FU/FA and Irinotecan or Oxaliplatin is more effective than than 5FU/FA alone (Christopoulou, 2004).

Irinotecan or Oxaliplatin, when used as a neoadjuvant treatment with 5-FU—folinic acid (FUFA), can give a percentage of colorectal cancer patients hope for long-term survival because the treatments make originally unresectable liver or lung metastases of colorectal cancer respectable. For patients with Stage IV colorectal cancer, Irinotecan combined with 5-FU is necessary for palliative sequential chemotherapy. The longest progression-free and overall survival for metastatic colorectal patients in the palliative setting can be achieved with sequential FOLFIRI before or after FOLFOX combination. Sequential use of both 5-FU, Irinotecan and Oxaliplatin is necessary to attain maximum survival time. The French GERCOR Group reported a 26-month median overall survival in stage IV colorectal cancer patients who received sequential use of continuous infusional FUFA, Oxaliplatin and Irinotecan combinations. In large phase III trials employing 5-FU, Irinotecan, and Oxaliplatin, a higher percentage of patients who were treated with all three drugs had longer overall survival (Lang and Hitre, 2004).

The oral Fluoropyrimidine Capecitabine is an alternative to bolus Fluorouracil plus Leucovorin as first-line therapy for metastatic colorectal cancer. Twelves, et al. (2005) analyzed Capecitabine as adjuvant treatment for stage III colon cancer. They randomly assigned 1,987 patients with resected stage III colon cancer to receive oral Capecitabine or bolus Fluorouracil plus Leucovorin for 24 weeks. The results indicated that patients receiving Capecitabine had a better relapse-free survival rate and fewer adverse events than patients treated with bolus Fluorouracil plus Leucovorin.

For rectal cancer, investigators in phase I/II clinical trials are evaluating the effectiveness of integrating Irinotecan into pre-operative combined-modality therapy regimens. These clinical trials reveal that continuous infusion Fluorouracil (5-FU), Irintecan, and pelvic radiation is the recommended therapy for patients who get Irinotecan-based combined-modality therapy. Capecitabine is being substituted for continuous infusion of 5-FU in new trials that analyze preoperative combined-modality regimens (Minsky, 2004).

Epidermal growth factor inhibitors, vascular endothelial growth factor (VEGF) inhibitors, and cyclooxygenase 2 inhibitors are new agents under investigation (Christopoulou, 2004). Beva-cizumab, the VEGF inhibitor, has been shown to increase the effec-tiveness of first-line Irinotecan treatment. Evidence also indicates that in the second-line treatment of stage IV colorectal cancer, the addition of Cetuximab brings back Irinotecan sensitivity (Lang and Hitre, 2004).

With regard to the treatment of elderly patients, Lang and Hitre (2004) note that the toxicity and efficacy of Irinotecan is not significantly different from the toxicity and efficacy reported in a younger population.

Skin Cancer

Treatment results for metastatic melanoma continue to be unfavorable (Buzaid, 2004). Response rates from 8% to 15% are produced by single-agent chemotherapy and combination chemotherapy obtains a response rate from 10% to 30% (Buzaid, 2004; O'Day, et al., 2002). However, these responses are not gener-ally sustained. Immunotherapy, especially high-dose Interleukin (IL)-2 (Proleukin) also has produced a low response rate (about 15%), but it is frequently more durable. The combination of Cis-platin-based chemotherapy with IL-2 and Interferon-Alpha (known as biochemotherapy) has demonstrated responses rates from 40% to 60% in phase II research, and 8% to 10% of patients have had sustained complete remissions (Buzaid, 2004; Flaherty, 2000).

A phase II study of neoadjuvant biochemotherapy for stage III melanoma discovered that neoadjuvant biochemotherapy seemed to be promising (Gibbs, et al., 2002). However, phase III trials have obtained predominantly negative findings. Buzaid (2004) believes that these inconsistencies in results are due to the use of different treatment regimens, selection of patients, and physician selection.

Effective treatments for basal cell carcinoma have been developed. An immune response modifier, Imiquimod, has been demonstrated to be efficacious in the treatment of basal cell carcinoma (Peris, et al., 2005).

Chemoprevention offers hope in preventing photoaging and cancer development (Uliasz and Spencer, 2004). Chemoprevention involves employing natural or synthetic agents that slow down, block or reverse carcinogenesis (Uliasz and Spencer, 2004; Gupta and Mukhtar, 2002). Since both photoaging and carcinogenesis are multi-stage in nature, tumor development can be stopped at several intervention points. Vitamins, diet, aspirin and non-steroidal anti-inflammatory drugs, and topical agents are novel chemoprevention agents under analysis (Uliasz and Spencer, 2004). Various agents under investigation are present in food and are supplemented or topically applied to prevent different stage of skin cancer. The effects of retinoid on preventing human skin cancer are being analyzed. A polyphenolic fraction isolated from green tea and silymarin, a flavonoid present in artichoke are also being evaluated for their chemopreventive potential using different stages of mouse skin cancer (Gupta and Mukhtar, 2002).

Psychosocial Interventions with Cancer Patients

A randomized clinical trial by Andersen, et al. (2004) tested the hypothesis that a psychological intervention would lower psychosocial distress, enhance health behaviors, improved dose-intensity of chemotherapy, and immune responses. Based on a sample of 227 women who were surgically treated for regional breast cancer, the researchers evaluated the effects of a 4-month, weekly small group session consisting of strategies to lower stress, improve mood, change health behaviors, and maintain adherence to the cancer regimen. The results of the clinical trial indicated that cancer patients who participated in the psychological intervention had significantly lower anxiety levels, improved levels of perceived social support, improved nutritional patterns, and reductions in smoking. Cancer patients in the psychological intervention had improved dose-intensity measures and immune responses.

On the basis of a sample of 174 patients, aged 18 to 74 years, with a malignant disease, Greer, et al. (1992) reported that patients who received the therapy had significant improvements in different psychological measures than control patients at the 8-week follow-up period. Patients in the therapy group scored significantly higher in fighting spirit and lower in helplessness, anxious preoccupation, fatalism, anxiety, and psychological symptoms than control patients. After the 4-month follow-up, patients in the therapy group had lower anxiety, psychological symptoms, and psychological distress than the control patients. In the therapy group, the percentage of severely anxious patients went down from 46% at baseline to 20% at eight weeks and 20% at four months. In the control group, the proportion dropped from 48% at baseline to 41% at eight weeks and to 43% at four months. In the therapy group, the percentage of patients suffering depression went down from 40% at baseline to 13% at eight weeks, and 18% at four months and 30%, 29%, and 23%, respectively, in the control group.

Other research has examined the effects of tricyclic antidepressants, serotonin reuptake inhibitors, and norepinephrine reuptake inhibitors in cancer patients. Reboxetine has been found to be effective safe and effective in the treatment of patients suffering depression, including those with Parkinson's disease and HIV. However, more research is needed to determine its usefulness in the treatment of major depressive disorder among breast cancer patients. An open, prospective 8-week clinical trial evaluated the effects of Reboxetine, a norepinephrine reuptake inhibitor, in 20 breast cancer patients (Grassi, et al., 2004). At the 8-week follow-up, breast cancer patients in the treatment group showed improvement in the severity of depression (based on the 17-item Hamilton Scale for Depression), psychiatric symptoms (using the Brief Symptom Inventory), and 2 coping styles: feelings of hopelessness and anxious preoccupation (using the Mini-Mental Adjustment to Cancer Scale). Breast cancer patients in the treatment group also showed improvement in emotional, cognitive, dyspnea, sleep, and global dimensions of the European Organization for Research and Treatment of Cancer Quality-of-Life Questionnaire. One breast cancer patient had to discontinue the medication because of hypo-manic switch and another patient had to discontinue it because of two side effects: tachycardia and tension. Seven patients developed transient side effects: mild anxiety, insomnia, and sweating. The investigators concluded that Reboxetine was well tolerated in this small group and has the potential to improve depressive symptoms, quality of life and dysfunctional coping styles.

Cancer Patient Education and Self-Management

Cancer patient education and self-management programs have several goals. One goal is to determine the best ways to inform patients about the need for cancer screening (Volk, et al., 2003; Ruthman and Ferrans, 2004). Patient education is essential to teach patients about their risks for certain cancers and inform them of effective cancer screening procedures.

When the efficacy of cancer screening is uncertain, patient education interventions seek to promote informed decision making about cancer screening. For example, the efficacy of screening for prostate cancer among primary care patients has been viewed as problematic (Volk, et al., 2003). Volk, et al. (2003) studied the impact of an educational videotape on developing informed patient decisions about prostate cancer screening practices. Using a random-ized controlled trial of 160 men, ages 45 to 70 years, without a history of prostate cancer, the authors discovered that patients who viewed the educational videotape had greater knowledge about prostate screening than those in the control group, although these differences were reduced within 1 year. Patient satisfaction with the screening decision did not differ between patients in the videotape group and patients in the control group. The researchers suggest that these aids can foster informed decision making.

Ruthman and Ferrans (2004) found similar support for the use of an educational videotape to facilitate informed decisions about prostate cancer screening. Using a quasi-experimental design with 52 men who viewed an educational videotape and 52 men who received usual care only, they found that patients who viewed the instructional videotape were more likely to prefer prostate-specific antigen (PSA) screening than those in the usual care group. Moreover, patient knowledge about prostate screening increased for patients in the experimental group compared to those in the control group.

A second goal of cancer patient education programs is to develop programs to decrease patient's anxieties over diagnostic testing. Patients can experience significant anxiety over initial abnormal diagnostic test results, and patient education interventions seek to minimize these anxieties. In a controlled trial of 2,390 women who received an abnormal mammogram (e.g., one with a recommendation for follow-up), the investigators found that patients who had an immediate reading of abnormal mammograms by a radiologist experienced less anxiety compared to patients in an educational intervention (e.g., taught skills to cope with anxiety) and in a control group (Barton, et al., 2004).

A third goal is to find the most effective ways to assist cancer patients in participating in their treatment decisions. Targeted treatment education has the potential to help cancer patients better participate in their treatment decisions, enhance patient compliance, and deal with treatment side effects. One investigation by Dunn, et al. (2004) used a quasi-experimental design to evaluate the impact of targeted treatment education materials (an educational videotape) about radiation therapy on patients' coping with breast and head and neck cancer. No differences were found between the experimental and control groups in terms of primary outcomes (psychological distress, knowledge about radiation therapy, and self-efficacy about coping with radiation therapy and symptoms). However, 90% of the patients in the intervention group reported that some or all of the information on the instructional videotape was new to them. Moreover, patients in the experimental group were satisfied with the instructional videotape and would recommend it to others preparing for radiation therapy.

A fourth goal is to develop the most effective ways to help patients increase their knowledge of cancer diagnosis and treatment and empower themselves by accessing the Internet and other sources of information (Eng, et al., 2003; Ziebland, et al., 2004; Pitts, 2004). Patients may seek cancer-related information from a variety of sources. Some patients may wish to know as much as possible about all of the treatment effects, while other patients may not want to know about all of the side effects associated with a treatment.

Researchers are exploring ways to evaluate the informational needs of cancer patients and design educational interventions based on these assessments. Skalla, et al. (2004) met with a focus group of 51 patients and 14 spouses of patients who had completed chemotherapy or radiation therapy for cancer to assess their preferences for information about the side effects of treatment. They found that patients and their spouses are interested in getting information about how to get treatment, possible side effects, and the impact of treatment on their daily activities. While patients rely on a variety of informational sources, they often found other patients to be the best sources of information. A majority of the patients preferred to get as much information as possible, but some preferred not to know about possible treatment effects. They identified the following obstacles to obtaining information: difficulties in accessing clinicians, in communicating with practitioners, having information overload, and difficulties in retaining information.

Cancer patient education research is underway to evaluate patient use of the internet to obtain information on cancer diagnosis and treatment. On the basis of semi-structured interviews with 175 men and women aged 19–83 years with one of five cancers (prostate, testicular, breast, cervical, or bowel), Ziebland, et al. (2004) discovered that Internet use, either direct or through friends or family members, was highly prevalent. Patients reported extensive use of the Internet at every stage of cancer care. They accessed the Internet for a variety of purposes, including obtaining a second opinion, receiving support and advice from other patients, interpreting symptoms, and seeking information about diagnoses and treatments. Cancer patients also accessed the Internet to secretly verify their physicians' advice and to become expert on their type of cancer so that they can deal intelligently with their serious health condition.

Pitts (2004) suggests that women with breast cancer are visiting the personal Web pages of breast cancer survivors to negotiate identity and acquire practical knowledge about their disease.

An important area of patient education research is determining the extent to which cancer patients seek information about complementary and alternative medicine and use these therapies. Clinicians can use these findings to provide cancer patients with reliable information on complementary and alternative medicine.

Eng, et al. (2003), using a mail survey, evaluated the prevalence and use of complementary and alternative medicine by 1,108 men newly diagnosed with prostate cancer. Based on a 42% response rate, the investigators discovered that 39% of the patients used complementary and alternative medicine therapies in an attempt to improve their immune systems and to prevent recurrence. The most common therapies used included herbal supplements (saw palmetto), vitamins (vitamin E), and minerals (selenium). Fifty-eight percent of the users of complementary and alternative medicine therapies informed their physicians about their use of these therapies. Users of complementary and alternative medicine therapies were less likely to rely on their family physician (15%) or oncologist (7%) for information about these therapies. They were more likely to consult their friends or family (39%) or the Internet (19%) for this information. More research is needed to evaluate the prevalence, use, and effectiveness of complementary and alternative medicine therapies by cancer patients.

A fifth goal is to develop patient education programs that help prevent cancer by promoting healthy lifestyle changes (Robinson and Rigel, 2004). Patient education interventions need to use curricula designed to achieve essential lifestyle changes, such as correcting individuals' erroneous perceptions of their cancer and emphasizing those factors that increase their cancer risks. People continue to believe that having a suntan is beneficial instead of being a precursor to skin cancer. Information about the correct use of the newer sunscreens is essential to reducing the risk of skin cancer. In addition, the increased risks of cancer, such as obesity, inadequate nutrition, and sedentary lifestyles need to be emphasized.

Robinson and Rigel (2004) evaluated sun protection attitudes and behaviors of 200 solid-organ transplant recipients and 1,091 randomly selected individuals in the United States. According to the survey findings, a larger percentage of solid-organ transplant recipients felt that people with suntans looked healthier compared to the general population, and 88% of the solid-organ transplant recipients were unaware that they were at increased risk of acquiring skin cancer. Thirty-five percent of the transplant recipients reported using sunscreens, as their primary protection. Thirty-five percent of transplant recipients reported sun burning, a rate similar to that reported by the general population. In addition, solid-organ transplant recipients wear less protective apparel and stay in the shade less than the general population. Clinicians need to be aware of the attitudes and behaviors of high-risk individuals towards sun protection and customize their patient education interventions accordingly.

A sixth goal is to develop patient education programs that help patients cope with the psychosocial impact of cancer, such as impaired quality of life, emotional distress, loss of social support, and decreased occupational and educational opportunities (Scura, et al., 2004). Studies are underway to develop and evaluate cost-effective programs that provide both social support and education for cancer patients.

References

Aaron, L.A., Bradley, L.A., Alarcon, G.S., et al. (1997). Perceived physical and emotional trauma as precipitating events in fibromyalgia. Associations with health care seeking and disability status but not pain severity. Arthritis Rheum, 40 (3), 453–60.

Acton, R.T., Go, R.C., Roseman, J.M. (2004). Genetics and cardiovascular disease. Ethn Dis, 14 (4), S2–8–16.

Adjadj, E., Rubino, C., Shamsaldim, A., et al. (2003). The risk of multiple primary breast and thyroid carcinomas. Cancer, 98 (6), 1309–17.

Ahlbom, C., Cardis, E., Green, A., et al. (2001). ICNIRP (International Commission for Non-Ionizing Radiation Protection) Standing Committee on Epidemiology. Environ Health Perspect, 109 Suppl 6, 911–13.

Akechi, T., Okuyama, T., Imoto, S., et al. (2001). Biomedical and psychosocial determinants of psychiatric morbidity among postoperative ambulatory breast cancer patients. Breas Cancer Res Treat, 65 (3), 195–202.

Akimoto, M., Fukunishi, I., Kanno, K., et al. (2004). Psychosocial predictors of relapse among diabetes patients: a 2-year follow-up after inpatient diabetes education. Psychosomatics, 45 (4), 343–9.

Al-Otaibi, S.T. (2004). Evaluation of disability of occupational illness claims for workers' compensation. Saudi Med J, 25 (2), 145–9.

Alavanja, M.C., Brownson, R.C., Lubin, J.H., et al. (1994). Residential radon exposure and lung cancer among nonsmoking women. J Natl Cancer Inst, 86 (24), 1829–37.

Albus, C., De Backer, G., Bages, N., et al. (2005). Psychosocial factors in coronary heart disease—scientific evidence and recommendations for clinical practice. Gesundheitswesen, 67 (1), 1–8.

Aldana, S.G., Greenlaw, R., Thomas, D., et al. (2004). The influence of an intense cardiovascular disease risk factor modification program. Prev Cardiol, 7 (1), 19–25.

Aldwin, C.M., Yancura, L.A., "Coping and health: A comparison of the stress and trauma literatures. In: Schnurr, P.P., Green, B.L. Physical health consequences of exposure to extreme stress. Washington, D.C.: American Psychological Association (in press).

Allegra, C., Sargent, D.J. (2005). Adjuvant therapy for colon cancer—the pace quickens. New Eng J Med, 352 (26), 2746–8.

Allen, J.K. (2000). Genetics and cardiovascular disease. Nurs Clin North Am, 35 (3), 653–62.

Allen, N.E., Roddam, A.W., Allen, D.S., et al. (2005). A prospective study of serum insulin-like growth factor-I (IGF-I), IGF-II, IGF-binding protein-3 and breast cancer risk. Br J Cancer, 92 (7), 1283–7.

Almahroos, M., Kurban, A.K. (2004). Ultraviolet carcinogenesis in nonmelanoma skin cancer part II: review and update on epidemiologic correlations. Skinmed, 3 (3), 132–9.

Altaf, F.J., Abdullah, L.S., Jamal, A.A. (2004). Frequency of benign and preinvasive breast disease. Saudi Med J, 25 (4), 493–7.

American Cancer Society, http://www.cancer.org.

American Medical Association (1999). Health literacy: report of the Council on Scientific Affairs. Ad Hoc Committee on Health Literacy for the Council on Scientific Affairs, American Medical Association. JAMA, 281 (6), 552–7.

American Obesity Association. Health effects of obesity. AOA Fact Sheets, (http://www.obesity.org).

Amos, A.F., McCarty, D.J., Zimmet, P. (1997). The rising global burden of diabetes and its complications: estimates and projections to the year 2010. Diabet Med, 14 Suppl 5, S1–85.

Amouyel, P. (1998). The contribution of genetics in the evaluation of cardiovascular risk. Arch Mal Coeur Vaiss, 91 (Suppl), 13–18.

Andersen, A., Glatte, E., Johansen, B.V. (1993). Incidence of cancer among lighthouse keepers exposed to asbestos in drinking water. Am J Epidemiol, 138 (9), 682–7.

Andersen, B.L., Farrar, W.B., Golden-Kreutz, D.M., et al. (2004). Psychological, behavioral, and immune changes after a psychological intervention: a clinical trial. J Clin Oncol, 22 (17), 3570–80.

Anderson, R.J., Freedland, K.E., Clouse, R.E., Lustman, P.J. (2001). The prevalence of co morbid depression in adults with diabetes. Diabetes Care, 24 (6), 1069–78.

Andrus, M.R., Roth, M.T. (2002). Health literacy: a review. Pharmacotherapy, 22 (3), 282–302.

Araki, A., Izumo, Y., Inoue, J., et al. (1995). Factors associated with increased diabetes burden in elderly diabetic patients. Nippon Ronen Igakkai Zasshi, 32 (12), 797–803.

Archenholtz, B., Nordberg, E., Bremell, T. (2001). Lower level of education in young adults with arthritis starting in the early adulthood. Scand J Rheumatol, 30 (6), 353–5.

Ardizzoni, A., Tiseo, M. (2004). Second-line chemotherapy in the treatment of advanced non-small cell lung cancer (NSCLC). J Chemother, 16 (Suppl 4), 104–7.

Armstrong, B.K., Kricker, A., English, D.R. (1997). Sun exposure and skin cancer. Australas J Dermatol, 38 (Suppl 1), S1–6.

Armstrong, B.K., Kricker, A. (2001). The epidemiology of UV induced skin cancer. J Photochem Photobiol B, 63 (1–3), 8–18.

Arnold, L.M., Hudson, J.I., Hess, E.V. (2004). Family study of fibromyalgia. Arthritis Rheum, 50 (3), 944–52.

Aronoff, G.M., Livengood, J.M. (2003). Pain: psychiatric aspects of impairment and disability. Curr Pain Headache Rep, 7 (2), 105–15.

Arthur, H.M., Smith, K.M., Kodis, J., et al. (2002). A controlled trial of hospital versus home-based exercise in cardiac patients. Med Sci Sports Exerc, 34 (10), 1544–50.

Artinian, N.T., Magnan, M., Christian, W., et al. (2002). What do patients know about their heart failure? Appl Nurs Res, 15 (4), 200–8.

Asbring, P., Narvanen, A.L. (2002). Women's experiences of stigma in relation to chronic fatigue syndrome and fibromyalgia. Qual Health Res, 12 (2), 148–60.

Assendelft, W.J., Morton, S.C., Yu, E.I., et al. (2003). Spinal manipulative therapy for low back pain. A meta-analysis of effectiveness relative to other therapies. Ann Intern Med, 138 (11), 871–81.

Astin, J.A., Berman, B.M., Bausell, B., et al. (2003). The efficacy of mindfulness meditation plus Qigong movement therapy in the treatment of fibromyalgia: a randomized controlled trial. J Rheumatol, 30 (10), 2257–62.

Atienza, A.A., Collins, R., King, A.C. (2001). The mediating effects of situational control on social support and mood following a stressor: a prospective study of dementia caregivers in their natural environments. J Gerontol B Psychol Sci Soc Sci, 56 (3), S129–39.

Atlas, S.J., Wasiak, R., van den Ancker, M., et al. (2004). Primary care involvement and outcomes of care in patients with a workers' compensation claim for back pain. Spine, 29 (9), 1041–8.

Aure, O.F., Nilsen, J.H., Vasselgen, O. (2003). Manual therapy and exercise therapy in patients with chronic low back pain: a randomized, controlled trial with 1-year follow-up. Spine, 28, 525–31.

Austenfeld, J.L., Stanton, A.L. (2004). Coping through emotional approach: a new look at emotion, coping, and health-related outcomes. J Pers, 72 (6), 1335–64.

Azizi, E., Modan, M., Fuchs, Z., et al. (1990). Skin cancer risk of Israeli workers exposed to sunlight. Harefuah, 118 (9), 508–11.

Azizi, F., Mirmiran, P., Azadbakht, L. (2004). Predictors of cardiovascular risk factors in Tehranian adolescents: Tehran Lipid and Glucose Study. Int J Vitam Nutr Res, 74 (5), 307–12.

Backman, C.L. (2004). Employment and work disability in rheumatoid arthritis. Curr Opin Rheumatol, 16 (2), 148–52.

Badley, E.M., Ibanez, D. (1994). Socioeconomic risk factors and musculoskeletal disability. J Rheumatol, 21 (3), 515–22.

Baecklund, E., Askling, J., Rosenquist, R., et al. (2004). Rheumatoid arthritis and malignant lymphomas. Curr Opin Rheumatol, 16 (3), 254–61.

Baird, C.L., Schmeiser, D., Yehle, K.T. (2003). Self-caring of women with osteoarthritis living at different levels of independence. Health Care Women Int, 24 (7), 617–34.

Bakris, G.L. (2004). The importance of blood pressure control in the patient with diabetes. American Journal of Medicine, 116 (Suppl 5A), 30S–38S.

Balagopal, P., George, D., Patton, N., et al. (2005). Lifestyle-only intervention attenuates the inflammatory state associated with obesity: a randomized controlled study in adolescents. J Pediatr, 146 (3), 342–8.

Banaszkiewicz, P.A., Kader, D., Wardlaw, D. (2003). The role of caudal epidural injections in the management of low back pain. Bull Hosp Jt Dis, 61 (3–4), 127–31.

Barlow, J.H., Wright, C.C., Wright, S. (2003). Development of job-seeking ability in people with arthritis: evaluation of a pilot program. Int J Rehabil Res, 26 (4), 329–33.

Baron, J.A., Gerhardsson de Verdier, M. Ekbom, A. (1994). Coffee, tea, tobacco, and cancer of the large bowel. Cancer Epidemiol Biomarkers Prev, 3 (7), 565–70.

Barrera, M., D'Agostino, N.M., Gibson, J., et al. (2004). Predictors and mediators of psychological adjustment in mothers of children newly diagnosed with cancer. Psychooncology, 13 (9), 630–41.

Barton, M.B., Morley, D.S., Moore, S., et al. (2004). Decreasing women's anxieties after abnormal mammograms: a controlled trial. J Natl Cancer Inst, 96 (7), 529–38.

Baselga, J., Carbonell, X., Castaneda-Soto, N.J., et al. (2005). Phase II study of efficacy, safety, and pharmacokinetics of trastuzumab monotherapy administered on a 3-weekly schedule. J Clin Oncol, 23 (10), 2162–71.

Bataille, V., Winnett, A., Sasieni, P., et al. (2004). Exposure to the sun and sunbeds and the risk of cutaneous melanoma in the UK: a case-control study. Eur J Cancer, 40 (3), 429–35.

Ben-Zur, H., Gilbar, O., Lev, S. (2001). Coping with breast cancer: patient, spouse, and dyad models. Psychosom Med, 63 (1), 32–9.

Berger, J.P., Akiyama, T.E., Meinke, P.T. (2005). PPARs: therapeutic targets for metabolic disease. Trends Pharmacol Sci, 26 (5), 244–51.

Bernard, A.L., Prince, A., Edsall, P. (2000). Quality of life issues for fibromyalgia patients. Arthritis Care Res, 13 (1), 42–50.

Bernstein, J.L., Langholz, B., Haile, R.W., et al. (2004). Study design: evaluating gene-environment interactions in the etiology of breast cancer—the WECARE study. Breast Cancer Res, 6 (3), R199–214. Epub 2004 Mar 09.

Berto, P., Degli Esposti, E., Ruffo, P. (2002). The Pandora project: cost of hypertension from a general practitioner database. Blood Press, 11 (3), 151–6.

Berwick, M., Orlow, I., Mahabir, S., et al. (2004). Estimating the relative risk of developing melanoma in INK4A carriers. Eur J Cancer Prev, 13 (1), 65–70.

Bhutra, S. (2001). Back pain: management & controversies. http://www.theiaforum.org/apr2001.htm

Biffi, R.G., Mamede, M.V. (2004). Social support in the rehabilitation of mastectomized women: the role of the sexual partner. Rev Esc Enferm USP, 38 (3), 262–9.

Bishop, S.R., Warr, D. (2003). Coping, catastrophizing and chronic pain in breast cancer. J Behav Med, 26 (3), 265–81.

Blask, D.E., Dauchy, R.T., Sauer, L.A., et al. (2002). Light during darkness, melatonin suppression and cancer protection. Neuro Endocrinol Lett, 23 (Suppl 2), 52–6.

Blot, W.J., Xu, Z.Y., Boice, J.D., Jr., et al. (1990). Indoor radon and lung cancer in China. J Natl Cancer Inst, 82 (12), 1025–30.

Blum, C.A., Muller, B., Huber, P., et al. (2005). Low-grade inflammation and estimates of insulin resistance of insulin resistance during the menstrual cycle in lean and overweight women. J Clin Endocrinol Metab, March 29 (Epub ahead of print).

Blumenauer, B., Coyle, D., Tugwell, P. (2002). Pharmacoeconomics of long-term treatment of rheumatoid arthritis. Expert Opin Pharmacother, 3 (4), 417–22.

Blumenstiel, K., Eich, W. (2003). Psychosomatic aspects in the diagnosis and treatment of fibromyalgia. Schmerz, 17 (6), 399–404.

Boccardo, F., Campisi, C. (2002). Disability and lymphadema. Ann Ital Chir, 73 (5), 485–8.

Boden-Albala, B., Sacco, R.L. (2000). Lifestyle factors and stroke risk: exercise, alcohol, diet, obesity, smoking, drug use, and stress. Curr Atheroscler Rep, 2 (2), 160–6.

Body, J.J., Gaich, G.A., Scheele, W.H., et al. (2002). A randomized double-blind trial to compare the efficacy of teriparatide (recombinant human parathyroid hormone 1–34) with alendronate in postmenopausal women with osteoporosis. J Clin Endocrinol Metab, 87 (10), 4528–35.

Boffetta, P., Nyberg, F. (2003). Contribution of environmental factors to cancer risk. Br Med Bull, 68, 71–94.

Bolen, J.C., Rhodes, L., Powell-Griner, E.E. (2000). State-specific prevalence of selected health behaviors, by race and ethnicity—Behavioral Risk Factor Surveillance System. MMWR CDC Surveill Summ, 49 (2), 1–60.

Bordea, C., Wojnarowska, F., Millard, P.R., et al. (2004). Skin cancers in renal-transplant recipients occur more frequently than previously recognized in a temperate climate. Tranplantation, 77 (4), 574–9.

Borenstein, D. (2004). Does osteoarthritis of the lumbar spine cause chronic low back pain? Curr Rheumatol Rep, 6 (1), 14–19.

Borenstein, D. (1995). Prevalence and treatment outcome of primary and secondary fibromyalgia in patients with spinal pain. Spine, 20 (7), 796–800.

Borgstrom, F., Johnell, O., Kanis, J.A., et al. (2004). Cost effectiveness of raloxifene in the treatment of osteoporosis in Sweden: an economic evaluation based on the MORE study. Pharmacoeconomics, 22 (17), 1153–65.

Borissova, A.M., Tankova, T.I., Koev, D.J. (2004). Insulin secretion, peripheral insulin sensitivity and insulin-receptor binding in subjects with different degrees of obesity. Diabetes Meab, 30 (5), 425–31.

Borodulin, K., Laatikainen, T., Lahti-Koski, M., et al. (2005). Associations between estimated aerobic fitness and cardiovascular risk factors in adults with different levels of abdominal obesity. Eur J Cardiovasc Prev Rehabil, 12 (2), 126–31.

Bos, G., Dekker, J.M., Feskens, E.J., et al. (2005). Ineractions of dietary fat intake and the hepatic lipase −580C→T polymorphism in determining hepatic lipase activity: the Hoorn Study. Am J Clin Nutr, 81 (4), 911–15.

Boukhors, Y., Rabasa-Lhoret, R., Langelier, H., et al. (2003). The use of information technology for the management of intensive insulin therapy in type 1 diabetes mellitus. Diabetes Metab, 29 (6), 619–27.

Boulay, P., Prud'homme, D. (2004). Health-care consumption and recurrent myocardial infarction after 1 year of conventional treatment versus short- and long-term cardiac rehabilitation. Prev Med, 38 (5), 586–93.

Boyapati, S.M., Shu, X.O., Gao, Y.T., et al. (2004). Correlation of blood sex steroid hormones with body size, body fat distribution, and other known risk factors for breast cancer in post-menopausal Chinese women. Cancer Causes Control, 15 (3), 305–11.

Boyle, J.P., Honeycutt, A.A., Narayan, K.M., et al. (2001). Projection of diabetes burden through 2050: impact of changing demography and disease prevalence in the U.S. Diabetes Care, 24 (11), 1936–40.

Braaten, T., Weiderpass, E., Kumle, M., et al. (2004). Education and risk of breast cancer in the Norwegian-Swedish women's lifestyle and health cohort study. Int J Cancer, 110 (4), 579–83.

Brauer, W., Merkesdal, S., Mau, W. (2002). Long-term follow-up and prognosis of work capacity in the early stage of chronic polyarthritis. Z Rheumatol, 61 (4), 426–34.

Bray, F., Tyczynski, J.E., Parkin, D.M. (2004). Going up or down? The changing phases of the lung cancer epidemic from 1967 to 1999 in the 15 European Union countries. Eur J Cancer, 40 (1), 96–125.

Breedveld, F.C. (2004). Osteoarthritis—the impact of a serious disease. Rheumatology (Oxford), 43 (Suppl 1), 14–18.

Brezinka, V., Kittle, F. (1996). Psychosocial factors of coronary heart disease in women: a review. Soc Sci Med, 42 (10), 1351–65.

Briggs, A., Scott, E., Steele, K. (1999). Impact of osteoarthritis and analgesic treatment on quality of life of an elderly population. Ann Pharmacother, 33 (11), 1154–9.

Brixen, K.T., Christensen, P.M., Ejersted, C., et al. (2004). Teriparatide (biosynthetic human parathyroid hormone 1–34): a new paradigm in the treatment of osteoporosis.

Bronfort, G., Haas, M., Evans, R.L., et al. (2004). Efficacy of spinal manipulation and mobilization for low back pain and neck pain: a systematic review and best evidence synthesis. Spine J, 4 (3), 335–56.

Browne, M.L., Varadarajulu, D., Lewis-Michl, E.L., et al. (2005). Cancer incidence and asbestos in drinking water, Town of Woodstock, New York, 1980–1998. Environ Res, 98 (2), 224–32.

Brummett, B.H., Mark, D.B., Siegler, I.C., et al. (2005). Perceived social support as a predictor of mortality in coronary patients: effects of smoking, sedentary behavior, and depressive symptoms. Psychosom Med, 67 (1), 40–5.

Bruusgaard, D., Evensen, A.R., Bjerkedal, T. (1993). Fibromyalgia—a new cause for disability pension. Scand J Soc Med, 21 (2), 116–19.

Buchbinder, R., Jolley, D., Wyatt, M. (2001). Population based intervention to change back pain beliefs and disability: three part evaluation. Br Med J, 322, 1516–20.

Buckwalter, J.A., Lane, N.E. (1997). Athletics and osteoarthritis. Am J Sports Med, 25 (6), 873–81.

Buckwalter, J.A., Lappin, D.R. (2000). The disproportionate impact of chronic arthralgia and arthritis among women. Clin Orthop Relat Res, (372), 159–68.

Budde, L.S., Hanna, N.H. (2005). Antimetabolites in the management of non-small cell lung cancer. Curr Treat Options Oncol, 6 (1), 83–93.

Burckhardt, C.S. (2002). Nonpharmacologic management strategies in fibromyalgia. Rheum Dis Clin North Am, 28 (2), 291–304.

Burdorf, A., Naaktgeboren, B., deGroot, H.C. (1993). Occupational risk factors for low back pain among sedentary workers. J Occup Med, 35 (12), 1213–20.

Burge, R.T., King, A.B., Balda, E., et al. (2003). Methodology for estimating current and future burden of osteoporosis in state populations: application to Florida in 2000 through 2025. Value Health, 6 (5), 574–83.

Burger, M., Mensink, G., Bronstrup, A., et al. (2004). Alcohol consumption and its relation to cardiovascular risk factors in Germany. Eur J Clin Nutr, 58 (4), 605–14.

Burke, M., Flaherty, M.J. (1993). Coping strategies and health status of elderly arthritic women. J Adv Nurs, 18 (1), 7–13.

Burker, E.J., Evon, D.M., Sedway, J.A., et al. (2004). Appraisal and coping as predictors of psychological distress and self-reported physical disability before lung transplantation. Prog Transplant, 14 (3), 222–32.

Burkman, R., Schlesselman, J.J., Zieman, M. (2004). Safety concerns and health benefits associated with oral contraception. Am J Obstet Gynecol, 190 (Suppl 4), S5–22.

Burns, D.M. (2003). Tobacco-related diseases. Semin Oncol Nurs, 19 (4), 244–9.

Burton, A.K., Waddell, G., Tillotson, K.M., et al. (1999). Information and advice to patients with back pain can have a positive effect: a randomized controlled trial of a novel educational booklet in primary care. Spine, 24, 2484–91.

Buzaid, A.C. (2004). Management of metastatic cutaneous melanoma. Oncology (Huntingt). 18 (11), 1443–40; discussion 1457–9.

Centers for Disease Control and Prevention (2001). CDC fact book 2000/2001, Atlanta, Georgia.

Calle, E.E., Miracle-McMahill, H.L., Thun, M.J. (1994). Cigarette smoking and risk of fatal breast cancer. Am J Epidemiol, 139 (10), 1001–7.

Carey, T.S., Garrett, J., Jackman, A., et al. (1995). The outcomes and costs of care for acute low back pain among patients seen by primary care practitioners, chiropractors, and orthopedic surgeons. The North Carolina Back Pain Project. N Engl J Med, 333, 913–17.

Carmona, L., Ballina, J., Gabriel, R., et al. (2001). The burden of musculoskeletal diseases in the general population of Spain: results from a national survey. Ann Rheum Dis, 60 (11), 1040–5.

Carr, A., Hewlett, S., Hughes, R., et al. (2003). Rheumatology outcomes: the patient's perpective. J Rheumatol, 30 (4), 880–3.

Carter, M.L. (2004). Spinal cord stimulation in chronic pain: a review of the evidence. Anaesth Intensive Care, 32 (1), 11–21.

Castaneda, C. (2003). Diabetes control with physical activity and exercise. Nutr Clin Care, 6 (2), 89–96.

CDC, National Center for Chronic Disease Prevention and Health Promotion, p. 1, http://www.cdc.gov/needphp/overview.htm.

Cettour-Rose, P., Samec, S., Russell, A.P., et al. (2005). Redistribution of glucose from skeletal muscle to adipose tissue during catch-up fat: a link between catch-up growth and later metabolic syndrome. Diabetes, 54 (3), 751–6.

Chang, H.J., Mehta, P.S., Rosenberg, A., et al. (2004). Concerns of patients actively contemplating total knee replacement: differences by race and gender. Arthritis Rheum, 51 (1), 117–23.

Chao, A., Thun, M.J., Connell, C.J., et al. (2005). Meat consumption and risk of colorectal cancer. JAMA 293 (2), 172–82.

Cheah, J. (2000). Clinical pathways—an evaluation of its impact on the quality of care in an acute care general hospital in Singapore. Singapore Med J, 41 (7), 335–46.

Chen, M.F., Ma, F.C. (2004). Symptom distresses and coping strategies in breast cancer women with mastectomy. Hu Li Za Zhi, 51 (4), 37–44.

Chen, R., Rabinovitch, P.S., Crispin, et al. (2005). The initiation of colon cancer in a chronic inflammatory setting. Carcinogenesis, Apr 28; (Epub ahead of print).

Cherkin, D.C., Deyo, R.A., Street, J.H., et al. (1996). Pitfalls of patient education: limited success of a program for back pain in primary care. Spine, 21, 345–55.

Cherry, J.C., Moffatt, T.P., Rodrigquez, C., et al. (2002). Diabetes disease management program for an indigent population empowered by telemedicine technology. Diabetes Technol Ther, 4 (6), 783–91.

Childs, J.D., Piva, S.R., Erhard, R.E. (2004). Immediate improvements in side-to-side weight bearing and iliac symmetry after manipulation in patients with low back pain. J Manipulative Physiol Ther, 27 (5), 306–13.

Cho, E., Smith-Warner, S.A., Ritz, J., et al. (2004). Alcohol intake and colorectal cancer: a pooled analysis of 8 cohort studies. Ann Intern Med, 140 (8), 603–13.

Choi, H.K. (2005). Dietary risk factors for rheumatic diseases. Curr Opin Rheumatol, 17 (2), 141–6.

Christopoulou, A. (2004). Chemotherapy in metastatic colorectal cancer. Tech Coloproctol, 8 (Suppl 1), S43–6.

Chupkovich, P.J. (1993). Statutory caps: an involuntary contribution to the medical malpractice insurance crisis or a reasonable mechanism for obtaining affordable health care? J Contemp Health Law Policy, 9, 337–75.

Cirera, L., Tormo, N.J., Chirlaque, M.D., et al. (1998). Cardiovascular risk factors and educational attainment in Southern Spain: a study of a random sample of 3091 adults. Eur J Epidemiol, 14 (8), 755–63.

Clarke, P., Marshall, V., Black, S.E., et al. (2002). Well-being after stroke in Canadian seniors: findings from the Canadian Study of Health and Aging. Stroke, 33 (4), 1016–21.

Cleland, L.G., James, M.J., Keen, H., et al. (2005). Fish oil—an example of an anti-inflammatory food. Asia Pac J Clin Nutr, 14 (Suppl), S66–71.

Cleveland Clinic. A vicious cycle: chronic illness and depression. The Cleveland Clinic Health Information Center, 2003.

Cliff, A.M., MacDonagh, R.P. (2000). Psychosocial morbidity in prostate cancer: II. A comparison of patients and partners. BJU Int, 86 (7), 834–9.

Cockerill, W., Lunt, M., Silman, A.J., et al. (2004). Health-related quality of life and radiographic vertebral fracture. Osteoporos Int, 15 (2), 113–19. Epub 2003 Nov 13.

Cohen, A.J., Roe, F.J. (2000). Review of risk factors for osteoporosis with particular reference to a possible aetiological role of dietary salt. Food Chem Toxicol, 38 (2–3), 237–53.

Colditz, G.A., Rosner, B.A., Chen, W.Y., et al. (2004). Risk factors for breast cancer according to estrogen and progesterone receptor status. J Natl Cancer Inst, 96 (3), 218–28.

Collado Cruz, A., Torres I Mata, X., Arias I Gassol, A., et al. (2001). Efficiency of multidisciplinary treatment of chronic pain with locomotor disability. Med Clin (Barc), 117 (11), 401–5.

Collins, L.G., Nash, R., Round, T., et al. (2004). Perceptions of upper-body problems during recovery from breast cancer treatment. Support Care Cancer, 12 (2), 106–13. Epub 2003 Oct 31.

Colomer, R. (2004). Gemcitabine and paclitaxel in metastatic breast cancer: a review. Oncology (Huntingt). 18 (14 Suppl 12), 8–12.

Contreras, I., Parra, D. (2000). Estrogen replacement therapy and the prevention of coronary heart disease in postmenopausal women. Am J Health Syst Pharm, 57 (21), 1963–8.

Corella, D., Ordovas, J.M. (2004). Single nucleotide polymorphisms that influence lipid metabolism: Interaction with dietary factors. Annu Rev Nutr, May 21 (Epub ahead of print).

Cormier, Y., Israel-Assayag, E. (2004). Chronic inflammation induced by organic dust and related metabolic cardiovascular disease risk factors. Scand J Work Environ Health, 30 (6), 438–44.

Corona, R. Epidemiology of nonmelanoma skin cancer: a review. Ann Ist Super Sanita, 32 (1): 37–42.

Costa, A., Conget, I., Gomis, R. (2002). Impaired glucose tolerance: is there a case for pharmacologic intervention? Treat Endocrinol, 1 (4), 205–10.

Costacou, T., Mayer-Davis, E.J. (2003). Nutrition and prevention of type 2 diabetes. Annual Review of Nutrition, 23, 147–70, Epub 2003 Feb 21.

Cowan, P., Morewitz, S. (1995). Encouraging discussion of psychosocial issues at student health visits. J of Amer College Health, March, Vol. 43, pp. 197–200.

Criswell, L.A., Merlino, L.A., Cerhan, J.R., et al. (2002). Cigarette smoking and the risk of rheumatoid arthritis among postmenopausal women: results from the Iowa Women's Health Study. Am J Med, 112 (6), 465–71.

Croft, P., Coggon, D., Cruddas, M., et al. (1992). Osteoarthritis of the hip: an occupational disease in farmers. BMJ, 304 (6837), 1269–72.

Cuomo, G., Di Micco, P., Niglio, A., et al. (2004). Atherosclerosis and rheumatoid arthritis: relationships between intima-media thickness of the common carotid arteries and disease activity and disability. Reumatismo, 56 (4), 242–6.

Cutler, R.B., Fishbain, D.A. Rosomoff, H.L., et al. (1994). Does nonsurgical pain center treatment of chronic pain return patients to work? A review and meta-analysis of the literature. Spine, 19, 643–52.

Cymet, T.C. (2003). A practical approach to fibromyalgia. J Natl Med Assoc, 95 (4), 278–85.

Czene, K., Tiikkaja, S., Hemminki, K. (2003). Cancer risks in hairdressers: assessment of carcinogenicity of hair dyes and gels. Int J Cancer, 105 (1), 108–12.

Da Costa, D., Dobkin, P.L., Fitzcharles, M.A., et al. (2000). Determinants of health status in fibromyalgia: a comparative study with systemic lupus erythematosus. J Rheumatol, 27 (2), 365–72.

Dai, S.M., Han, X.H., Zhao, D.B., et al. (2003). Prevalence of rheumatic symptoms, rheumatoid arthritis, ankylosing spondylitis, and gout in Shanghai, China: a COPCORD study. Journal of Rheumatology, 30 (10), 2245–51.

Damush, T.M., Weinberger, M., Perkins, S.M., et al. (2003). The long-term effects of a self-management program for inner-city primary care patients with acute low back pain. Arch Intern Med, 163 (21), 2632–8.

Dandona, P., Aljada, A., Chaudhuri, A., et al. (2003). The potential influence of inflammation and insulin resistance on the pathogenesis and treatment of atherosclerosis-related complications in type 2 diabetes. J Clin Endocrinol Metab, 88, 2422–9.

Dangelser, G., Besson, S., Gatina, J.H., et al. (2003). Amputations among diabetics in Reunion Island. Diabetes Metab, 29 (6), 628–34.

Dankner, R., Chetrit, A., Lubin, F., et al. (2004). Life-style habits and homocysteine levels in an elderly population. Aging Clin Exp Res, 16 (6), 437–42.

Darby, S., Hill, D., Auvinen, A., et al. (2005). Radon in homes and risk of lung cancer: collaborative analysis of individual data from 13 European case-control studies. BMJ, 330 (7485), 223. Epub 2004 Dec 21.

Das, U.N. (2005). A defect in the activity of Delta6 and Delta5 desaturases may be a factor predisposing to the development of insulin resistance syndrome. Prostaglandins Leukot Essent Fatty Acids, 72 (5), 343–50.

Davidson, P.M., Daly, J., Hancock, K., et al. (2003). Perceptions and experiences of heart disease: a literature review and identification of a research agenda in older women. Eur J Cardiovsc Nurs, 2 (4), 255–64.

Davies, E., Hall, S., Clarke, C. (2003). Two year survival after malignant cerebral glioma: patient and relative reports of handicap, psychiatric symptoms and rehabilitation. Disabil Rehabil, 25 (6), 259–66.

Daviglus, M.L., Liu, K., Yan, L.L., et al. (2004). Relation of body mass index in young adulthood and middle age to Medicare expenditures in older age. JAMA, 292 (22), 2743–9.

Davis, M.C., Zautra, A.J., Reich, J.W. (2001). Vulnerability to stress among women in chronic pain from fibromyalgia and osteoarthritis. Ann Behav Med, 23 (3), 215–26.

Davis, S., Mirick, D.K., Steven, R.G. (2001). Night shift work, light at night, and risk of breast cancer. J Natl Cancer Inst, 93 (20), 1557–67.

De Bacquer, D., Pelfrene, E., Clays, E., et al. (2005). Perceived job stress and incidence of coronary events: 3-year follow-up of the Belgian Job Stress Project cohort. Am J Epidemiol, 161 (5), 434–41.

Debiais, F. (2003). Efficacy data on teriparatide (parathyroid hormone) in patients with postmenopausal osteoporosis. Joint Bone Spine, 70 (6), 465–70.

de Buck, P.D., Schoones, J.W., Allaire, S.H. (2002). Vocational rehabilitation in patients with chronic rheumatic diseases: a systematic literature review. Semin Arthritis Rheum, 32 (3), 196–203.

Dedert, E.A., Studts, J.L., Weissbecker, I., et al. (2004). Religiosity may help preserve the cortisol rhythm in women with stress-related illness. Int J Psychiatry Med, 34 (1), 61–77.

D'Eramo-Melkus, G., Spollett, G., Jefferson, V., et al. (2004). A culturally competent intervention of education and care for black women with type 2 diabetes. Appl Nurs Res, 17 (1), 10–20.

De Filippis, L., Gulli, S., Caliri, A., et al. (2004). Epidemiology and risk factors in osteoarthritis: literature review data from "OASIS" study. Reumatismo, 56 (3), 169–84.

de Gaetano, G., Di Castelnuovo, A., Donati, M.B., et al. (2003). The Mediterranean lecture: wine and thrombosis—from epidemiology to physiology and back. Pathophysiol Haemost Thromb, 33 (5–6), 466–71.

DeGroot, M., Anderson, R., Freedland, K., et al. Association of depression and diabetes complications. Psychosomatic Medicine, 2001.

DeLeo, D., Spanthonis K. Suicide and euthanasia in late life. Aging and Clinical Experimental Research, 2003.

De Luca, D.E., Boccini, A. (2003). Cardiovascular diseases and risk factors. Ann Ig, 15 (6), 1051–6.

Delbruck, H. (1997). Assessment of work capacity and occupational rehabilitation in curatively treated tumor patients. Versicherungsmedizin, 49 (5), 167–72.

DeLellis, K., Rinaldi, S., Kaaks, R.J., et al. (2004). Dietary and lifestyle correlates of plasma insulin-like growth factor-I (IGF-I) and IGF binding protein-3 (IGFBP-3): the multiethnic cohort. Cancer Epidemiol Biomarkers Prev, 13 (9), 1444–51.

Devereux, J.J., Buckle, P.W., Vlachonikolis, I.G. (1999). Interactions between physical and psychosocial risk factors at work increase the risk of back disorders: an epidemiological approach. Occup Environ Med, 56 (5), 343–53.

Devroey, D., De Swaef, N., Coigniez, P., et al. (2004). Correlation between lipid levels and age, gender, glycemia, obesity, diabetes, and smoking. Endocr Res, 30 (1), 83–93.

Diabetesliving.com (2004). Diabetes living—economics of diabetes. http://www.diabetesliving.com/basics/bsc_econ.htm

Dickinson, J.K., O'Reilly, M.M. (2004). The lived experience of adolescent females with type 1 diabetes. Diabetes Educ, 30 (1), 99–107.

Dixey, J., Solymossy, C., Young, A., et al. (2004). Is it possible to predict radiological damage in early rheumatoid arthritis (RA)? A report on the occurrence, progression, and prognostic factors of radiological erosions over the first 3 years in 866 patients from the Early RA Study (ERAS). J Rheumatol Suppl, 69, 48–54.

Dobnig, H. (2004). A review of teriparatide and its clinical efficacy in the treatment of osteoporosis. Expert Opin Pharmacother, 5 (5), 1153–62.

Doedel, R.C., Haacke, C., Zamzow, K., et al. (2004). Resource utilization and costs of stroke unit care in Germany. Value Health, 7 (2), 144–52.

Doeglas, D., Suurmeijer, T., Krol, B., et al. (1994). Social support, social disability, and psychological well-being in rheumatoid arthritis. Arthritis Care Res, 7 (1), 10–5.

Dominick, K.L., Ahern, F.M., Gold, C.H., et al. (2004a). Health-related quality of life and health service use among older adults with osteoarthritis. Arthritis Rheum, 51 (3), 326–31.

Dominick, K.L., Ahern, F.M., Gold, C.H., et al. (2004b). Health-related quality of life among older adults with arthritis. Health Qual Life Outcome, 2 (1), 5.

Donnelly, J.E., Smith, B., Jacobsen, D.J., et al. (2004). The role of exercise for weight loss and maintenance. Best Pract Res Clin Gastroenterol, 18 (6), 1009–29.

Donnelly, P., Cooke, D. (1982). A study of the combined effect of ACTH (gel) and D-penicillamine on the functional disability of patients with rheumatoid disease. J Rheumatol, 9 (6), 867–72.

Downe-Wamboldt, B. (1991). Stress, emotions, and coping: a study of elderly women with osteoarthritis. Health Care Women Int, 12 (1), 85–98.

Downe-Wamboldt, B. (1991b). Coping and life satisfaction in elderly women with osteoarthritis. J Adv Nurs, 16 (11), 1328–35.

Dowsett, M., Ebbs, S.R., Dixon, J.M., et al. (2005). Biomarker changes during neoadjuvant anastrozole, tamoxifen, or the combination: influence of hormonal status and HER-2 in breast cancer—a study from the IMPACT trialists. J Clin Oncol, 23 (11), 2477–92. Epub 2005 Mar 14.

Dreiser, R.L., Marty, M., Ionescu, E., et al. (2003). Relief of acute low back pain with diclofenac-K 12.5 mg tablets: a flexible dose, ibuprofen 200 mg and placebo-controlled clinical trial. Int J Clin Pharmacol Ther, 41 (9), 375–85.

Duggleby, W., Wright, K. (2004). Elderly palliative care cancer patients' descriptions of hope-fostering strategies. Int J Palliat Nurs, 10 (7), 352–9.

Duncan, A.M. (2004). The role of nutrition in the prevention of breast cancer. AACN Clin Issues, 15 (1), 119–35.

Duncan, G.E., Li, S.M., Zhou, X.H. (2004). Prevalence and trends of a metabolic syndrome phenotype among U.S. adolescents, 1999–2000. Diabetes Care, 27, 2438–43.

Dunn, J., Steginga, S.K., Rose, P., et al. (2004). Evaluating patient education materials about radiation therapy. Patient Educ Couns, 52 (3), 325–32.

Dunn, S.M., Beeney, L.J., Hoskins, P.L. (1990). Knowledge and attitude change as predictors of metabolic improvement in diabetes education. Soc Sci Med, 31 (10), 1135–41.

Durai, R., Yang, W., Gupta, S., et al. (2005). The role of the insulin-like growth factor system in colorectal cancer: review of current knowledge. Int J Colorectal Dis, 20 (3), 203–20. Epub 2005 Jan 14.

Dykes, P.C., Currie, L., Bakken, S. (2004). Patient Education and Recovery Learning System (PEARLS) pathway: a tool to drive patient centered evidence-based practice. J Health Inf Manag, 18 (4), 67–73.

Eaker, E.D., Sullivan, L.M., Kelly-Hayes, M., et al. (2004). Does job strain increase the risk for coronary heart disease or death in men and women? The Framingham Offspring Study. Am J Epidemiol, 159 (10), 950–8.

Eckel, R.H., Wassef, M., Chait, A., et al. (2002). Prevention Conference VI: diabetes and cardiovascular disease. Writing Group II: pathogenesis of atherosclerosis in diabetes. Circulation, 105, E138–43.

Ehrlich, G.E. (2003a). Back pain. J Rheumatol Suppl, (67), 26–31.

Ehrlich, G.E. (2003b). Low back pain. Bull World Health Organ, 81 (9), 671–6.

Eisenmann, J.C. (2004). Physical activity and cardiovascular disease risk factors in children and adolescents: an overview. Canadian Journal of Cardiology, 20 (3), 295–301.

Ellis, S.E., Speroff, T., Dittus, R.S., et al. (2004). Diabetes patient education: a meta-analysis and meta-regression. Patient Educ Couns, 52 (1), 97–105.

Emanuel, E.J., Fairclough, D.L., Daniels, E.R. (1996). Euthanasia and physician-assisted suicide: attitudes and experiences of oncology patients, oncologists and the public. Lancet, 347 (9018), 1805–10.

Eneman, J.D., Wood, M.E., Muss, H.B. (2004). Selecting adjuvant endocrine therapy for breast cancer. Oncology (Huntingt), 18 (14), 1733–44, discussion 1744–5, 1748.

Eng, J., Ramsum, D., Verhoef, M., et al. (2003). A population-based survey of complementary and alternative medicine use in men recently diagnosed with prostate cancer. Integr Cancer Ther, 2 (3), 212–16.

Engelgau, M.M., Geiss, L.S., Saaddine, J.B., et al. (2004). The evolving diabetes burden in the United States. Ann Int Med, 140 (11), 945–50.

English, D.R., Armstrong, B.K., Kricker, A., et al. (1997). Sunlight and cancer. Cancer Causes Control, 8 (3), 271–83.

Erbagci, Z., Erkilic, S. (2002). Can smoking and/or occupational UV exposure have any role in the development of the morpheaform basal cell carcinoma? A critical role for peritumoral mast cells. Int J Dermatol, 41 (5), 275–8.

Erdmann, E. (2005). Diabetes and cardiovascular risk markers. Curr Med Res Opin, 21 (Suppl 1), 21–8.

Eriksen, W., Natvig, B., Bruusgaard, D. (1999). Smoking, heavy physical work and low back pain: a four-year prospective study. Occup Med (Lond), 49 (3), 155–60.

Ettinger, B., Black, D.M., Nevitt, M.C., et al. (1992). Contribution of vertebral deformities to chronic back pain and disability. The Study of Osteoporotic Fractures Research Group. J Bone Miner Res, 7 (4), 449–56.

Evans, W.J. (2002). Physical function in men and women with cancer. Effects of anemia and conditioning. Oncology (Huntingt), 16 (9 Suppl 10), 109–15.

Evers, A.W., Kraaimaat, F.W., Geenen, R., et al. (2003). Stress-vulnerability factors as long-term predictors of disease activity in early rheumatoid arthritis. J Psychosomatic Res, 55 (4), 293–302.

Eyre, H., Kahn, R., Robertson, R.M., et al. (2004). Preventing cancer, cardiovascular disease, and diabetes. A common agenda for the American Cancer Society, the American Diabetes Association, and the American Heart Association. Circulation, June 15 (Epub ahead of print).

Faas, A. (1997). Exercises: which ones are worth trying, for which patients, and when? Spine, 21, 2874–9.

Fairbank, J., Frost, H., Wilson-MacDonald, J., et al. (2005). Randomised controlled trial to compare surgical stabilisation of the lumbar spine with an intensive rehabilitation programme for patients with chronic low back pain: the MRC spine stabilisation trial. BMJ, 330 (7502), 1233. Epub 2005 May 23.

Fayad, F., Lefevre-Colau, M.M., Poiraudeau, S., et al. (2004). Chronicity, recurrence, and return to work in low back pain: common prognostic factors. Ann Readapt Med Phys, 47 (4), 179–89.

Feychting, M., Ahlbom, A., Kheifets, L. (2005). EMF and health. Annu Rev Public Health, 26, 165–89.

Felson, D.T. (2004). An update on the pathogenesis and epidemiology of osteoarthritis. Radiol Clin North Am, 42 (1), 1–9.

Ferchak, C.V., Meneghini, L.F. (2004). Obesity, bariatric surgery and type 2 diabetes—a systematic review. Diabetes Metab Res Rev, 20 (6), 438–45.

Field, R.W., Steck, D.J., Smith, B.J., et al. (2001). The Iowa radon lung cancer study—phase I: Residential radon gas exposure and lung cancer. Sci Total Environ, 272 (1–3), 67–72.

Fink, H.A., Ensrud, K.E., Nelson, D.B., et al. (2003). Disability after clinical fracture in postmenopausal women with low bone density: the fracture intervention trial (FIT). Osteoporos Int, 14 (1), 69–76.

Fishbain, D.A. (1999). The association of chronic pain and suicide. Seminars in Clinical Neuropsychiatry, 4 (3), 221–7.

Fishbain, D.A., Goldberg, M., Rosomoff, R.S., et al. (1991). Completed suicide in chronic pain. Clinical Journal of Pain, 7 (1), 29–36.

Fisher, B.J., Haythornthwaite, J.A., Heinberg, L.J., et al. (2001). Suicidal intent in patients with chronic pain. Pain, 89 (2–3), 199–206.

Fitzpatrick, R., Newman, S., Lamb, R., et al. (1988). Social relationships and psychological well-being in rheumatoid arthritis. Soc Sci Med, 27 (4), 399–403.

Flaherty, L.E. (2000). Rationale for intergroup trial E-3695 comparing concurrent biochemotherapy with cisplatin, vinblastine, and DTIC alone in patients with metastatic melanoma. Cancer J Sci Am, 6 (Suppl 1), S15–20.

Flor, H., Fydrich, T., Turk, D.C. (1992). Efficacy of multidisciplinary pain treatment centers: a meta-analytical review. Pain, 49: 221–30.

Follath, F. (2003). Depression, stress and coronary heart disease—epidemiology, prognosis and therapeutic sequelae. Ther Umsch, 60 (11), 697–701.

Ford, E.S., Giles, W.H., Mokdad, A.H. (2004). Increasing prevalence of the metabolic syndrome among U.S. adults. Diabetes Care, 27, 2444–9.

Forssen, U.M., Rutqvist, L.E., Ahlbom, A., et al. (2005). Occupational magnetic fields and female breast cancer: a case-control study using Swedish population registers and new exposure data. Am J Epidemiol, 161 (3), 250–9.

Frank, C., Smith, S. (1990). Stress and the heart: biobehavioral aspects of sudden cardiac death. Psychosomatics, 32 (1), 115–16.

Fransson, E.I., Alfredsson, L.S., de Faire, U.H., et al. (2003). Leisure time, occupational and household physical activity, and risk factors for cardiovascular disease in working men and women: the WOLF study. Scand J Public Health, 31 (5), 324–33.

Frattini, E., Lindsay, P., Kerr, E., et al. (1998). Learning needs of congestive heart failure patients. Prog Cardiovasc Nurs, 13 (2), 11–16, 33.

Frayn, K.N. (2002). Insulin resistance, impaired postprandial lipid metabolism and abdominal obesity. A deadly triad. Med Princ Pract, 11 (Suppl 2), 31–40.

Freedman, D.M., Sigurdson, A., Rao, R.S. (2003). Risk of melanoma among radiologic technologists in the United States. (2003). Int J Cancer, 103 (4), 556–62.

Freedman, O.C., Verma, S., Clemons, M.J. (2005). Using aromatase inhibitors in the neoadjuvant setting: evolution or revolution? Cancer Treat Rev, 31 (1), 1–17. Epub 2004 Nov 18.

Friedenreich, C.M., Bryant, H.E., Courneya, K.S. (2001). Case-control study of lifetime physical activity and breast cancer risk. Am J Epidemiol, 154 (4), 336–47.

Friedrich, M., Cermak, T., Heiller, I. (2000). Spinal troubles in sewage workers: epidemiological data and work disability due to low back pain. Int Arch Occup Environ Health, 73 (4), 245–54.

Frijling, B.D., Lobo, C.M., Keus, I.M., et al. (2004). Perceptions of cardiovascular risk among patients with hypertension or diabetes. Patient Educ Couns, 52 (1), 47–53.

Frisbie, S.H., Ortega, R., Maynard, D.M., et al. (2002). The concentrations of arsenic and other toxic elements in Bangladesh's drinking water. Environ Health Perspect, 110 (11), 1147–53.

Fritzell, P., Hagg, O., Jonsson, D., et al. (2004). Cost-effectieness of lumbar fusion and nonsurgical treatment for chronic low back pain in the Swedish Lumbar Spine Study: a multicenter, randomized controlled trial from the Swedish Spine Study Group. Spine, 29 (4), 421–34; discussion Z3.

Fritzsche, K., Liptai, C., Henke, M. (2004). Psychosocial distress and need for psychotherapeutic treatment in cancer patients undergoing radiotherapy. Radiother Oncol, 72 (2), 183–9.

Froom, P., Cohen, C., Rashcupkin, J., et al. (1999). Referral to occupational medicine clinics and resumption of employment after myocardial infarction. J Occup Environ Med, 41 (11), 943–7.

Frost, H., Lamb, S.E., Doll, H.A., et al. (2004). Randomized controlled trial of physiotherapy compared with advice for low back pain. BMJ, 329 (7468), 708. Epub 2004 Sept 17.

Frykberg, R.G., Armstrong, D.G., Giurini, J., et al. (2000). Diabetic foot disorders: a clinical practice guideline. American College of Foot and Ankle Surgeons. J Foot Ankle Surg, 39 (5 Suppl), S1–60.

Frymoyer, J.W. (1988). Back pain and sciatica. New Eng J Med, 318 (5), 291–300.

Fu, F.H., Fung, L. (2004). The cardiovascular health of residents in selected metropolitan cities in China. Prev Med, 38 (4), 458–67.

Fung, T., Hu, F.B., Fuchs, C., et al. (2003). Major dietary patterns and the risk of colorectal cancer in women. Arch Intern Med, 163 (3), 309–14.

Fung, T.T., Hu, F.B., Pereira, M.A., et al. (2002). Whole-grain intake and the risk of type 2 diabetes: a prospective study in men. American Journal of Clinical Nutrition, 76 (3), 535–40.

Gaillard, T.R., Schuster, D.P., Bossetti, B.M., et al. (1997). The impact of socioeconomic status on cardiovascular risk factors in African-Americans at high risk for type II diabetes. Implications for syndrome X. Diabees Care, 20 (5), 745–52.

Gaillard, T.R., Schuster, D.P., Osei, K. (1998). Gender differences in cardiovascular risk factors in obese, nondiabetic first degree relatives of African Americans with type 2 diabetes mellitus. Ethn Dis, 8 (3), 319–30.

Gallagher, R.P., Bajdik, C.D., Fincham, S., et al. (1996). Chemical exposures, medical history, and risk of squamous and basal cell carcinoma of the skin. Cancer Epidemiol Biomarkers Prev, 5 (6), 419–24.

Garcia, A.M. (2003). Pesticide exposure and women's health. Am J Ind Med, 44 (6), 584–94.

Garland, C.F., Garland, F.C., Gorham, E.D. (1993). Rising trends in melanoma. An hypothesis concerning sunscreen effectiveness. Ann Epidemiol, 3 (1), 103–10.

Gaudet, M.M., Britton, J.A., Kabat, G.C., et al. (2004). Fruits, vegetables, and micronutrients in relation to breast cancer modified by menopause and hormone receptor status. Cancer Epidemiol Biomarkers Prev, 13 (9), 1485–94.

Gavard, J.A., Lustman, P.J., Clouse, R.E. (1993). Prevalence of depression in adults with diabetes. Diabetes Care, 16 (8), 1167–78.

Gavin, J.R. (2004). Slowing cardiovascular disease progression in African-American patients: diabetes management. Journal of Clinical Hypertension, 6 (4 Suppl 1), 26–33.

Geller, A.C., Annas, G.D. (2003). Epidemiology of melanoma and nonmelanoma skin cancer. Semin Oncol Nurs, 19 (1), 2–11.

Gibbs, P., Anderson, C., Pearlman, N., et al. (2002). A phase II study of neoadjuvant biochemotherapy for stage III melanoma. Cancer, 94 (2), 470–6.

Gibson, J.N., Waddell, G., Grant, I.C. (2000). Surgery for degenerative lumbar spondylosis. Cochrane Database Syst Rev, 3, CD001352.

Gies, P., Wright, J. (2003). Measured solar ultraviolet radiation exposure of outdoor workers in Queensland in the building and construction industry. Photochem Photobiol, 78 (4), 342–8.

Giesecke, T., Williams, D.A., Harris, R.E. (2003). Subgrouping of fibromyalgia patients on the basis of pressure-pain thresholds and psychological factors. Arthritis Rheum, 48 (10), 2916–22.

Gignac, M.A., Cott, C., Badley, E.M. (2000). Adaptation to chronic illness and disability and its relationship to perceptions of independence and dependence. J Gerontol B Psychol Sci Soc Sci, 55 (6), P362–72.

Gilden, J.L., Hendryx, M.S., Clar, S., et al. (1992). Diabetes support groups improve health care of older diabetic patients. J Am Geriatr Soc, 40 (2), 147–50.

Gillard, M.L., Nwanko, R., Fitzgerald, J.T., et al. (2004). Informal diabetes education: impact on self-management and blood glucose control. Diabetes Educ, 30 (1), 136–42.

Gilworth, G., Chamberlain, M.A., Harvey, A. (2003). Development of work instability scale for rheumatoid arthritis. Arthritis Rheum, 49 (3), 349–54.

Giovannucci, E. (2001). Insulin, insulin-like growth factors and colon cancer: a review of the evidence. J Nutr, 131 (11 Suppl), 3109S–20S.

Giovannucci, E. (2002). Modifiable risk factors for colon cancer. Gastroenterol Clin North Am, 31 (4), 925–43.

Giovannucci, E. (2003). Diet, body weight, and colorectal cancer: a summary of the epidemiologic evidence. J Womens Health (Larchmt), 12 (2), 173–82.

Giovannucci, E., Rimm, E.B., Ascherio, A., et al. (1995). Alcohol, low-methionine—low folate diets, and risk of colon cancer in men. J Natl Cancer Inst, 87 (4), 265–73.

Giraudet-Le Quintrec, J.S., Coste, J., Vastel, L., et al. (2003). Positive effect of patient education for hip surgery: a randomized trial. Clin Orthop, 414, 112–20.

Glassman, A., Shapiro, P. (1998). Depression and the course of coronary artery disease. American Journal of Psychiatry, 155 (1), 4–11.

Glew, R.H., Conn, C.A., Vanderjagt, T.A., et al. (2004). Risk factors for cardiovascular disease and diet of urban and rural dwellers in northern Nigeria. J Health Popul Nutr, 22 (4), 357–69.

Godefroi, R., Klementowicz, P., Pepler, C., et al. (2005). Levels of, and factors associated with C-reactive protein in employees attending a company-sponsored cardiac screening program. Cardiology, 103 (4), 180–4.

Gohlke, H. (2004). Lifestyle modification—is it worth it? Herz, 29 (1), 139–44.

Gold, D.T. (1996). The clinical impact of vertebral fractures: quality of life in women with osteoporosis. Bone, 18 (3 Suppl), 185S–9S.

Gold, D.T. (2001). The nonskeletal consequences of osteoporotic fractures. Psychologic and social outcomes. Rheum Dis Clin North Am, 27 (1), 255–62.

Gold, D.T., Bales, C.W., Lyles, K.W., et al. (1989). Treatment of osteoporosis. The psychological impact of a medical education program on older patients. J Am Geriatr Soc, 37 (5), 417–22.

Goldbohm, R.A., Van den Brandt, P.A., Van den Veer, P., et al. (1994). Prospective study on alcohol consumption and the risk of cancer of the colon and rectum in the Netherlands. Cancer Causes Control, 5 (2), 95–104.

Goldenberg, D.L. (1999). Fibromyalgia syndrome a decade later: what have we learned? Arch Internal Med, 159 (8), 777–85.

Gonzales, G.R. (1995). Central pain: diagnosis and treatment strategies. Neurology, 45 (12 Suppl 9), S11–16; discussion S35–6.

Gonzalez, B., Lupon, J., Parajon, T., et al. (2004). Nurse evaluation of patients in a new multidisciplinary Heart Failure Unit in Spain. Eur J Cardiovasc Nurs, 3 (1), 61–9.

Goodstine, S.L., Zheng, T., Holford, T.R., et al. (2003). Dietary (n – 3)/(n – 6) fatty acid ratio: possible relationship to premenopausal but not postmenopausal breast cancer risk in U.S. women. J Nutr, 133 (5), 1409–14.

Gordon, D.A. (1999). Chronic widespread pain as a medio-legal issue. Baillieres Best Pract Res Clin Rheumatol, 13 (3), 531–43.

Gore, E. (2004). Celecoxib and radiation therapy in non-small-cell lung cancer. Oncology (Huntingt), 18 (14 Suppl), 10–4.

Goya Wannamethee, S., Gerald Shaper, A., Whincup, P.H., et al. (2004). Overweight and obesity and the burden of disease and disability in elderly men. Int J Obes Relat Metab Disorder, 28 (11), 1374–82.

Gracely, R.H., Geisser, M.E., Giesecke, T., et al. (2004). Pain catastrophizing and neural responses to pain among persons with fibromyalgia. Brain, 127 (Pt 4), 835–43.

Grainger, R., Cicuttini, F.M. (2004). Medical management of osteoarthritis of the knee and hip joints. Med J Aust, 180 (5), 232–6.

Grant, P.J. (2005). Inflammatory, atherothrombotic aspects of type 2 diabetes. Curr Med Res Opin, 21 (Suppl 1), 5–12.

Grassi, L., Biancosino, B., Marmai, L., et al. (2004a). Effect of reboxetine on major depressive disorder in breast cancer patients: an open-label study. J Clin Psychiatry, 65 (4), 515–20.

Grassi, L., Rossi, E., Sabato, S., et al. (2004b). Diagnostic criteria for psychosomatic research and psychosocial variables in breast cancer patients. Psychosomatics, 45 (6), 483–91.

Grassi, L., Travado, L., Moncayo, F.L., et al. (2004c). Psychosocial morbidity and its correlates in cancer patients of the Mediterranean area: findings from the Southern European Psycho-Oncology Study. J Affect Disord, 83 (2–3), 243–8.

Greenfield, S., Fitzcharles, MA., Esdaile, J.M. (1992). Reactive fibromyalgia syndrome. Arthritis Rheum, 35 (6), 678–81.

Greer, S., Moorey, S., Baruch, J.D., et al. (1992). Adjuvant psychological therapy for patients with cancer: a prospective randomized trial. BMJ, 304 (6828), 675–80.

Grodstein, F., Manson, J.E., Stampfer, M.J. (2001). Postmenopausal hormone use and secondary prevention of coronary events in the nurses' health study. A prospective, observational study. Ann Intern Med, 135 (1), 1–8.

Gruber, A.J., Hudson, J.I. (1996). The management of treatment-resistant depression in disorders on the interface of psychiatry and medicine. Psychiatric Clinics North America, 19 (2), 351–69.

Gruber, U., Fegg, M., Buchmann, M., et al. (2003). The long-term psychosocial effects of haematopoetic stem cell transplantation. Eur J Cancer Care (Engl), 12 (3), 249–56.

Guenel, P., Laforest, L., Cyr, D., et al. (2001). Occupational risk factors in ultraviolet radiation, and ocular melanoma: a case-control study in France. Cancer Causes Control, 12 (5), 451–9.

Guerreiro da Silva, J.B., Nakamura, M.U., Cordeiro, J.A., et al. (2004). Acupuncture for low back pain in pregnancy—a prospective, quasi-randomised controlled study. Acupuncture Med, 22 (2), 60–7.

Gulliford, M.C., Sedgwick, J.E., Pearce, A.J. (2003). Cigarette smoking, health status, socio-economic status and access to health care in diabetes mellitus: a cross-sectional survey. BMC Health Serv Res, 3 (1), 4.

Gupta, R., Gupta, V.P., Sarna, M., et al. (2003). Serial epidemiological surveys in an urban Indian population demonstrate increasing coronary risk factors among the lower socioeconomic strata. J Assoc Physicians India, 51, 470–7.

Gupta, S., Mukhtar, H. (2002). Chemoprevention of skin cancer: current status and future prospects. Cancer Metastasis Rev, 21 (3–4), 363–80.

Guralnik, J.M., Ferrucci, L., Balfour, J.L., et al. (2001). Progressive versus catastrophic loss of the ability to walk: implications for the prevention of mobility loss. J Am Geriatr Soc, 49 (11), 1463–70.

Guzman, J., Esmail, R., Karjalainen, K., et al. (2001). Multidisciplinary rehabilitation for chronic low back pain: systematic review. Br Med J, 322, 1511–16.

Haase, J.E., Phillips, C.R. (2004). The adolescent/young adult experience. J Pediatr Oncol Nurs, 21 (3), 145–9.

Hadjistavropoulos, G.J.G., Asmundson, D.L., LaChapelle, A.Q. (2002). The role of health anxiety among patients with chronic pain in determining response to therapy. Pain Research and Management, 7 (3), 127–33.

Haffner, S.J., Cassells, H. (2003). Hyperglycemia as a cardiovascular risk factor. American Journal of Medicine, 115 (Suppl 8A), 6S–11S.

Hahn, R.A., Heath, G.W., Chang, M.H. (1998). Cardiovascular disease risk factors and preventive practices among adults—United States, 1994: a behavioral risk factor atlas. Behavior Risk Factor Surveillance System State Coordinators. MMWR CDC Surveillance Summ, 47 (5), 35–69.

Hakkinen, A., Sokka, T., Lietsalmi, A.M., et al. (2003). Effects of dynamic strength training on physical function, Valpar 9 work sample test, and working capacity in patients with recent-onset rheumatoid arthritis. Arthritis Rheum, 49 (1), 71–7.

Haldeman, S. (1999). Low back pain: current physiologic concepts. Neurol Clin, 17 (1), 1–15.

Haley, W.E. (2003). Family caregivers of elderly patients with cancer: understanding and minimizing the burden of care. J Support Oncol, 1 (4 Suppl 2), 25–9.

Hamdy, O. (2005). Lifetyle modification and endothelial function in obese subjects. Expert Rev Cardiovasc Ther, 3 (2), 231–41.

Hammar, N., Alfredsson, L., Johnson, J.V. (1998). Job strain, social support at work, and incidence of myocardial infarction. Occup Environ Med, 55 (8), 548–53.

Hammerlid, E., Ahlner-Elmqvist, M., Bjordal, K., et al. (1999). A prospective multicentre study in Sweden and Norway of mental distress and psychiatric morbidity in head and neck cancer patients. Br J Cancer, 80 (5–6), 766–74.

Han, D.F., Zhou, X., Hu, M.B., et al. (2004). Sulfotransferase 1A1 (SULT1A1) polymorphism and breast cancer risk in Chinese women. Toxicol Lett, 150 (2), 167–77.

Han, W.T., Collie, K., Koopman, C. (2004). Breast cancer and problems with medical interactions: Relationships with traumatic stress, emotional self-efficacy, and social support. Psychooncology, Epub ahead of print.

Hansen, L.B., Vondracek, S.F. (2004). Prevention and treatment of nonpostmenopausal osteoporosis. Am J Health Syst Pharm, 61 (24), 2637–54.

Harding, A.H., Day, N.E., Khaw, K.T., et al. (2004). Dietary fat and the risk of clinical type 2 diabetes: the European prospective investigation of Cancer-Norfolk study. American Journal of Epidemiology, 159 (1), 73–82.

Harris, J.E., Thun, M.J., Mondul, A.M., et al. (2004). Cigarette tar yields in relation to mortality from lung cancer in the cancer prevention study II prospective cohort, 1982–8. BMJ, 328 (7431), 72.

Harrison, B.J. (2002). Influence of cigarette smoking on disease outcome in rheumatoid arthritis. Curr Opin Rheumatol, 14 (2), 93–7.

Hart, L.G., Deyo, R.A., Cherkin, D.C. (1995). Physician office visits for low back pain. Frequency, clinical evaluation, and treatment patterns from a U.S. national survey. Spine, 20, 11–19.

Harwood, K.V. (2004). Advances in endocrine therapy for breast cancer: considering efficacy, safety, and quality of life. Clin J Oncol Nurs, 8 (6), 629–37.

Hashimoto, A., Sato, H., Nishibayahi, Y., et al. (2002). A multicenter cross-sectional study on the health related quality of life of patients with rheumatoid arthritis using a revised Japanese version of the arthritis impact measurement scales version 2 (AIMS 2), focusing on the medical care costs and their associative factors. Ryumachi, 42 (1), 23–39.

Hasserius, R., Karlsson, M.K., Nilsson, B.E., et al. (2003). Prevalent vertebral deformities predict increased mortality and increased fracture rate in both men and women: a 10-year population-based study of 598 individuals from the Swedish cohort in the European Vertebral Osteoporosis Study. Osteoporos Int, 14 (1), 61–8.

Hay, E.K. (1991). That old hip. The osteoporosis process. Nur Clin North Am, 26 (1), 43–51.

Hay, E.M. (2005). Comparison of physical treatments versus a brief pain-management programme for back pain in primary care: a randomized clinical trial in physiotherapy practice. Lancet, 365 (9476), 2024–30.

Hayashi, T., Tsumura, K., Suematsu, C., et al. (1999). High normal blood pressure, hypertension, and the risk of type 2 diabetes in Japanese men. The Osaka Health Survey. Diabetes Care, 22 (10), 1683–7.

Haywood, L.J., Ell, K., deGuman, M., et al. (1993). Chest pain admissions: characteristics of black, Latino, and white patients in low- and mid-socioeconomic strata. J Natl Med Assoc, 85 (10), 749–57.

Hazard, R.G., Reid, S., Haugh, L.D., et al. (2000). A controlled trial of an educational pamphlet to prevent disability after occupational low back injury. Spine, 25, 1419–23.

Healy, W.L., Ayers, M.E., Iorio, R., et al. (1998). Impact of a clinical pathway and implant standardization on total hip arthroplasty: a clinical and economic study of short-term patient outcome. J Arthroplasty, 13 (3), 266–76.

Heller, S. (2004). Weight gain during insulin therapy in patients with type 2 diabetes mellitus. Diabetes Res Clin Pract, 65 (Suppl 1), S23–7.

Hemingway, H., Shipley, M.J., Stansfeld, S. (1997). Sickness absence from back pain, psychosocial work characteristics and employment grade among office workers. Scand J Work Environ Health, 23 (2), 121–9.

Henriksson, C., Liedberg, G. (2000). Factors of importance for work disability in women with fibromyalgia. J Rheumatol, 27 (5), 1271–6.

Hersh, W.R., Wallace, J.A., Patterson, P.K., et al. (2001). Telemedicine for the Medicare population: pediatric, obstetric, and clinician-indirect home interventions. Evid Rep Technol Assess (Summ), (24 Suppl), 1–32.

Hevey, D., Brown, A., Cahill, A., et al. (2003). Four-week multidisciplinary cardiac rehabilitation produces similar improvements in exercise capacity and quality of life to a 10-week program. J Cardiopulm Rehabil, 23 (1), 17–21.

Hewitt, M., Rowland, J.H., Yancik, R. (2003). Cancer survivors in the United States: age, health, and disability. J Gerontol A Biol Sci Med Sci, 58 (1), 82–91.

Higashi, Y., Chayama, K. (2002). Renal endothelial dysfunction and hypertension. J Diabetes Complications, 16 (1), 103–7.

Hill, C.L., Parsons, J., Taylor, A., et al. (1999). Health related quality of life in a population sample with arthritis. J Rheumatol, 26 (9), 2029–35.

Hill-Briggs, F., Cooper, D.C., Loman, K., et al. (2003). A qualitative study of problem solving and diabetes control in type 2 diabetes self-management. Diabetes Educ, 29 (6), 1018–28.

Holmboe, E.S., Meehan, T.P., Radford, M.J., et al. (1999). Use of critical pathways to improve the care of patients with acute myocardial infarction. Am J Med, 107 (4), 324–31.

Honkanen, R., Tuppurainen, M., Kroger, H., et al. (1998). Relationships between risk factors and fractures differ by type of fracture: a population-based study of 12,192 perimenopausal women. Osteoporos Int, 8 (1), 25–31.

Hoogendoorn, W.E., Bongers, P.M., de Vet, H.C., et al. (2000). Flexion and rotation of the trunk and lifting at work are risk factors for low back pain: results of a prospective cohort study. Spine, 25 (23), 3087–92.

Hoogendoorn, W.E., Bongers, P.M., de Vet, H.C., et al. (2001). Psychosocial work characteristics and psychological strain in relation to low-back pain. Scand J Work Environ Health, 27 (4), 258–67.

Hoogendoorn, W.E., Bongers, P.M., de Vet, H.C., et al. (2002). Comparison of two different approaches for the analysis of data from a prospective cohort study: an application of data from a prospective cohort study: an application to work related risk factors for low back pain. Occup Environ Med, 59 (7), 459–65.

Horne, B.D., Muhlestein, J.B., Lappe, D.L., et al. (2004). Less affluent area of residence and lesser-insured status predict an increased risk of death or myocardial infarction after angiographic diagnosis of coronary disease. Ann Epidemiol, 14 (2), 143–50.

Horsten, M., Mittleman, M.A.,Wamala, S.P., et al. (2000). Depressive symptoms and lack of social integration in relation to prognosis of CHD in middle-aged women. The Stockholm Female Coronary Risk Study. Eur Heart J, 21 (13), 1072–80.

Horwitz, E.B., Thorell, T., Anderberg, U.M. (2003). Fibromyalgia patients' own experiences of video self-interpretation: a phenomenological-hermeneutic study. Scand J Caring Sci, 17 (3), 257–64.

Hossain, M.A., Sengupta, M.K., Ahmed, S., et al. (2005). Ineffectiveness and poor reliability of arsenic removal plants in West Bangal. Environ Sci Technol, 39 (11), 4300–6.

Howard, V.J., Acker, J., Gomez, C.R., et al. (2004). An approach to coordinate efforts to reduce the public health burden of stroke: the Delta States Stroke Consortium. Prev Chronic Dis, 1 (4), A19, Epub 2004 Sep 15.

Howe, H.L. Wolfgang, P.E., Burnett, W.S., et al. (1989). Cancer incidence following exposure to drinking water with asbestos leachate. Public Health Rep, 104 (3), 251–6.

Hsu, V.M., Patella, S.J., Sigal, L.H. (1993). "Chronic Lyme disease" as the incorrect diagnosis in patients with fibromyalgia. Arthritis Rheum, 36 (11), 1493–500.

Hu, F.B. (2003). Sedentary lifestyle and risk of obesity and type 2 diabetes. Lipids, 38 (2), 103–8.

Hu, F.B., Grodstein, F. (2002). Postmenopausal hormone therapy and the risk of cardiovascular disease: the epidemiologic evidence. Am J Cardiol, 90 (1A), 26F–29F.

Hu, F.B., Manson, J.E., Stampfer, M.J., et al. (2001). Diet, lifestyle, and the risk of type 2 diabetes. New England Journal of Medicine, 345 (11), 790–7.

REFERENCES

265

Hu, F.B., van Dam, R.M., & Liu, S. (2001). Diet and risk of Type II diabetes: the role of types of fat and carbohydrate. Diabetologia, 44 (7), 805–17.

Huang, C., Ross, P.D., Wasnich, R.D. (1996). Vertebral fracture and other predictors of physical impairment and health care utilization. Arch Intern Med, 156 (21), 2469–75.

Huang, M.H., Chen, C.H., Chen, T.W., et al. (2000). The effect of weight reduction on the rehabilitation of patients with knee osteoarthritis and obesity. Arthritis Care Res, 13 (6), 398–405.

Hughes, S.L., Seymour, R.B., Campbell, R., et al. (2004). Impact of the fit and strong intervention on older adults with osteoarthritis. Gerontologist, 44 (2), 217–28.

Hulley, S., Grady, D., Bush, T., et al. (1998). Randomized trial of estrogen plus progestin for secondary prevention of coronary heart disease in postmenopausal women. Heart and Estrogen/progestin Replacement Study (HERS) Research Group. JAMA, 280 (7), 605–13.

Humphreys, C.G., Eck, J.C., Hodges, S.D. (2002). Neuroimaging in low back pain. American Family Physician, 65 (11), 1–12, http://www.aafp.org/afp/2002061/2299.html.

Hung, J., McQuillan, B.M., Chapman, C.M., et al. (2005). Elevated interleukin-18 levels are associated with the metabolic syndrome independent of obesity and insulin resistance. Arterioscler Thromb Vasc Biol, March 24 (Epub ahead of print).

Hurwitz, E.L., Morgenstern, H., Harber, P., et al. (2002). A randomized trial of medical care with and without physical therapy and chiropractic care. Spine, 27 (20), 2193–204.

Hydrie, M.Z., Basit, A., Ahmedani, M.Y., et al. (2005). Comparison of risk factors for diabetes in children of different socioeconomic status. J Coll Physicians Surg Pak, 15 (2), 74–7.

Imaginis, Breast Cancer Treatment- Sentinel lymph node biopsy, http://imaginis.com.

Indahl, A., Haldorsen, E.M.H., Holm, S., et al. (1998). Five-year follow-up study of a controlled clinical trial using light mobilization and an informative approach to low back pain. Spine, 23, 2625–30.

Indahl, A., Velund, L., Reikeraas, O., et al. (1995). Good prognosis for low back pain when left untampered: a randomized clinical trial. Spine, 20, 473–77.

Irons, B.K., Mazzolini, T.A., Greene, R.S. (2004). Delaying the onset of type 2 diabetes mellitus in patients with prediabetes. Pharmacotherapy, 24 (3), 362–71.

Ismail, A.A., Cockerill, W., Cooper, C., et al. (2001). Prevalent vertebral deformity predicts incident hip though not distal forearm fracture: results from the European Prospective Osteoporosis Study. Osteoporos Int, 12 (2), 85–90.

Iwasaki, Y., Butcher, J. (2004). Coping with stress among middle-aged and older women and men with arthritis. The Int J of Psychosocial Rehabilitation, 8, 179–208.

Izawa, K., Hirano, Y., Yamada, S., et al. (2004). Improvement in physiological outcomes and health-related quality of life following cardiac rehabilitation in patients with acute myocardial infarction. Circ J, 68 (4), 315–20.

Izquierdo, R.E., Knudson, P.E., Meyer, S., et al. (2003). A comparison of diabetes education administered through telemedicine versus in person. Diabetes Care, 26 (4), 1002–7.

Jaar, B.G., Astor, B.C., Berns, J.S., et al. (2004). Predictors of amputation and survival following lower extremity revascularization in hemodialysis patients. Kidney Int, 65 (2), 613–20.

Jacob, T., Baras, M., Zeev, A., et al. (2004). A longitudinal, community-based study of low back pain outcomes. Spine, 29 (16), 1810–17.

Jakes, R.W., Day, N.E., Khaw, K.T., et al. (2003). Television viewing and low participation in vigorous recreation are independently associated with obesity and markers of cardiovascular disease risk: EPIC-Norfolk population-based study. Eur J Clin Nutr, 57 (9), 1089–96.

James, P.T., Rigby, N., Leach, R., et al. (2004). The obesity epidemic, metabolic syndrome and future prevention strategies. Eur J Cardiovasc Prev Rehabil, 11 (1), 3–8.

Jemal, A., Tiwari, R.C., Murray, T., et al. (2004). Cancer statistics. CA Cancer J Clin, 54 (1), 8–29.

Jensen, M.P., Nielson, W.R., Turner, J.A., et al. (2003). Readiness to self-manage pain is associated with coping and with psychological and physical functioning among patients with chronic pain. Pain, 104 (3), 529–37.

Jernstrom, H., Lerman, C., Ghadirian, P., et al. (1999). Pregnancy and risk of early breast cancer in carriers of BRCA1 and BRCA2. Lancet, 354 (9193), 1846–50.

Jernstrom, H., Lubinski, J., Lynch, H.T., et al. (2004). Breast-feeding and the risk of breast cancer in BRCA1 and BRCA2 mutation carriers. J Natl Cancer Inst, 96 (14), 1094–8.

Johansen, C. (2004). Electromagnetic fields and health effects—epidemiologic studies of cancer, diseases of the central nervous system and arrhythmia-related heart disease. Scand J Work Environ Health, 30 (Suppl 1), 1–30.

Journal of Bone Mineral Res (April 2002). Incidence of vertebral fracture in Europe: results from the European Prospective Osteoporosis Study. 17 (4), 716–24.

Journal of Bone Mineral Res (December 2002). The relationship between bone density and incident vertebral fracture in men and women. 17 (12), 2214–21.

Journal of Medical Practice Management (July–August 2004). Medical malpractice litigation raises health-care cost, reduces access, and lower quality of care. 20 (1), 44–51.

Ju, W.D., Krupa, D.A., Walters, D.J., et al. (2001). (211) a placebo-controlled trial of rofecoxib in the treatment of chronic low back pain. Pain Med, 2 (3), 242–3.

Kaaks, R. Lukanova, A. (2002). Effects of weight control and physical activity in cancer prevention: role of endogenous hormone metabolism. Ann N Y Acad Sci, 963, 268–81.

Kadam, U.T., Jordan, K., Croft, P.R. (2004). Clinical comorbidity in patients with osteoarthritis: a case-control study of general practice consulters in England and Wales. Ann Rheum Dis, 63 (4), 408–14.

Kaleta Stasiolek, D., Kwasniewska, M., Drygas, W. (2003). Selected risk factors and primary prevention of colorectal cancer. Przegl Lek, 60 (3), 170–5.

Kapidzic-Basci, N., Seleskovic, H., Mulic, S. (2004). Criteria for work capacity evaluation in rheumatoid arthritis. Med Arc, 58 (1), 39–41.

Kaplan, M.S., Huguet, N., Newsom, J.T., et al. (2003). Characteristics of physically inactive older adults with arthritis: results of a population-based study. Prev Med, 37 (1), 61–7.

Karjalainen, K., Malmivaara, A., van Tulder, M., et al. (2001). Multidisciplinary biopsychosocial rehabilitation for subacute low back pain among working age adults. (Cochrane review) Spine, 26, 262–9.

Karoff, M., Roseler, S., Lorenz, C., et al. (2000). Intensified after-care—a method for improving occupational reintegration after myocardial infarct and/or bypass operation. Z Kardiol, 89 (5), 423–33.

Katz, M.R., Irish, J.C., Devins, G.M. (2004). Development and pilot testing of a psychoeducational intervention for oral cancer patients. Psychooncology, 13 (9), 642–53.

Katz, N., Rodgers, D.B., Krupa, D., et al. (2004). Onset of pain relief with rofecoxib in chronic low back pain: results of two four-week, randomized, placebo-controlled trials. Curr Med Res Opin, 20 (5), 651–8.

Kaur, S., Cohen, A. Dolor, R., et al. (2004). The impact of environmental tobacco smoke on women's risk of dying from heart disease: a meta-analysis. J Womens Health (Larchmt), 13 (8), 888–97.

Keck, M. (2000). Optimization of the transition from phase I to III of cardiac rehabilitation. Rehabilitation, 39 (2), 101–5.

Kelsey, J.L., White, A.A., 3rd (1980). Epidemiology and impact of low back pain. Spine, 5, 133–42.

Kerns, R.D., Otis, J.D. (2003). Family therapy for persons experiencing pain: evidence for its effectiveness. Seminars in Pain Medicine.

Kerns, R.D., Otis, J.D. (2004). Family therapy for persons with chronic pain. Pain Clinic Perspectives.

Kerns, R.D., Otis, J.D., Wise, E. (2002). Treating families of chronic pain patients: application of a cognitive-behavioral transactional model. In RJ Gatchel and DC Turk, Psychological Approaches to Pain Management, 2nd edition, New York: Guilford Press.

Ketola, E., Sipila, R., Makela, M. (2000). Effectiveness of individual lifestyle interventions in reducing cardiovascular disease and risk factors. Ann Med, 32 (4), 239–51.

Khang, Y.H., Lynch, J.W., Kaplan, G.A. (2004). Health inequalities in Korea: age- and sex-specific educational differences in the 10 leading causes of death. Int J Epidemiol, 33 (2), 299–308.

Khor, G.L. (2004). Dietary fat quality: a nutritional epidemiologist's view. Asia Pac J Clin Nutr, 13 (Suppl), S22.

Kim, H.S. (2003). The comparison of the stress and coping methods of cancer patients and their caregivers. Taehan Kanho Hakhoe Chi, 33 (5), 538–43.

Kimble, L.P., McGuire, D.B., Dunbar, S.B., et al. (2003). Gender differences in pain characteristics of chronic stable angina and perceived physical limitation in patients with coronary artery disease. Pain, 101 (1–2), 45–53.

King, R.B. (1981). Neuropharmacology of depression, anxiety and pain. Clinical Neuro-surgery, 28, 116–36.

Kington, R.S., Smith, J.P. (1997). Socioeconomic status and racial and ethnic differences in functional status associated with chronic diseases. Am J Public Health, 87 (5), 805–10.

Kiortsis, D.N., Filippatos, T.D., Elisaf, M.S. (2005). The effects of orlistat on metabolic parameters and other cardiovascular risk factors., Diabetes Metab, 31 (1), 15–22.

Kirkhorn, S., Greenlee, R.T., Reeser, J.C. (2003). The epidemiology of agriculture-related osteoarthritis and its impact on occupational disability. WMJ, 102 (7), 38–44.

Kirman, I., Poltoratskaia, N., Sylla, P., et al. (2004). Insulin-like growth factor-binding protein 3 inhibits growth of experimental colocarcinoma. Surgery, 136 (2), 205–9.

Kissel, W., Mahnig, P. (1998). Fibromyalgia (generalized tendomyopathy) in expert assessment. Analysis of 158 cases. Schweiz Rudnsch Med Prax, 87 (16), 538–45.

Kliukiene, J. Tynes, T., Andersen, A. (2004). Residential and occupational exposures to 50-Hz magnetic fields and breast cancer in women: a population-based study. Am J Epidemiol, 159 (9), 852–61.

Koes, B.W., Assendelft, W.J., van der Heijden, G.J., et al. (1996). Spinal manipulation for low back pain. An updated systematic review of randomized clinical trials. Spine, 21, 2860–73.

Koes, B.W., Scholten, R.J., Mens, J.M., et al. (1995). Efficacy of epidural steroid injections for low back pain and sciatica: a systematic review of randomized clinical trials. Pain, 63, 279–88.

Koes, B., van Tulder, M., van der Windt, W.M., et al. (1994). The efficacy of back schools: a review of randomized clinical trials. J Clin Epidemiol, 47, 851–62.

Koh-Banerjee, P., Chu, N.F., Spiegelman, D., et al. (2003). Prospective study of the association of changes in dietary intake, physical activity, alcohol consumption, and smoking with 9-y gain in waist circumference among 16,587 US men. American Journal of Clinical Nutrition, 78 (4), 719–27.

Kollbrunner, J., Zbaren, P., Quack, K. (2001). Quality of life stress in patients with large tumors of the mouth. 2: Dealing with the illness: coping, anxiety and depressive symptoms. HNO, 49 (12), 998–1007.

Konecny, G.E., Pegram, M.D. (2004). Gemcitabine in combination with trastuzumab and/or platinum salts in breast cancer cells with HER2 overexpression. Oncology (Huntingt), 18 (14 Suppl 12), 32–6.

Koster, A., Bosma, H., Kempen, G.I., et al. (2004). Socioeconomic inequalities in mobility decline in chronic disease groups (asthma/COPD, heart disease, diabetes mellitus, low back pain): only a minor role for disease severity and comorbidity. J Epidemiol Community Health, 58 (10), 862–9.

Koukouli, S., Vlachonikolis, I.G., Philalithis, A. (2002). Socio-demographic factors and self-reported functional status: the significance of social support. BMC Health Serv Res, 2 (1), 20.

Kozek, E., Gorska, A., Fross, K., et al. (2003). Chronic complications and risk factors in patients with type 1 diabetes mellitus—retrospective analysis. Przegl Lek, 60 (12), 773–7.

Kraemer, K.H., Lee, M.M., Andrew, A.D., et al. (1994). The role of sunlight and DNA repair in melanoma and nonmelanoma skin cancer. The xeroderma pigmentosum paradigm. Arch Dermatol, 130 (8), 1018–21.

Kralik, D., Koch, T., Price, K., et al. (2004). Chronic illness self-management: taking action to create order. J Clin Nurse, 13 (2), 259–67.

Krause, N., Ragland, D.R., Greiner, B.A., et al. (1997). Psychosocial job factors associated with back and neck pain in public transit operators. Scand J Work Environ Health, 23 (3), 179–86.

Krewski, D., Lubin, J.H., Zielinski, J.M., et al. (2005). Residential radon and risk of lung cancer: a combined analysis of 7 North American case-control studies. Epidemiology, 16 (2) 137–45.

Kricker, A., Armstrong, B.K., English, D.R., et al. (1995). A dose-response curve for sun exposure and basal cell carcinoma. Int J Cancer, 60 (4), 482–8.

Krieger, N., Quesenberry, C. Jr., Peng, T., et al. (1999). Social class, race/ethnicity, and incidence of breast, cervix, colon, lung, and prostate cancer among Asian, Black, Hispanic, and White residents of the San Francisco Bay Area, 1988–92 (United States), Cancer Causes Control, 10 (6), 525–37.

Kriegsman, D.M., Deeg, D.J., Stalman, W.A. (2004). Comorbidity of somatic chronic diseases and decline in physical functioning: the Longitudinal Aging Study Amsterdam. J Clin Epdemiol, 57 (1), 55–65.

Krishnan, E., Sokka, T., Hannonen, P. (2003). Smoking-gender interaction and risk for rheumatoid arthritis. Arhtritis Res Ther, 5 (3), R158–62.

Krousel-Wood, M.A., Muntner, P., He, J., et al. (2004). Primary prevention of essential hypertension. Med Clin North Am, 88 (1), 223–38.

Kuehn, T., Bembenek, A., Decker, T., et al. (2005). A concept for the clinical implementation of sentinel lymph node biopsy in patients with breast carcinoma with special regard to quality assurance. Cancer, 103 (3), 451–61.

Kuller, L.H. (2004). Ethnic differences in atherosclerosis, cardiovascular disease and lipid metabolism. Curr Opin Lipidol, 15 (2), 109–13.

Kumari, M., Head, J., Marmot, M., et al. (2004). Prospective study of social and othr risk factors for incidence of type 2 diabetes in the Whitehall II study. Arch Int Med, 164 (17), 1873–80.

Kuper, H., Marmot, M. (2003). Job strain, job demands, decision latitude, and risk of coronary heart disease within the Whitehall II study. J Epidemiol Community Health, 57 (2), 147–53.

Kurihara, T., Tomiyama, H., Hashimoto, H., et al. (2004). Excessive alcohol intake increases the risk of arterial stiffening in men with normal blood pressure. Hypertens Res, 27 (9), 669–73.

Kushnir, T., Luria, O. (2002). Supervisors' attitudes toward return to work after myocardial infarction or coronary artery bypass graft. J Occup Environ Med, 44 (4), 331–7.

Kwan, J., Sandercock, P. (2004). In-hospital care pathways for stroke. Cochrane Database Syst Rev, 4, CD002924.

Kyngas, H. (2003). Patient education: perspective of adolescents with a chronic disease. J Clin Nurs, 12 (5), 744–51.

Labreche, F., Goldberg, M.S., Valois, M.F., et al. (2003). Occupational exposures to extremely low frequency magnetic fields and postmenopausal breast cancer. Am J In Med, 44 (6), 643–52.

Lacey, E.A., Musgrave, R.J., Freeman, J.V., et al. (2004). Psychological morbidity after myocardial infarction in an area of deprivation in the UK: evaluation of a self-help package. Eur J Cardiovasc Nurs, 3 (3), 219–24.

Lambert, C.E., Jr., Lambert, V.A. (1999). Psychological hardiness: state of the science. Holistic Nurs Pract, 13 (3), 11–19.

Lambert, V.A., Lambert, C.E., Klipple, G.L. (1990). Relationships among hardiness, social support, severity of illness, and psychological well-being in women with rheumatoid arthritis. Health Care Women Int, 11 (2), 159–73.

Lane, D., Carroll, D., Ring, C., et al. (2000). Effects of depression and anxiety on mortality and quality-of-life 4 months after myocardial infarction. J Psychosom Res, 49 (4), 229–38.

Lang, I., Hitre, E. (2004). Recent results in irinotecan therapy in colorectal cancer. Magy Onkol, 48 (4), 281–8. Epub 2005 Jan 17.

Langer, F., Helsberg, K., Schutte, W.H., et al. (2005). Gemcitabine in the first line therapy of advanced and metastatic non-small-cell lung carcinoma (NSCLC): review of the results of phase III studies. Onkologie, 28 (Suppl 1), 1–28. Epub 2005 Mar 30.

Langer, H.E., Ehlebracht-Konig, I., Mattussek, S. (2003). Quality assurance of rheumatologic patient education. Z Arztl Fortbild Qualitatssich, 97 (6), 357–63.

Larsson, S.C., Rafter, J., Holmberg, L., et al. (2005). Red meat consumption and rik of cancers of the proximal colon, distal colon and rectum: the Swedish Mammography Cohort. Int J Cancer, 113 (5), 829–34.

Latza, U., Pfahlberg, A., Gefeller, O. (2002). Impact of repetitive manual materials handling and psychosocial work factors on the future prevalence of chronic low-back pain among construction workers. Scand J Work Environ Health, 28 (5), 314–23.

Laufer, E.M., Hartman, T.J., Baer, D.J., et al. (2004). Effects of moderate alcohol consumption on folate and vitamin B (12) status in postmenopausal women. Eur J Clin Nutr, May 12 (Epub ahead of print).

Lavery, L.A., Ashry, H.R., van Houtum, W., et al. (1996). Variation in the incidence and proportion of diabetes-related amputations in minorities. Diabetes Care, 19 (1), 48–52.

Le, H., Dahle, S., Kang, J., et al. (2002). African-American/White differences in hypertension and ankle pain among insulin-dependent diabetics. (abstract) Diabetes, 51, Supplement 2, #2082.

Lean, M.E., Han, T.S., Seidell, J.C. (1999). Impairment of health and quality of life using new US federal guidelines for the identification of obesity. Arch Intern Med, 159 (8), 837–43.

Lee, J.R., Paultre, F., Mosca, L. (2005). The association between educational level and risk of cardiovascular disease fatality among women with cardiovascular disease. Womens Health Issues, 15 (2), 80–8.

Lee, J.T., Kim, H., Cho, Y.S., et al. (2003). Air pollution and hospital admissions for ischemic heart diseases among individuals 64+ years of age residing in Seoul, Korea. Arch Environ Health, 58 (10), 617–23.

Leiter, L.A. (2005). Diabetic dyslipidaemia: Effective management reduces cardiovascular risk. Atheroscler Suppl, 6 (2), 37–43.

Lemaire, J.P., Skalli, W., et al. (1997). Invertebral disc prothesis. Results and prospects for the year 2000. Clin Orthop, 337, 64–76.

Lerner, D., Reed, J.I., Massarotti, E., et al. (2002). The Work Limitations Questionnaire's validity and reliability among patients with osteoarthritis. J Clin Epidemiol, 55 (2), 197–208.

Lethbridge-Cejku, M., Helmick, C.G., Popovic, J.R. (2003). Hospitalizations for arthritis and other rheumatic conditions: data from the 1997 National Hospital Discharge Survey. Med Care, 41 (12), 1367–73.

Leveille, S.G. (2004). Musculoskeletal aging. Curr Opin Rheumatol, 16 (2), 114–18.

Li, J.J., Chen, J.L. (2005). Inflammation may be a bridge connecting hypertension and atherosclerosis. Med Hypotheses, 64 (5), 925–9.

Liedberg, G.M. Henriksson, C.M. (2002). Factors of importance for work disability in women with fibromyalgia: an interview study. Arthritis Rheum, 47 (3), 266–74.

Lightwood, J. (2003). The economics of smoking and cardiovascular disease. Prog Cardiovasc Dis, 46 (1), 39–78.

Lim, J., Morewitz, S., Dintcho, A., Babros, D., St.Louis, J. (2002). Ankle joint symptoms among insulin-dependent and non-insulin-dependent diabetics. (abstract) Diabetes, 51, Supplement 2, #2235.

Lim, J.G., Kang, H.J., Stewart, K.J. (2004). Type 2 diabetes in Singapore: the role of exercise training for its prevention and management. Singapore Medical Journal, 45 (2), 62–8.

Lin, Y.K., Su, J.Y., Lin, G.T., et al. (2002). Impact of a clinical pathway for total knee arthroplasty. Kaohsiung J Med Sci, 18 (3), 134–40.

Lindelof, B., Granath, F., Dal, H. (2003). Sun habits in kidney transplant recipients with skin cancer: a case-control study of possible causative factors. Acta Derm Venereol, 83 (3), 189–93.

Lindsay, R., Scheele, W.H., Neer, R., et al. (2004). Sustained vertebral fracture risk reduction after withdrawal of teriparatide in postmenopausal women with osteoporosis. Arch Intern Med, 164 (18), 2024–30.

Lindstrom, I., Ohlund, C., Eek, C., et al. (1992). Mobility, strength, and fitness after a graded activity program for patients with subacute low back pain. Spine, 17, 641–52.

Linnemeier, G., Rutter, M.K., Barsness, G., et al. (2003). Enhanced External Counterpulsation for the relief of angina in patients with diabetes: safety, efficacy and 1-year clinical outcomes. Am Heart J, 146 (3), 453–8.

Linton, S.J. (1997). A population-based study of the relationship between sexual abuse and back pain: establishing a link. Pain, 73 (1), 47–53.

Linton, S.J., Gotestam, K.G. (1985). Relations between pain, anxiety, mood and muscle tension in chronic pain patients. Psychotherapy Psychosomatics, 43 (2), 90–5.

Linton S., Hellsing, A.L., Larsson, I. (1997). Bridging the gap: support groups do not enhance long-term outcome in chronic back pain. Clin J Pain, 13, 221–8.

Lippuner, K. (2003). Medical treatment of vertebral osteoporosis. Eur Spine J, 12 (Suppl 2), S13–41.

Liu, K., Xu, L., Berger, J.P., et al. (2005). Discovery of a novel series of peroxisome proliferators-activated receptor alpha/gamma dual agonists for the treatment of type 2 diabetes and dyslipidemia. J Med Chem, 48 (7), 2262–5.

Lobo, C.M., Frijling, B.D., Hulscher, M.E., et al. (2004). Effect of a comprehensive intervention program targeting general practice staff on quality of life in patients at high cardiovascular risk: a randomized controlled study. Qual Life Res, 13 (1), 73–80.

Loisel, P., Abenhaim, L., Durand, P., et al. (1997). A population-based, randomized clinical trial on back pain management. Spine, 22, 2911–8.

Loisel, P., Lemaire, J., Poitras, S., et al. (2002). Cost-benefit and cost-effectiveness analysis of disability prevention model for back pain management: a six year follow up study. Occup Environ Med, 59, 807–15.

Loman, N., Johannsson, O., Kristoffersson, U., et al. (2001). Family history of breast and ovarian cancers and BRCA1 and BRCA2 mutations in a population-based series of early-onset breast cancer. J Natl Cancr Inst, 93 (16), 1215–23.

Loomis, D., Browning, S.R., Schenck, A.P., et al. (1997). Cancer mortality among electric utility workers exposed to polychlorinated biphenyls. Occup Environ Med, 54 (10), 720–8.

Lowe, R., Vedhara, K., Bennett, P., et al. (2003). Emotion-related primary and secondary appraisals, adjustment and coping: associations in women awaiting breast disease diagnosis. Br J Health Psychol, 8 (Pt 4), 377–91.

Lu, W.Q., Resnick, H.E., Jablonski, K.A. (2004). Effects of glycaemic control on cardiovascular disease in diabetic American Indians: the Strong Heart Study. Diabet Med, 21 (4), 311–7.

Lubin, J.H., Boice, J.D., Jr. (1997). Lung cancer risk from residential radon: meta-analysis of eight epidemiologic studies. J Natl Cancer Inst, 89 (1), 49–57.

Lubin, J.H., Boice, J.D., Jr., Edling, C., et al. (1995). Lung cancer in radon-exposed miners and estimation of risk from indoor exposure. J Natl Cancer Inst, 87 (11), 817–27.

Lucia, A., Earnest, C., Perez, M. (2003). Cancer-related fatigue: can exercise physiology assist oncologists? Lancet Oncol, 4 (10), 616–25.

Lund, K.E., Lund, M. (2005). Smoking and social inequality in Norway 1998–2000. Tidsskr Nor Laegeforen, 125 (5), 560–3.

Lund, M.B., Kongerud, J., Boe, J., et al. (1996). Cardiopulmonary sequelae after treatment for Hodgkin's disease: increased risk in females? Ann Oncol, 7 (3), 257–64.

Lunt, M., O'Neill, T.W., Felsenberg, D., et al. (2003). Characteristics of a prevalent vertebral deformity predict subsequent vertebral fracture: results from the European Prospective Osteoporosis Study. Bone, 33 (4), 505–13.

Ma, J., Giovannucci, E., Pollak, M., et al. (2004). A prospective study of plasma C-peptide and colorectal cancer risk in men. J Ntl Cancer Inst, 96 (7): 546–53.

MacFarlane, B.V., McBeth, J., Silman, A.J. (2001). Widespread body pain and mortality: prospective population based study. British Medical Journal, 323 (7314), 662–5.

MacFarlane, B.V., Wright, A., O'Callaghan, J. (1997). Chronic neuropathic pain and its control by drugs. Pharmacology Therapy, 75 (1), 1–19.

MacFarlane, G.J., Thomas, E., Papageorgiou, A.C., et al. (1997). Employment and physical work activities as predictors of future low back pain. Spine, 22 (10), 1143–9.

Machold, K.P., Nell, V.P., Stamm, T.A., et al. (2003). The Austrian Early Arthritis Registry. Clin Exp Rheumatol, 21 (5 Suppl 31), S113–7.

Magni, G. Rigatti-Luchini, S., Fracca, F., et al. (1998). Suicidality in chronic abdominal pain. Pain, 76 (1–2), 137–44.

Magni, G. (1987). On the relationship between chronic pain and depression when there is no organic lesion. Pain, 31 (1), 1–21.

Magro Lopez, A.M., Molinero de Miguel, E., Saez Meabe, Y., et al. (2003). Prevalence of main cardiovascular risk factors in women from Biscay. Rev Esp Cardiol, 56 (8), 783–8.

Mailis-Gagnon, A., Furlan, A.D., Sandoval, J.A., et al. (2004). Spinal cord stimulation for chronic pain. Cochrane Database Syst Rev, 3, CD003783.

Maillefert, J.F., Combe, B., Goupille, P., et al. (2004). The 5-yr HAQ-disability is related to the first year's changes in the narrowing, rather than erosion score in patients with recent-onset rheumatoid arthritis. Rheumatology (Oxford), 43 (1), 79–84. Epub 2003 Nov 17.

Major, G.C., Piche, M.E., Bergeron, J., et al. (2005). Energy expenditure from physical activity and the metabolic risk profile at menopause. Med Sci Sports Exerc, 37 (2), 204–12.

Makela, M., Heliovaara, M., Sievers, K., et al. (1993). Musculoskeletal disorders as determinants of disability in Finns aged 30 years or more. J Clin Epidemiol, 46 (6), 549–59.

Manios, Y., Antonopoulou, S., Kaliora, A.C., et al. (2005). Dietary intake and biochemical risk factors for cardiovascular disease in two rural regions of Crete. J Physiol Pharmacol, 56 (Suppl 1), 171–81.

Mannisto, S., Smith-Warner, S.A., Spiegelman, D., et al. (2004). Dietary carotenoids and risk of lung cancer in a pooled analysis of seven cohort studies. Cancer Epdiemiol Biomarkers Prev, 13 (1), 40–8.

Mantzoros, C., Petridou, E., Dessypris, N., et al. (2004). Adiponectin and breast cancer risk. J Clin Endocrinol Metab, 89 (3), 1102–7.

Mao, Y., Pan, S., Wen, S.W., et al. (2003). Physical activity and the risk of lung cancer in Canada. Am J Epidemiol, 158 (6), 564–75.

Mao, Y., Pan, S., Wen, S.W., et al. (2003). Physical inactivity, energy intake, obesity and the risk of rectal cancer in Canada. Int J Cancer, 105 (6), 831–7.

March, L.M., Bagga, H. (2004). Epidemiology of osteoarthritis. Medical Journal of Australia, 180 (5 Suppl), S6–S10.

Marchionni, N., Fattirolli, F., Fumagalli, S., et al. (2003). Improved exercise tolerance and quality of life with cardiac rehabilitation of older patients after myocardial infarction: results of a randomized, controlled trial. Circulation, 107 (17), 2201–6. Epub 2003 Apr 21.

Markenson, J.A. (1991). Worldwide trends in the socioeconomic impact and long-term prognosis of rheumatoid arthritis. Semin Arthritis Rheum, 21 (2 Suppl 1), 4–12.

Marks, R. (1995). An overview of skin cancers. Incidence and causation. Cancer, 75 (2 Suppl): 607–12.

Marks, R., Allegrante, J.P. (2002). Comorbid disease profiles of adults with end-stage hip osteoarthritis. Med Sci Monit, 8 (14), CR305–9.

Martin-Du, Pan R. (2003). Prevention of cardiovascular and degenerative diseases: II. Hormones and/or Mediterranean diet. Rev Med Suisse Romande, 123 (3), 183–9.

Martinez, D.A., Aguayo, J., Morales, G., et al. (2004). Impact of a clinical pathway for the diabetic foot in a general hospital. An Med Interna, 21 (9), 420–4.

Martinez, J.E., Cruz, C.G., Aranda, C., et al. (2003). Disease perceptions of Brazilian fibromyalgia patients: do they resemble perceptions from other countries? Int J Rehabil Res, 26 (3), 223–7.

Marugame, T., Sobue, T., Nakayama, T., et al. (2004). Filter cigarette smoking and lung cancer risk; a hospital-based case-control study in Japan. Br J Cancer, 90 (3), 646–51.

Masini, C., Fuchs, P.G., Gabrielli, F., et al. (2003). Evidence for the association of human papillomavirus infection and cutaneous squamous cell carcinoma in immunocompetent individuals. Arch Dermatol, 139 (7), 890–4.

Matsui, H., Maeda, A., Tsuji, H., et al. (1997). Risk indicators of low back pain among workers in Japan. Association of familial and physical factors with low back pain. Spine, 22 (11), 1242–7, discussion 1248.

Matteucci, E., Passerai, S., Mariotti, M., et al. (2005). Dietary habits and nutritional biomarkers in Italian type 1 diabetes families: evidence of unhealthy diet and combined-vitamin deficient intakes. Eur J Clin Nutr, 59 (1), 114–22.

Mattison, I., Wirfalt, E., Wallstrom, P., et al. (2004). High fat and alcohol intake are risk factors of postmenopausal breast cancer: A prospective study from the Malmo diet and cancer cohort. Int J Cancer, 110 (4), 589–97.

Maunsell, E., Brisson, C., Dubois, L., et al., (1999). Work problems after breast cancer: an exploratory qualitative study. Psychooncology, 8 (6), 467–73.

Max, W., Sinnot, P., Kao, C., et al. (2002). The burden of osteoporosis in California, 1998. Osteoporos Int, 13 (6), 493–500.

Mayfield, J.A., Deb, P., Whitecotton, L. (1999). Work disability and diabetes. Diabetes Care, 22 (7), 1105–9.

McCracken, L.M., Turk, D.C. (2002). Behavioral and cognitive-behavioral treatment for chronic pain: outcome, predictors of outcome, and treatment process. Spine, 27, 2564–73.

McGruder, H.F., Malarcher, A.M., Antoine, T.L., et al. (2004). Racial and ethnic differences in cardiovascular risk factors among stroke survivors: United States 1999 to 2001. Stroke, 35 (7), 1557–61, Epub 2004 Jun 10.

Mcintyre, S., Mutrie, N. (2004). Socio-economic differences in cardiovascular disease and physical activity: stereotypes and reality. J R Soc Health, 124 (2), 66–9.

McPherson, R. (2000). Is hormone replacement therapy cardioprotective? Decision-making after the heart and estrogen/progestin replacement study. Can J Cardiol, 16 Suppl A, 14A–19A.

McQuade, D.V. (2002). Negative social perception of hypothetical workers with rheumatoid arthritis. J Behav Med, 25 (3), 205–217.

McVeigh, G.E., Cohn, J.N. (2003). Endothelial dysfunction and the metabolic syndrome. Curr Diab Rep, 3 (1), 87–92.

Meigs, J.B., Mittleman, M.A., Nathan, D.M., et al. (2000). Hyperinsulinemia, hyperglycemia, and impaired hemostasis: the Framingham Offspring Study. JAMA, 283 (2), 221–8.

Melanoma Cancer Treatment Information (2005). Melanoma Cancer Treatment & Prevention. http://patient.cancerconsultants.com.

Melanson, P.M., Downe-Wamboldt, B. (2003). Confronting life with rheumatoid arthritis. J Adv Nurs, 42 (2), 125–33.

Mellick, E., Buckwalter, K.C., Stolley, J.M. (1992). Suicide among elderly white men: development of a profile. Journal of Psychosocial Nursing, 30 (2), 29–34.

Mengshoel, A.M. Haugen, M. (2001). Health status in fibromyalgia—a follow-up study. J Rheumatol, 28 (9), 2085–9.

Mennen, L.I., Sapinho, D., de Bree, A., et al. (2004). Consumption of foods rich in flavonoids is related to a decreased cardiovascular risk in apparently healthy French women. J Nutr, 134 (4), 923–6.

Mera, S.L. (1994). Diet and disease. Br J Biomed Sci, 51 (3), 189–206.

Michaud, K., Messer, J., Choi, H.K. (2003). Direct medical costs and their predictors in patients with rheumatoid arthritis: a three-year study of 7,527 patients. Arthritis Rheum, 48 (10), 2750–62.

Michaels, A.D., Barsness, G.W., Soran, O., et al. (2005). Frequency and efficacy of repeat enhanced external counterpulsation for stable angina pectoris (from the International EECP Patient Registry). Am J Cardiol, 95 (3), 394–7.

Michaels, A.D., Linnemeier, G., Soran, O., et al. (2004). Two-year outcomes after enhanced external counterpulsation for stable angina pectoris (from the International EECP Patient Registry, IEPR). 93 (4), 461–4.

Michels, K.B., Willett, W.C., Fuchs, C.S., et al. (2005). Coffee, tea and caffeine consumption and incidence of colon and rectal cancer. J Natl Cancer Inst, 97 (4), 282–92.

Mikulis, T.R. (2003). Co-morbidity in rheumatoid arthritis. Best Pract Res Clin Rheumatol, 17 (5), 729–59.

Mili, F., Helmick, C.G., Zack, M.M. (2002). Prevalence of arthritis: analysis of data from the US Behavioral Risk Factor Surveillance System, 1996–99. Journal of Rheumatology, 29 (9), 1981–8.

Miles, T.P., Flegal, K., Harris, T. (1993). Musculoskeletal disorders: time trends, comorbid conditions, self-assessed health status, and associated activity limitations. Vital Health Stat 3, (27), 275–88.

Millar, W.J. (2002). Hip and knee replacement. Health Rep, 14 (1), 37–50.

Miller, A.B., Altenburg, H.P., Bueno-de-Mesquita, B., et al. (2004). Fruits and vegetables and lung cancer: Findings from the European Prospective Investigation into Cancer and Nutrition. Int J Cancer, 108 (2), 269–76.

Millikan, R.C., Player, J., De Cotret, A.R., et al. (2004). Manganese superoxide dismutase Ala-9Val polymorphism and risk of breast cancer in a population-based case-control study of African Americans and whites. Breast Cancer Res, 6 (4), R264–74. Epub 2004 Apr 07.

Minnock, P., Fitzgerald, O., Bresnihan, B. (2003). Quality of life, social support, and knowledge of disease in women with rheumatoid arthritis. Arthritis Rheum, 49 (2), 221–7.

Minor, M.A. (1999). Exercise in the treatment of osteoarthritis. Rheum Dis Clin North Am, 25 (2), 397–415, viii.

Minsky, B.D. (2004). Combined-modality therapy of rectal cancer with irinotecan-based regimens. Oncology (Huntingt), 18 (14 Suppl 14), 49–55.

Mishra, G.D., Malik, N.S., Paul, A.A. (2003). Childhood and adult dietary vitamin E intake and cardiovascular risk factors in mid-life in the 1946 British Birth Cohort. Eur J Clin Nutr, 57 (11), 1418–25.

MMWR (2001). Mortality from coronary heart disease and acute myocardial infarction— United States, 1998. MMWR Morb Mort Wkly Rep, 50 (06), 90–3.

MMWR (2003). Direct and indirect costs of arthritis and other rheumatic conditions—United States, 1997. MMWR Morb Mort Wkly Rep, 52 (46), 1124–7.

MMWR (2003). Public health and aging: projected prevalence of self-reported arthritis or chronic joint symptoms among persons aged >65 years—United States, 2005–2030. MMWR Morb Mortal Wkly Rep, 52 (21), 489–91.

MMWR (2005). Differences in disability among black and white stroke survivors—United States, 2000–2001. MMWR Morb Mort Wkly Rep, 54 (1), 3–6.

Mobley, C.C. (2004). Lifestyle interventions for "diabesity": the state of the science. Compend Contin Educ Dent, 25 (3), 207–8, 211–2, 214–8, quiz 220.

Moffroid, M.T. (1997). Endurance of trunk muscles in persons with chronic low back pain: assessment, performance, training. J Rehabil Res Dev, 34, 440–7.

Mohan, V., Shanthirani C.S., Deepa, R. (2003). Glucose intolerane (diabetes and IGT) in a selected South Indian population with special reference to family history, obesity and lifestyle factors—the Chennai Urban Population Study (CUPS 14).

Mohrschladt, M.F., van der Sman-de Beer, F., Hofman, M.K., et al. (2005). TaqIB polymorphism in CETP gene: the influence on incidence of cardiovascular disease in statin-treated patients with familial hypercholesterolemia. Eur J Hum Genet, Apr 27 (Epub ahead of print).

Mokdad, A.H., Bowman, B.A., Ford, E.S., et al. (2001). The continuing epidemics of obesity and diabetes in the United States. JAMA, 286 (10), 1195–200.

Moldofsky, H. (2001). Sleep and pain. Sleep Med Rev, 5 (5), 385–396.

Moore, H., Summerbell, C., Hooper, L. et al. (2004). Dietary advice for treatment of type 2 diabetes mellitus in adults. Cochrane Database Syst Rev 3, CD003097.

Moore, J.E., Chaney, E.F. (1985). Outpatient group treatment of chronic pain: effects of spouse involvement. Journal of Consulting and Clinical Psychology, 53 (3), 326–34.

Moran, E.M. (1992). Epidemiological factors of cancer in California. J Environ Pathol Toxicol Oncol, 11 (5–6), 303–7.

Morewitz, S. (2002a). Socioeconomic differences among Hispanics who suffer both stroke and heart attack. (abstract) Circulation, online, P130.

Morewitz, S. (2002b). Gender, racial, and socioeconomic differences in persons with colon cancer. (abstract) Cancer Epidemiology, Biomarkers & Prevention, 11 (Suppl.): C213.

Morewitz, S. Dintcho, A., Lim, J., et al. (2002). Impairment from arthritis among diabetics and non-diabetics with ankle pain and stiffness. (abstract) Annals of Behavioral Medicine, (24), Supplement, #B–10, p. 25.

Morewitz, S., Shamtoub, S., Ky, N., Saito, N., Reber, L., Kuy, S. (2002). Anxiety and ankle pain symptoms among Whites and African-Americans. (abstract) Annals of Behavioral Medicine, 24, Supplement, #B–9, p. 25.

Morewitz, S., Tse, J., Lee, R., Muhl, K., Risch, S. (2002). Gender differences in hypertension and toe pain in insulin-dependent diabetics. (abstract), Diabetes, 51, Supplement 2, #2086.

Morewitz, S. (2003a). Arthritis impairment and socioeconomic differences among persons with non-insulin-dependent diabetes. (abstract) Psychosomatic Medicine, #1089.

Morewitz, S. (2003b). Vigorous activity among persons with hypertension: The role of race and socioeconomic factors. (abstract) Circulation, online, P57.

Morewitz, S. (2004a). Duration of heart problems among persons with non-insulin-dependent diabetes: socioeconomic differences. (abstract) Proceedings of the American Association for the Advancement of Science, Pacific Division, 85th Annual Meeting of the AAAS: Pacific Division, (23), Part 1, p. 33.

Morewitz, S. (2004b). Hypertension impairment: the role of gender and socioeconomic status factors. (abstract) Circulation, online, 109 (20), P88, p. 18.

Morewitz, S. (2004c). Coronary heart disease impairment and patients' ability to afford and access prescription drugs. (abstract) Circulation, online, 109 (20), P1, p. 1.

Morewitz, S. (2004d). Marital status as a risk factor for hypertension impairment. (abstract) Circulation, online, 109 (20), P89, p. 18.

Morewitz, S. (2005a). African-American/white differences in recent feelings of sadness among persons with diabetes: A population-based study. (abstract) Diabetes, June, Vol. 54, Supplement 1, #2368-PO, p. A571.

Morewitz, S. (2005b). Gender differences in low back pain: Analysis of the National Health Interview Survey. (abstract) Psychosomatic Medicine, online, March, Vol. 67, No. 1, #1179.

Morewitz, S. (2005c). Psychosocial impairment as a risk factor for radiating lower extremity pain. (abstract) Psychosomatic Medicine, online, March 5, 2005, Vol. 67, No. 1, #1277.

Morewitz, S. (2005d). African-American and white differences in hypertension history among pregnant women. Circulation, online, May, #13.

Morewitz, S. (2005e). Income and racial/ethnic differences in use of the emergency department among persons with self-reported hypertension impairment. Circulation, online, May, #10.

Mozaffarian, D., Longstreth, W.T., Jr., Lemaitre, R.N., et al. (2005). Fish consumption and stroke risk in elderly individuals: the cardiovascular health study. Arch Int Med, 165 (2), 200–6.

Muhl, K., Morewitz, S., Lee, R., et al. (2002). African-American/White differences in perceived weight impairment and desirable body weight among insulin-dependent and non-insulin-dependent diabetics. (abstract) Diabetes, 51, Supplement 2, #2508.

Mukhtar, H., Argarwal, R. (1996). Skin cancer chemoprevention. J Investig Dermatol Symp Proce, 1 (2), 209–14.

Mullan, R.H., Bresnihan, B. (2003). Disease-modifying anti-rheumatic drug therapy and structural damage in early rheumatoid arthritis. Clin Exp Rheumatol, 21 (5 Suppl 31), S158–64.

Mullins, C.D., Shaya, F.T., Flowers, L.R., et al. (2004). Health care cost of analgesic use in hypertensive patients. Clin Ther, 26 (2), 285–93.

Mullins, S., Morewitz, S., Palma, I., Mukker, J. (2002). Gender differences in perceived weight impairment and exercise in insulin-dependent diabetics. (abstract) Diabetes, 51, Supplement 2, #2221.

Murata, G.H., Shah, J.H., Wendel, C.S., et al. (2003). Risk factor management in stable, insulin-treated patients with Type 2 diabetes: the Diabetes Outcomes in Veterans Study. J Diabetes Complications, 17 (4), 186–91.

Musgrave, D.S., Vogt, M.T., Nevitt, M.C., et al. (2001). Back problems among post-menopausal women taking estrogen replacement therapy: the study of osteoporotic fractures. Spine, 26 (14), 1606–12.

Must, A., Spadano, J., Coakley, E.H., et al. (1999). The disease burden associated with overweight and obesity. JAMA, 282 (16), 1523–9.

Nafstad, P., Haheim, L.L., Oftedal, B., et al. (2003). Lung cancer and air pollution: a 27-year follow-up of 16,209 Norwegian men. Thorax, 58 (12), 1071–6.

Nahit, E.S., Pritchard, C.M., Cherry, N.M., et al. (2001). The influence of work related psychosocial factors and psychological distress on regional musculoskeletal pain: a study of newly employed workers. J Rheumatol, 28 (6), 1378–84.

Nakanishi, N., Nakamura, K., Matsuo, Y., et al. (2000). Cigarette smoking and risk for impaired fasting glucose and type 2 diabetes in middle-aged Japanese men. Annals of Internal Medicine, 133 (3), 183–91.

Narod, S.A., Dube, M.P., Klijn, J., et al. (2002). Oral contraceptives and the risk of breast cancer in BRCA1 and BRCA2 mutation carriers. J Natl Cancer Inst, 94 (23), 1773–9.

National Cancer Institute (2005). Treatment statement for health professionals. Small cell lung cancer. Med News, http://www.meb.uni-bonn.de/cancer.gov.

National Center for Complementary and Alternative Medicine. Research report—About chiropractic and its use in treating low-back pain. http://nccam.nih.gov/health/chiropractic/

Nelemans, P.J., de Bie, R.A., de Vet, H., et al. (2000). Injection therapy for subacute and chronic benign low back pain. Cochrane Database Syst Rev, 2, CD001824.

Nevitt, M.C., Ross, P.D., Palermo, L., et al. (1999). Association of prevalent fractures, bone density, and alendronate treatment with incident vertebral fractures: effect of number and spinal location of fractures. The Fracture Intervention Trial Research Group. Bone, 25 (5), 613–9.

Nevitt, M.C., Thompson, D.E., Black, D.M., et al. (2000). Effect of alendronate on limited-activity days and bed-disability days caused by back pain in postmenopausal women with existing vertebral fractures. Fracture Intervention Trial Research Group. Arch Int Med, 160 (1), 77–85.

Nicassio, P.M., Schuman, C., Kim, J., et al. (1997). Psychosocial factors associated with complementary treatment use in fibromyalgia. J Rheumatol, 24 (10), 2008–13.

Niemisto, L., Sarna, S., Lahtinen-Suopanki, T., et al. (2004). Predictive factors for 1-year outcome of chronic low back pain following manipulation, stabilizing exercises, and physician consultation or physician consultation alone. J Rehabil Med, 36 (3), 104–9.

Nishimura, F., Soga, Y., Iwamoto, Y., et al. (2005). Peridontal disease as part of the insulin resistance syndrome in diabetic patients. J Int Acad Periodontol, 7 (1), 16–20.

Nkondjock, A., Ghadirian, P. (2004). Intake of specific carotenoids and essential fatty acids and breast cancer risk in Montreal, Canada. Am J Clin Nutr, 79 (5), 857–64.

Nkondjock, A., Receveur, O. (2003). Fish-seafood consumption, obesity, and risk of type 2 diabetes: an ecological study. Diabetes and Metabolism, 29 (6), 635–42.

Noguchi, S., Koyama, H., Uchino, J., et al. (2005). Postoperative adjuvant therapy with tamoxifen, tegafur plus uracil, or both in women with node-negative breast cancer: a pooled analysis of six randomized controlled trials. J Clin Oncol, 23 (10), 2172–84.

Noller, V., Sprott, H. (2003). Prospective epidemiological observations on the course of the disease in fibromyalgia patients. J Negat Results Biomed, 2, 4.

Norris, S.L., Zhang, X., Avnell, A., et al. (2004a). Efficacy of pharmacotherapy for weight loss in adults with type 2 diabetes mellitus: a meta-analysis. Arch Intern Med, 164 (13), 1395–404.

Norris, S.L., Zhang, X., Avnell, A., et al. (2004b). Long-term effectiveness of lifestyle and behavioral weight loss interventions in adults with type 2 diabetes: a meta-analysis. Am J Med, 117 (10), 762–74.

Northern California Cancer Center (2004). NCCC news—NCCC study finds alcohol consumption increases breast cancer risk among women taking hormone replacement therapy (http://www.nccc.org/news/breastcancer_study_042704.html).

Nyiendo, J., Haas, M. Goodwin, P. (2000). Patient characteristics, practice activities, and one-month outcomes for chronic, recurrent low-back pain treated by chiropractors and family medicine physicians: a practice-based feasibility study. J Manipulative Physiol Ther, 23 (4), 239–45.

O'Connor, P.J., Crabtree, B.F., Abourizk, N.N. (1992). Longitudinal study of a diabetes education and care intervention: predictors of improved glycemic control. J Am Board Fam Pract, 5 (4), 381–7.

O'Day, S.J., Kim, C.J., Reintgen, D.S. (2002). Metastatic melanoma: chemotherapy to biochemotherapy. Cancer Control, 9(1), 31–8.

Oestreicher, N., White, E., Malone, K.E., et al. (2004). Hormonal factors and breast tumor proliferation: Do factors that affect cancer risk also affect tumor growth? Breast Cancer Res Treat, 85 (2), 133–42.

Ohara-Hirano, Y., Kaku, T., Hirakawa, T., et al. (2004). Uterine cervical cancer: a holistic approach to mental health and it's socio-psychological implications. Fukuoka Igaku Zasshi, 95 (8), 83–94.

Ohnaka, T. (1993). Health effects of ultraviolet radiation. Ann Physiol Anthropol, 12 (1), 1–10.

Oka, R.K., Szuba, A., Giacomini, J.C., et al. (2004). Predictors of physical function in patients with peripheral arterial disease and claudication. Prog Cardiovasc Nurs, 19 (3), 89–94.

Okosun, I.S., Choi, S., Dent, M.M. (2001). Abdominal obesity defined as a larger than expected waist girth is associated with racial/ethnic differences in risk of hypertension. J Hum Hypertens, 15 (5), 307–12.

Okosun, I.S., Cooper, R.S., Rotimi, C.N., et al. (1998). Association of waist circumference with risk of hypertension and type 2 diabetes in Nigerians, Jamaicans, and African-Americans. Diabetes Care, 21 (11), 1836–42.

Oleske, D.M., Neelakantan, J., Andersson, G.B. (2004). Factors affecting recovery from work-related low back disorders in autoworkers. Arch Phys Med Rehabil, 85 (8), 1362–4.

Olsson, A.R., Skogh, T., Axelson, O., et al. (2004). Occupations and exposures in the work environment as determinants for rheumatoid arthritis. Occup Environ Med, 61 (3), 233–8.

Olstad, R., Sexton, H., Sogaard, A.J. (2001). The Finnmark Study. A prospective population study of the social support buffer hypothesis, specific stressors and mental distress. Soc Psychiatry Psychiatr Epidemiol, 36 (12), 582–9.

O'Meara, S., Riemsma, R., Shirran, L., et al. (2001). A rapid and systematic review of the clinical effectiveness and cost-effectiveness of orlistat in the management of obesity. Health Technol Assess, 5 (18), 1–81.

Onal, A.E., Erbil, S., Ozel, S. (2004). The prevalence of and risk factors for hypertension in adults living in Istanbul. Blood Press, 13 (1), 31–6.

O'Neill, T.W., Cockerill, W., Matthis, C., et al. (2004). Back pain, disability, and radiographic vertebral fracture in European women: a prospective study. Osteoporos Int, 15 (9), 760–5. Epub 2004 May 12.

Orchard, T.J., Temprosa, M. Goldberg, R., et al. (2005). The effect of metformin and intensive lifestyle intervention on the metabolic syndrome: the Diabetes Prevention Program randomized trial. Ann Intern Med, 142 (8), 611–9.

Orsini, L.S., Rousculp, M.D., Long, S.R., et al. (2005). Health care utilization and expenditures in the United States: a study of osteoporosis-related fractures. Osteoporos Int, 16 (4), 359–71. Epub 2004 Sep 1.

Orstavik, R.E., Haugeberg, G., Mowinckel, P. (2004). Vertebral deformities in rheumatoid arthritis: a comparison with population-based controls. Archives of Internal Medicine, 164 (4), 420–5.

Osborne, R.H., Elsworth, G.R., Kissane, D.W., et al. (1999). The Mental Adjustment to Cancer (MAC) scale: replication and refinement in 632 breast cancer patients. Psychol Med, 29 (6), 1335–45.

Osborne, R.H., Spinks, J.M., Wicks, I.P. (2004). Patient education and self-management programs in arthritis. Med J Aust, 180 (5 Suppl): S23–6.

Ostadal, P., Alan, D., Hajek, P., et al. (2005). Fluvastatin in the therapy of acute coronary syndrome: Rationale and design of a multicenter, randomized, double-blind, placebo-controlled trial (The FACS Trial). Curr Control Trials Cardiovasc Med, 6 (1), 4.

Ozguler, A., Loisel, P., Boureau, F., et al. (2004). Effectiveness of interventions for low back pain sufferers: the return to work criterion. Revue d'Epidemiologie et de Sante Publique, 52 (2), 1–19 (http://www.e2med.com/index).

Paier, G.S. (1996). Specter of the crone: the experience of vertebral fracture. ANS Adv Nurs Sci, 18 (3), 27–36.

Pan, S.Y., Johnson, K.C., Ugnat, A.M., et al. (2004). Association of obesity and cancer risk in Canada. Am J Epidemiol, 159 (3), 259–68.

Panagiotakos, D.B., Pitsavos, C., Zeimbekis, A., et al. (2005). The association between lifestyle-related factors and plasma homocysteine levels in healthy individuals from the "ATTICA" Study. Int J Cardiol, 98 (3), 471–7.

Pao, W., Miller, V.A. (2005). Epidermal growth factor receptor mutations, small-molecule kinase inhibitors, and non-small-cell lung cancer: current knowledge and future directions. J Clin Oncol, 23 (11), 2556–68. Epub 2005 Mar 14.

Papageorgiou, A.C., Croft, P.R., Thomas, E., et al. (1998). Psychosocial risks for low back pain: are these related to work. Ann Rheum Dis, 57 (8), 500–2.

Park, H.S., Oh, S.W., Cho, S.I. (2004). The metabolic syndrome and associated lifestyle factors among South Korean adults. Int J Epidemiol, 33 (2), 328–36.

Parker, J.C., Smarr, K.L., Buckelew, S.P., et al. (1995). Effects of stress management on clinical outcomes in rheumatoid arthritis. Arthritis Rheum, 38 (12), 1807–18.

Pasetto, L.M., Jirillo, A., Iadicicco, G., et al. (2005). FOLFOX versus FOLFIRI: a comparison of regimens in the treatment of colorectal cancer metastases. Anticancer Res, 25 (1B), 563–76.

Patel, J.D., Bach, P.B., Kris, M.G. (2004). Lung cancer in U.S. women: a contemporary epidemic. JAMA, 291 (14), 1763–8.

Patout, C.A., Jr., Birke, J.A., Wilbright, W.A., et al. (2001). A decision pathway for the staged management of foot problems in diabetes mellitus. Arch Phys Med Rehabil, 82 (12), 1724–8.

Pauley, S.M. (2004). Lighting for the human circadian clock: recent research indicates that lighting has become a public health issue. Med Hypotheses, 63 (4), 588–96.

Pearce, J., Boyle, P. (2005). Examining the relationship between lung cancer and radon in small areas across Scotland. Health Place, 11 (3), 275–82.

Pelfrene, E., Leynen, F., Mak, R.P., et al. (2003). Relationship of perceived job stress to total coronary risk in a cohort of working men and women in Belgium. Eur J Cardiovasc Prev Rehabil, 10 (5), 345–54.

Pelliccia, F., Cartoni, D., Verde, M., et al. (2004). Critical pathways in the emergency department improve treatment modalities for patients with ST-elevation myocardial infarction in a European hospital. Clin Cardiol, 27 (12), 698–700.

Pennello, G., Devesa, S., Gail, M. (2000). Association of surface ultraviolet B radiation levels with melanoma and nonmelanoma skin cancer in United States blacks. Cancer Epidemiol Biomarkers Prev, 9 (3), 291–7.

Penninx, B.W., Messier, S.P., Rejeski, W.J., et al. (2001). Physical exercise and the prevention of disability in activities of daily living in older persons with osteoarthritis. Arch Intern Med, 161 (19), 2309–16.

Penrod, J.R., Bernatsky, S., Adam, V., et al. (2004). Health services costs and their determinants in women with fibromyalgia. J Rheumatol, 31 (7), 1391–8.

Penttinen, J. (1995). Back pain and risk of suicide among Finnish farmers. American Journal of Public Health, 85 (10), 1452–3.

Perez-Gomez, B., Pollan, M., Gustavsson, P., et al. (2004). Cutaneous melanoma: hints from occupational risks by anatomic site in Swedish men. Occup Environ Med, 61 (2), 117–26.

Peris, K., Campione, E., Micantonio, T., et al. (2005). Imiquimod treatment of superficial and nodular basal cell carcinoma: 12-week open-label trial. Dematol Surg, 31 (3), 318–23.

Perry, I.J. (2002). Healthy diet and lifestyle clustering and glucose intolerance. Proceedings of Nutrition Soc, 61 (4), 543–51.

Peter, W.L., Khan, S.S., Ebben, J.P. (2004). Chronic kidney disease: The distribution of health care dollars. Kidney Int, 66 (1), 313–21.

Peters, G.J., Smorenburg, C.H., Van Groeningen, C.J. (2004). Prospective clinical trials using a pharmacogenetic/pharmacogenomic approach. J Chemother, 16 (Suppl) 4, 25–30.

Peters, T.J., Sanders, C., Dieppe, P., et al. (2005). Factors associated with change in pain and disability over time: a community-based prospective observational study of hip and knee osteoarthritis. Br J Gen Pract, 55 (512), 205–11.

Peyrot, M., McMurry, J.F., Jr., Kruger, D.F. (1999). A biopsychosocial model of glycemic control in diabetes: stress, coping and regimen adherence. J Health Soc Behav, 40 (2), 141–58.

Pfingsten, M., Leibing, E., Harter, W., et al. (2001). Fear-avoidance behavior and anticipation of pain in patients with chronic low back pain: a randomized controlled study. Pain Med, 2 (4), 259–66.

Pfund, A., Putz, J., Wendland, G., et al. (2001). Coronary intervention and occupational rehabilitation—a prospective, randomized intervention group. Z Kardiol, 90 (9), 655–60.

Philadelphia Panel (2001). Philadelphia Panel evidence-based clinical practice guidelines on selected rehabilitation interventions for knee pain. Phys Ther, 81 (10), 1675–700.

Philpott, S., Boynton, P.M., Fedar, G., et al. (2001). Gender differences in descriptions of angina symptoms and health problems immediately prior to angiography: the ACRE study. Appropriateness of Coronary Revascularisation study. Soc Sci Med, 52 (10), 1565–75.

Pincus, T., Sokka, T. (2003). Quantitative measures for assessing rheumatoid arthritis in clinical trials and clinical care. Best Pract Res Clin Rheumatol, 17 (5), 753–81.

Pincus, T., Sokka, T. (2003). Uniform databases in early arthritis: specific measures to complement classification criteria and indices of clinical change. Clin Exp Rheumatol, 21 (5 Suppl 31), S79–88.

Pinnington, M.A., Miller, J., Stanley, I. (2004). An evaluation of prompt access to physiotherapy in the management of low back pain in primary care. Fam Pract, 21 (4), 372–80.

Pinzur, M.S., Evans, A. (2003). Health-related quality of life in patients with Charcot foot. Am J Orthop, 32 (10), 492–6.

Pisters, K.M., Le Chevalier, T. (2005). Adjuvant chemotherapy in completely resected non-small-cell lung cancer. J Clin Oncol, 23 (14), 3270–8.

Pitts, V. (2004). Illness and Internet empowerment: writing and reading breast cancer in cyberspace. Health (London), 8 (1), 33–59.

Plach, S.K., Heidrich, S.M., Waite, R.M. (2003) Relationship of social role quality to psychological well-being in women with rheumatoid arthritis. ResNurs Health, 26 (3), 190–202.

Pletcher, M.J., Varosy, P., Kiefe, C.I., et al. (2005). Alcohol consumption, binge drinking, and early coronary calcification: findings from the Coronary Artery Risk Development in Young Adults (CARDIA) Study. Am J Epidemiol, 161 (5), 423–33.

Poiraudeau, S., Rannou, F., Lefevre Colau, M.M., et al. (2004). Rehabilitation on effort of low back pain. Functional restoration programs. Presse Med, 33 (6), 413–18.

Polissar, L., Severson, R.K., Boatman, E.S. (1984). A case-study of asbestos in drinking water and cancer risk. Am J Epidemiol, 119 (3), 456–71.

Pontiroli, A.E., Galli, L. (1998). Duration of obesity is a risk factor for non-insulin-dependent diabetes mellitus, not for arterial hypertension or for hyperlipidaemia. Acta Diabetol, 35 (3), 130–6.

Pradeepa, R., Mohan, V. (2002). The changing scenario of the diabetes epidemic: implications for India. Indian J Med Res, 116, 121–32.

Prince, M., Harwood, R., Thomas, A., et al. (1998). A prospective population-based cohort study of the effects of disablement and social milieu on the onset and maintenance of late-life depression. Psychological Medicine, 28 (2), 337–50.

Pucheu, S., Consoli, S.M., D'Auzac, C., et al. (2004). Do health causal attributions and coping strategies act as moderators of quality of life in peritoneal dialysis patients? J Psychosom Res, 56 (3), 317–22.

Pukkala, E., Aspholm, R., Auvinen, A., et al. (2002). Incidence of cancer among Nordic airline pilots over five decades: occupational cohort study. BMJ, 325 (7364), 567.

Puolakka, K., Kautiainen, H., Mottonen, T., et al. (2004). Impact of initial aggressive drug treatment with a combination of disease-modifying antirheumatic drugs on the development of work disability in early rheumatoid arthritis: a five-year randomized followup trial. Arthritis Rheum, 50 (1), 55–62.

Purushotham, A.D., Upponi, S., Klevesath, M.B., et al. (2005). Morbidity after sentinel lymph node biops in primary breast cncer: result from a randomized controlled trial. J Clin Oncol, 23 (19), 4312–21.

Quadrilatero, J., Hoffman-Goetz, L. (2003). Physical activity and colon cancer. A systematic review of potential mechanisms. J Sports Med Phys Fitness, 43 (2), 121–38.

Quinn, M.A., Emery, P. (2003). Window of opportunity in early rheumatoid arthritis: possibility of altering the disease process with early intervention. Clin Exp Rheumatol, 21 (5 Suppl 31), S154–7.

Raak, R., Hurtig, I., Wahren, L.K. (2003). Coping strategies and life satisfaction in sub-grouped fibromyalgia patients. Biol Res Nurse, 4 (3), 193–202.

Rafnsson, V., Hrafnkelsson, J., Tulinius, H., et al. (2003). Risk factors for cutaneous malignant melanoma among aircrews and a random sample of the population. Occup Environ Med, 60 (11), 815–20.

Rafnsson, V., Sulem, P., Tulinius, H., et al. (2003). Breast cancer risk in airline attendants: a nested case-control study in Iceland. Occup Environ Med, 60 (11), 807–9.

Ragnarson Tennvall, G., Apelqvist, J. (2000). Health-related quality of life in patients with diabetes mellitus and foot ulcers. J Diabetes Complications, 14 (5), 235–41.

Raina, P., Dukeshire, S., Lindsay, J., et al. (1998). Chronic conditions and disabilities among seniors: an analysis of population-based health and activity limitation surveys. Ann Epidemiol, 8 (6), 402–9.

Raitakari, O.T., Porkka, K.V., Rasanen, L., et al. (1994). Relations of life-style with lipids, blood pressure and insulin in adolescents and young adults. The Cardiovascular Risk in Young Finns Study. Atherosclerosis, 111 (2), 237–46.

Ramachandruni, S., Handberg, E., Sheps, D.S. (2004). Acute and chronic psychological stress in coronary disease. Curr Opin Cardiol, 19 (5), 494–9.

Rani, P.U., Naidi, M.U., Prasad, V.B. (1996). An evaluation of antidepressants in rheumatic pain conditions. Anesthesia, 83 (2), 371–5.

Rannou, F., Poiraudeau, S., Revel, M. (2001). Cartilage: from biomechanics to physical therapy. Ann Readapt Med Phys, 44 (5), 259–67.

Rauck, R.L., Gargiulo, C.A., Ruoff, G.E., et al. (1998). Chronic low back pain: new perspectives and treatment guidelines for primary care: Part II. Manag Care Interface, 11 (3), 71–5.

Ravert, R.D., Hancock, M.D., Ingersoll, G.M. (2004). Online forum messages posted by adolescents with type 1 diabetes. Diabetes Educ, 30 (5), 827–34.

Redaelli, A., Cranor, C.W., Okano, G.J., et al. (2003). Screening, prevention and socioeconomic costs associated with the treatment of colorectal cancer. Pharmacoeconomics, 21 (17), 1213–38.

Redekop, W.K., Koopmanschap, M.A., Stolk, R.P., et al. (2002). Health-related quality of life and treatment satisfaction in Dutch patients with type 2 diabetes. Diabetes Care, 25 (3), 458–63.

Redon, J. (2001). Hypertension in obesity. Nutr Metab Cardiovasc Dis, 11 (5), 344–53.

Redondo, J.R., Justo, C.M., Moraleda, F.V., et al. (2004). Long-term efficacy of therapy in patients with fibromyalgia: a physical exercise-based program and a cognitive-behavioral approach. Arthritis Rheum, 51 (2), 184–92.

Reginster, J.Y. (2002). The prevalence and burden of arthritis. Rheumatology, 41 (Suppl 1), 3–6.

Reich, J., Turpin, J.P., Abramowitz, S. (1983). Psychiatric diagnosis in chronic pain patients. American Journal of Psychiatry, 140 (11), 1495–8.

Reisine, S., Fifield, J., Walsh, S.J., et al. (2001). Factors associated with continued employment among patients with rheumatoid arthritis: a survival model. J Rheumatol, 28 (11), 2400–8.

Renehan, A.G., Zwahlen, M., Minder, C., et al. (2004). Insulin-like growth factor (IGF)-I IGF binding protein-3, and cancer risk: systematic review and meta-regression analysis. Lancet, 363 (9418), 1346–53.

Reynolds, P., Cone, J., Layefsky, M., et al. (2002). Cancer incidence in California flight attendants. Cancer Causes Control, 13 (4), 317–24.

Rhee, S.H., Parker, J.C., Smarr, K.L., et al. (2000). Stress management in rheumatoid arthritis: what is the underlying mechanism? Arthritis Care Res, 13 (6), 435–42.

Richardson, J. (2003). Gender differences associated with physical functioning in older persons with angina. Disabil Rehabil, 25 (17), 973–83.

Richter, E.D., Friedman, L.S., Tamir, Y., et al. (2003). Cancer risks in naval divers with multiple exposures to carcinogens. Environ Health Perspect, 111 (4), 609–17.

Rigas, J.R., Dragnev, K.H. (2005). Emerging role of rexinoids in non-small cell lung cancer: focus on bexarotene. Oncologist, 10 (1), 22–33.

Rissanen, A., Kalimo, H., Alaranta, H. (1995). Effect of intensive training on the isokinetic strength and structure of lumbar muscles in paients with chronic low back pain. Spine, 20, 333–40.

Rivera, M.P., Stover, D.E. (2004). Gender and lung cancer. Clin Chest Med, 25 (2), 391–400.

Rizzo, J.A., Simons, W.R. (1997). Variations in compliance among hypertensive patients by drug class: implications for health care costs. Clin Ther, 19 (6), 1446–57, 1424–5.

Roberto, K.A. (1988). Stress and adaptation patterns of older osteoporotic women. Women Health, 14 (3–4), 105–19.

Robertson, J.F., Come, S.E., Jones, S.E., et al. (2005). Endocrine treatment options for advanced breast cancer—the role of fulvestrant. Eur J Cancer, 41 (3), 346–56.

Robinson, J.K., Rigel, D.S. (2004). Sun protection attitudes and behaviors of solid-organ transplant recipients. Dermatol Surg, 30 (4 Pt 2), 610–15.

Robinson, L.E., Graham, T.E. (2004). Metabolic syndrome, a cardiovascular disease risk factor: role of adipocytokines and the impact of diet and physical activity. Can J Appl Physiol, 29 (6), 808–29.

Roos, E.M., Dahlberg, L. (2004). Physical activity as medication against arthrosis—training has a positive effect n the cartilage. Lakartidningen, 101 (25), 2178–81.

Rosal, M.C., Carbone, E.T., Goins, K.V. (2003). Use of cognitive interviewing to adapt measurement instruments for low-literate Hispanics. Diabetes Educ, 29 (6), 1006–17.

Roscoe, L.A., Malphurs, J.E., Dragovic, L.J., et al. (2003). Antecedents of euthanasia and suicide among older women. Journal of the American Medical Women's Association, 58 (1), 44–8.

Rosenson, R.S. (2005). New approaches in the intensive management of cardiovascular risk in the metabolic syndrome. Curr Probl Cardiol, 30 (5), 241–79.

Rosito, G.A., D'Agostino, R.B., Massaro, J., et al. (2004). Association between obesity and a prothrombotic state: the Framingham Offspring Study. 91 (4), 683–9.

Ross, P.D., Davis, J.W., Epstein, R.S., et al. (1994). Pain and disability associated with new vertebral factures and other spinal conditions. J Clin Epidemiol, 47 (3), 231–9.

Rossignol, M., Leclerc, A., Hilliquin, P., et al. (2003). Primary osteoarthritis and occupations: a national cross sectional survey of 10,412 symptomatic patients. Occup Environ Med, 60 (11), 882–6.

Roy, D.K., O'Neill, T.W., Finn, J.D., et al. (2003). Determinants of incident vertebral fracture in men and women: results from the European Prospective Osteoporosis Study. Osteoporos Int, 14 (1), 19–26.

Rozanski, A., Blumenthal, J.A., Davidson, K.W., et al. (2005). The epidemiology, pathophysiology, and management of psychosocial risk factors in cardiac practice: the emerging field of behavioral cardiology. J Am Coll Cardiol, 45 (5), 637–51.

Rozanski, A., Bumenthal, J.A., Kaplan, J. (1999). Impact of psychological factors on the pathogenesis of cardiovascular disease and implications for therapy. Circulation, 99 (16), 2192–217.

Rubin, R.J., Mendelson, D.N. (1994). How much does defensive medicine cost? J Am Health Policy, 4 (4), 7–15.

Ruland, S., Gorelick, P.B. (2005). Stroke in Black Americans. Curr Cardiol Rep, 7 (1), 29–33.

Ruland, S., Hung, E., Richardson, D., et al. (2005). Impact of obesity and the metabolic syndrome on risk factors in African American stroke survivors: a report from the AAASPS. Arch Neurol, 62 (3), 386–90.

Ruthman, J.L., Ferrans, C.E. (2004). Efficacy of a video for teaching patients about prostate cancer screening and treatment. Am J Health Promot, 18 (4), 292–5.

Rutledge, T., Reis, S.E., Olson, M., et al. (2003). Socioeconomic status variables predict cardiovascular disease risk factors and prospective mortality risk among women with chest pain. The WISE Study. Behav Modi, 27 (1), 54–67.

Ryerson, B., Tierney, E.F., Thompson, T.J., et al. (2003). Excess physical limitations among adults with diabetes in the U.S. population. Diabetes Care, 26 (1), 206–10.

Saarijarvi, S., Rytokowski, U., Alanen, E. (1991). A controlled study of couple therapy in chronic low back pain patients. Journal of Psychosomatic Research, 35 (6), 671–7.

Samanta, A., Samanta, J. (2004). Is epidural injection of steroids effective for low back pain? BMJ, 328, 1509–10.

Santoso, U., Iau, P.T., Lim, J., et al. (2002). The mastectomy clinical pathway: what has it achieved? Ann Acad Med Singapore, 31 (4), 440–5.

Satia-Abouta, J., Galanko, J.A., Martin, C.F., et al. (2004). Food groups and colon cancer risk in African-Americans and Caucasians. Int J Cancer, 109 (5), 728–36.

Satia-Abouta, J., Galanko, J.A., Potter, J.D., et al. (2003). Associations of total energy and macronutrients with colon cancer risk in African Americans and Whites: results from the North Carolina colon cancer study. American Journal of Epidemiology, 158 (10), 951–62.

Schacht, E. (2000). Osteoporosis in rheumatoid arthritis—significance of alfacalcidol in prevention and therapy. Z Rheumatol, 59 (Supplement 1), 10–20.

Schernhammer, E., Schulmeister, K. (2004). Light at night and cancer risk. Photochem Photobiol, 79 (4), 316–18.

Schernhammer, E.S., Holly, J.M., Pollak, M.N., et al. (2005). Circulating levels of insulin-like growth factors, their binding proteins, and breast cancer risk. Cancer Epidemiol Biomarkers Prev, 14 (3), 699–704.

Schneider, C.M., Dennehy, C.A., Roozeboom, M., et al. (2002). A model program: exercise intervention for cancer rehabilitation. Integr Cancer Ther, 1 (1), 76–82; discussion 82.

Schneiderman, N., Antoni, M.H., Saab, P.G., et al. (2001). Psychosocial and biobehavioral aspects of chronic disease management. Annual Review of Psychology, 52, 555–80.

Schonstein, E., Kenny, D.T., Keating, J., et al. (2003). Work conditioning, work hardening and functional restoration for workers with back and neck pain. Cochrane Database Syst Rev, 1, CD 001822.

Schulze, M.B., Rimm, E.B., Li, T. (2004). C-reactive protein and incident cardiovascular events among men with diabetes. Diabetes Care, 27 (4), 889–94.

Schwartz, A.G., Swanson, G.M. (1997). Lung carcinoma in African Americans and whites. A population-based study in metropolitan Detroit, Michigan. Cancer, 79 (1), 45–52.

Schwarzer, A.C., Spril, C.N., et al. (1995). The prevalence and clinical features of internal disc disruption in patients with chronic low back pain. Spine, 20 (17), 1878–83.

Scott, D.L., Smith, C., Kingsley, G. (2003). Joint damage and disability in rheumatoid arthritis: an updated systematic review. Clin Exp Rheumatol, 21 (5 Suppl 31), S20–7.

Scura, K.W., Budin, W., Garfing, E. (2004). Telephone social support and education for adaptation to prostate cancer: a pilot study. Oncol Nurs Forum, 31 (2), 335–8.

Scuteri, A., Najjar, S.S., Muller, D.C. (2004). Metabolic syndrome amplifies the age-associated increases in vascular thickness and stiffness. J Am Coll Cardiol, 43 (8), 1388–95.

Segal, L., Day, S.E., Chapman, A.B., et al. (2004). Can we reduce disease burden from osteoarthritis? Med J Aust, 180 (5 Suppl), S11–17.

Seidman, A.D. (2004). Gemcitabine and docetaxel in metastatic breast cancer. Oncology (Huntingt), 18 (14 Suppl 12), 13–16.

Seidman, J.J., Steinwachs, D., Rubin, H.R. (2003). Design and testing of a tool for evaluating the quality of diabetes consumer-information Web sites. J Med Intenet Res, 5 (4), e30.

Senez, B., Felicioli, P., Moreau, A., et al. (2004). Quality of life assessment of type 2 diabetic patients in general medicine. Presse Med, 33 (3), 161–6.

Shakir, Y.A., Samsioe, G., Nyberg, P., et al. (2004). Cardiovascular risk factors in middle-aged women and the association with use of hormone therapy: results from a population-based study of Swedish women. The Women's Health in the Lund Area (WHILA) Study. Climacteric, 7 (3), 74–83.

Sharma, S., Malarcher, A.M., Giles, W.H., et al. (2004). Racial, ethnic and socioeconomic disparities in the clustering of cardiovascular disease risk factors. Ethn Dis, 14 (1), 43–8.

Shaw, J.E., Chisholm, D.J. (2003). Epidemiology and prevention of type 2 diabetes and the metabolic syndrome. Medical Journal of Australia, 179 (10), 379–83.

Shaw, J.T., Purdie, D.M., Neil, H.A., et al. (1999). The relative risks of hyperglycaemia, obesity and dyslipidaemia in the rlatives of patients with Type II diabetes mellitus. Diabetologia, 42 (1), 24–7.

Shearn, M.A., Fireman, B.H. (1985). Stress management and mutual support groups in rheumatoid arthritis. Am J Med, 78 (5), 771–5.

Shera, A.S., Jawad, F., Maqsood, A., et al. (2004). Prevalence of chronic complications and associated factors in type 2 diabetes. J Pak Med Assoc, 54 (2), 54–9.

Shi, F., Gu, K., Lu, W., et al. (2003). Study on the prevalence of arthritis and relevant factors in Shanghai. Zhonghua Liu Xing Bing Xue Za Zhi, 24 (12): 1136–40.

Shrubsole, M.J., Gao, Y.T., Dai, Q., et al. (2004). Passive smoking and breast cancer risk among non-smoking Chinese women. Int J Cancer, 110 (4), 605–9.

Shuyler, K.S., Knight, K.M. (2003). What are patients seeking when they turn to the Internet? Qualitative content analysis of questions asked by visitors to an orthopaedics Web site. J Med Internet Res, 5 (4), e24.

Sidorov, J., Gabbay, R., Harris, R., et al. (2000). Disease management for diabetes mellitus: impact on hemoglobin A1c. Am J Manag Care, 6 (11), 1217–26.

Sidorov, J., Shull, R., Tomcavage, J., et al. (2002). Does diabetes disease management save money and improve outcomes? Diabetes Care, 25 (4), 684–9.

Simon, J., Mayer, O., Jr., Rosolova, H. (1999). Effect of folates, vitamin B12 and life style factors on mild hyperhomocysteinemia in a population sample. Cas Lek Cesk, 138 (21), 650–3.

Sinclair, V.G. (2001). Predictors of pain catastrophizing in women with rheumatoid arthritis. Arch Psychiatr Nurs, 15 (6), 279–88.

Sindrup, S.H., Gram, L.F., Brosen, K. The SSRI paroxetine is effective in the treatment of diabetic neuropathy symptoms. Pain, 1990.

Singer, R.B. (2003). Mortality in rheumatoid arthritis patients treated with or without methotrexate. J Insur Med, 35 (3–4), 144–9.

Singh, G., Miller, J.D., Lee, F.H., et al. (2002). Prevalence of cardiovascular disease risk factors among US adults with self-reported osteoarthritis: data from the Third National Health and Nutrition Examination Survey. Am J Manag Care, 8 (15 Suppl), S383–91.

Singh, G.K., Siahpush, M. (2002). Ethnic-immigrant differentials in health behaviors, morbidity, and cause-specific mortality in the United States: an analysis of two national data bases. Hum Biol, 74 (1), 83–109.

Sinha, S., Luben, R.N., Welch, A., et al. (2005). Fibrinogen and cigarette smoking in men and women in the European Prsopective Investigation into Cancer in Norfolk (EPIC-Norfolk) population. Eur J Cardiovasc Prev Rehabil, 12 (2), 144–50.

Skalla, K.A., Bakitas, M., Furstenberg, C.T., et al. (2004). Patients' need for information about cancer therapy. Oncol Nurs Forum, 31 (2), 313–19.

Skibinska, E., Sawicki, R., Lewczuk, A., et al. (2004). Homocysteine and progression of coronary artery disease. Kardiol Pol, 60 (3), 197–205.

Skurk, T., Hauner, H. (2005). Secretory activity of the adipocytes and comorbidities of obesity. MMW Fortschr Med, 147 (4), 41–3.

Slattery, M.L., Boucher, K.M., Caan, B.J., et al. (1998). Eating patterns and risk of colon cancer. Am J Epidemiol, 148 (1), 4–16.

Slattery, M.L., Curtin, K., Ma, K., et al. (2002). Diet, activity, and lifestyle associations with p53 mutations in colon tumors. Cancer Epidemiol Biomarkers Prev, 11 (6), 541–8.

Slattery, M.L., Edwards, S., Curtin, K., et al. (2003). Associations between smoking, passive smoking, GSTM-1, NAT2, and rectal cancer. Cancer Epidemiol Biomarkers Prev, 12 (9): 882–9.

Slattery, M.L., Levin, T.R., Ma, K., et al. (2003). Family history and colorectal cancer: predictors of risk. Cancer Causes Control, 14 (9), 879–87.

Slattery, M.L., Potter, J., Caan, B., et al. (1997). Energy balance and colon cancer—beyond physical activity. Cancer Res, 57 (1), 75–80.

Smith, J.A., Lumley, M.A., Longo, D.J. (2002). Contrasting emotional approach coping with passive coping for chronic myofascial pain. Ann Behav Med, 24 (4), 326–35.

Smith, M.T., Perls, M.L., Haythornthwaite, J.A. (2004). Suicidal ideation in outpatients with chronic musculoskeletal pain: an exploratory study in the role of sleep onset, insomnia and pain intensity. Clinical Journal of Pain, 20 (2), 111–18.

Sokka, T. (2003). Work disability in early rheumatoid arthritis. Clin Exp Rheumatol, 21 (5 Suppl 31), S71–4.

Sokka, T., Hakkinen, A., Krishnan, E., et al. (2004). Similar prediction of mortality by the general health assessment questionnaire in patients with rheumatoid arthritis and the general population. Ann Rheum Dis, 63 (5), 494–7.

Sokka, T., Willoughby, J., Yazici, Y., et al. (2003). Databases of patients with early rheumatoid arthritis in the USA. Clin Exp Rheumatol, 21 (5 Suppl 31), S146–53.

Solomon, L., Beighton, P., Valkenburg, H.A., et al. (1975). Rheumatic disorders in the South African Negro. Part I. Rheumatoid arthritis and ankylosing spondylitis. S Afr Med J, 49 (32), 1292–6.

Songer, T.J., LaPorte, R.E., Dorman, J.S., et al. (1989). Employment spectrum of IDDM. Diabetes Care, 12 (9), 615–22.

Sonmez, K., Pala, S., Mutlu, B., et al. (2004). Distribution of risk factors according to socioeconomic status in male and female cases with coronary artery disease. Anadolu Kardiyol Derg, 4 (4), 301–5.

Sorensen, H.T., Mellemkjaer, L., Nielsen, G.L., et al. (2004). Skin cancers and non-Hodgkin lymphoma among users of systemic glucocorticoids: a population-based cohort study. J Natl Cancer Inst, 96 (9), 709–11.

Spector, T.D., MacGregor, A.J. (2004). Risk factors for osteoarthritis: genetics. Osteoarthritis Cartilage, 12 (Suppl A), S39–44.

Spelten, E.R., Verbeek, J.H., Uitterhoeve, A.L., et al. (2003). Cancer, fatigue and the return of patients to work-a prospective cohort study. Eur J Cancer, 39 (11), 1562–7.

Spine-health.com, 1999–2005 (http://www.spine-health.com)

Spineuniverse.com (http://www.spineuniverse.com)

Stanton, W.R., Saleheen, H.N., O'Riordan, D., et al. (2003). Environmental conditions and variations in levels of sun exposure among children in child care. Int J Behav Med, 10 (4), 285–985.

Steenland, K., Stayner, L., Deddens, J. (2004). Mortality analyses in a cohort of 18,235 ethylene oxide exposed workers: follow up extended from 1987 to 1998. Occup Environ Med, 61 (1), 2–7.

Stellman, S.D., Chen, Y., Muscat, J.E., et al. (2003). Lung cancer risk in white and black Americans. Ann Epidemiol, 13 (4), 294–302.

Stelmach, W., Kaczmarczyk-Chalas, K., Bielecki, W., et al. (2005). How education, income, control over life and life style contribute to risk factors for cardiovascular disease among adults in a post-communist country. Public Helth, 119 (6), 498–508.

Stenager, E.N., Stenager, E., Jensen, K. (1994). Attempted suicide, depression and physical diseases: a 1-year follow-up study. Psychotherapy Psychosomatics, 61 (1–2), 65–73.

Stewart, D.E., Cheung, A.M., Duff, S., et al. (2001). Long-term breast cancer survivors: confidentiality, disclosure, effects on work and insurance Psychooncology, 10 (3), 259–63.

Stewart, S.L., King, J.B., Thompson, T.D., et al. (2004). Cancer mortality surveillance—United States, 1990–2000. MMWR Surveillance Summ, 53 (3), 1–108.

Steyn, N.P., Mann, J., Bennett, P.H., et al. (2004). Diet, nutrition and the prevention of type 2 diabetes. Public Health Nutrition, 7 (1A), 147–65.

Stolt, P., Bengtsson, C., Nordmark, B., et al. (2003). Quantification of the influence of cigarette smoking on rheumatoid arthritis: results from a population based case-control study, using incident cases. Ann Rheum Dis, 62 (9), 835–41.

Straaton, K.V., Maisiak, R., Wrigley, J.M., et al. (1996). Barriers to return to work among persons unemployed due to arthritis and musculoskeletal disorders. Arthritis Rheum, 39 (1), 101–9.

Strike, P.C., Steptoe, A. (2004). Psychosocial factors in the development of coronary artery disease. Prog Cardiovasc Dis, 46 (4), 337–47.

Strojek, K. (2003). Features of macrovascular complications in type 2 diabetic patients. Acta Diabetol, 40 (Suppl 2), S334–7.

Strom, S.S., Yamamura, Y. (1997). Epidemiology of nonmelanoma skin cancer. Clin Plast Surg, 24 (4), 627–36.

Su, L.J., Arab, L. (2001). Nutritional status of folate and colon cancer risk: evidence from NHANES I epidemiologic follow-up study. Ann Epidemiol, 11 (1), 65–72.

Suarez-Varela, M.M., Llopis Gonzalez, A., Ferrer Caraco, E. Non-melanoma skin cancer: a case-control study on risk factors and protective measures. J Environ Pathol Toxicol Oncol, 15 (2–4): 255–61.

Suehiro, T., Matsumata, T., Shikada, et al. (2005). Hyperinsulinemia in patients with colorectal cancer. Hepatogastroenterology, 52 (61), 76–8.

Sullivan, J., Sheppard, L., Schreuder, A., et al. (2005). Relation between short-term fine-particulate matter exposure and onset of myocardial infarction. Epidemiology, 16 (1), 41–8.

Sullivan, M.J., Reesor, K., Mikail, S., et al. (1992). The treatment of depression in low back pain: review and recommendations. Pain, 50 (1), 5–13.

Sultan, S., Fisher, D.A., Voils, C.I., et al. (2004). Impact of functional support on health-related quality of life in patients with colorectal cancer. Cancer, (Epub ahead of print).

Sundrarjun, T., Komindr, S., Archararit, N., et al. (2004). Effects of n-3 fatty acids on serum interleukin-6, tumor necrosis factor-alpha and soluble tumour necrosis factor receptor p55 in active rheumatoid arthritis. J Int Med Res, 32 (5), 443–54.

Symmons, D.P. (2003). Environmental factors and the outcome of rheumatoid arthritis. Best Pract Res Clin Rheumatol, 17 (5), 717–27.

Symonds, T.L., Burton, A.K., Tillotson, K.M., et al. (1995). Absence resulting from low back trouble can be reduced by psychosocial intervention at the work place. Spine, 20, 2738–45.

Syrigos, K.N., Tzannou, I., Katirtzoglou, N., et al. (2005). Skin cancer in the elderly. In Vivo, 19 (3), 643–52.

Tak, S.H., Laffrey, S.C. (2003). Life satisfaction and its correlates in older women with osteoarthritis. Orthop Nurs, 22 (3), 182–9.

Tallon, D., Chard, J., Dieppe, P. (2000). Exploring the priorities of patients with osteoarthritis of the knee. Arthritis Care Res, 13 (5), 312–19.

Tanvetyanon, T. (2005). Physician practices of bone density testing and drug prescribing to prevent or treat osteoporosis during androgen deprivation therapy. Cancer, 103 (2), 237–41.

Tavani, A., LaVecchia, C. (2004). Coffee, decaffeinated coffee, tea and cancer of the colon and rectum: a review of epidemiological studies, 1990–2003 Cancer Causes Control, 15 (8), 743–57.

Tavani, A., Pregnolato, A., La Vechia, C., et al. (1997). Coffee and tea intake and risk of cancers of the colon and rectum: a study of 3,530 cases and 7,057 controls. Int J Cancr, 73 (2), 193–7.

Teixeira, E., Conde, S., Alves, P., et al. (2003). Lung cancer and women. Rev Port Pneumol, 9 (3), 225–47.

Tengstrand, B., Carlstrom, K., Fellander-Tsai, L., et al. (2003). Abnormal levels of serum dehydroepiandrosterone, estrone, and estradiol in men with rheumatoid arthritis: high correlation between serum estradiol and current degree of inflammation. J Rheumatol, 30 (11), 2338–43.

Tenkate, T.D. (1999). Occupational exposure to ultraviolet radiation: a health risk assessment. Rev Environ Health, 14 (4), 187–209.

Terauchi, Y., Kadowaki, T. (2005). PPAR and diabetes. Nippon Rinsho, 63 (4), 623–9.

Terry, M.B., Gammon, M.D., Zhang, F.F., et al. (2004). Association of frequency and duration of aspirin use and hormone receptor status with breast cancer risk. JAMA, 291 (20), 2433–40.

Tessitore, L., Vizio, B., Pesola, D., et al. (2004). Adipocyte expression and circulating levels of leptin increase in both gynaecological and breast cancer patients. Int J Oncol, 24 (6), 1529–35.

Thelin, A., Vingard, E., Holmberg, S. (2004). Osteoarthritis of the hip joint and farm work. Am J Ind Med, 45 (2), 202–9.

Thomas, G.N., Ho, S.Y., and Lam, K.S., et al. (2004). Impact of obesity and body fat distribution on cardiovascular risk factors in Hong Kong Chinese. Obes Res, 12 (11), 1805–13.

Thune, I., Furberg, A.S. (2001). Physical activity and cancer risk: dose-response and cancer, all sites and site-specific. Med Sci Sports Exerc, 33 (6 Suppl), S530–50; discussion S609–10.

Tice, J.A. (2005). Artifical disc replacement for degenerative disc disease of the lumbar spine. San Francisco: California Technology Assessment Forum.

Touloumi, G., Samoli, E., Quenel, P., et al. (2005). Short-term effects of air pollution on total and cardiovascular mortality: the confounding effects of influenza epidemics. Epidemiology, 16 (1), 49–57.

Trief, P.M., Grant, W., Fredrickson, B. (2000). A prospective study of psychological predictors of lumbar surgery outcomes. Spine, 25 (20), 2616–21.

Tse, H.F., Lau, C.P. (2004). Future prospects for implantable devices for atrial defibrillation. Cardiol Clin, 22 (1), 87–100, ix.

Tsumura, K., Hayashi, T., Suematsu, C., et al. (1999). Daily alcohol consumption and the risk of type 2 diabetes in Japanese men: the Osaka Health Survey. Diabetes Care, 22 (9), 1432–7.

Tung, R.C., Vidimos, A.T. (2005). Non-melanoma skin cancer. The Cleveland Clinic, www.clevelandclinicmeded.com.

Turvey, C.L., Klein, D.M., Pies, C.J., et al. (2003). Attitudes about impairment and depression in elders suffering from chronic heart failure. Int J Psychiatry Med, 33 (2), 117–32.

Twelves, C., Wong, A., Nowacki, M.P., et al. (2005). Capecitabine as adjuvant treatment for stage III colon cancer. New Eng J Med, 352 (26), 2696–704.

Tyrer, J., Duffy, S.W., Cuzick, J. (2004). A breast cancer prediction model incorporating familial and personal risk factors. Stat Med, 23 (7), 1111–30.

Uebelhart, D., Frey, D., Frey-Rindova, P., et al. (2003). Therapy of osteoporosis: bisphosphonates, SERM's teriparatide and strontium. Z Rheumatol, 62 (6), 512–17.

Uhoda, I., Pierard-Franchimont, C., Pierard, G.E. (2002). Prevention of skin cancers with sunscreening agents. Rev Med Liege, 57 (8), 505–8.

Uliasz, A., Spencer, J.M. (2004). Chemoprevention of skin cancer and photoaging. Clin Dermatol, 22 (3), 178–82.

Ullman, T.A. (2005). Preventing neoplastic progression in ulcerative colitis. J Clin Gastroenterol, 39 (4 Suppl 2), S66–9.

Ullman, T., Croog, V., Harpaz, N., et al. (2003). Progression of flat low-grade dysplasia to advanced neoplasia in patients with ulcerative colitis. Gastroenterology, 125 (5): 1311–19.

U.S. Agency for Health Care Policy and Research (1994). Acute low back pain in adults: Assessment and treatment. Quick reference guide for clinicians. Clinical practice guideline # 14. http://www.chirobase.org/07Strategy/AHCPR/ahcprclinician.html.

U.S.D.H.H.S. (2003). Studies of the economics of cancer prevention, screening, and care (http://grants.hih.gov/grants/guide/pa-files/PA-04-017.html).

Ullrich, P.F. Treating chronic pain and depression from degenerative disc disease. Spine Health, 2000.

Unutzer, J., Patrick, D., Marmon, T., et al. (2002). Depressive symptoms and mortality in a prospective study of 2,558 older adults. American Journal of Geriatric Psychiatry, 10 (5), 521–30.

Valderrama-Gama, E., Damian, J., Ruigomez, A., et al. (2002). Chronic disease, functional status, and self-ascribed causes of disabilities among noninstitutionalized older people in Spain. J Gerontol A Biol Sci Med Sci, 57 (11), M716–21.

Valtola, A., Honkanen, R., Kroger, H., et al. (2002). Lifestyle and other factors predict ankle fractures in perimenopausal women: a population-based prospective cohort study. Bone, 30 (1), 238–42.

van Dam, R.M. (2003). The epidemiology of lifestyle and risk for type 2 diabetes. European Journal of Epidemiology, 18 (12), 1115–25.

Van der Hage, J.A., van den Broek, L.J., Legrand, C., et al. (2004). Overexpression of P70 S6 kinase protein is associated with increased risk of locoregional recurrence in node-negative premenopausal early breast cancer patients. Br J Cancer, 90 (8), 1543–50.

Van Nieuwenhuyse, A., Fatkhutdinova, L., Verbeke, G., et al. (2004). Risk factors for first-ever low back pain among workers in their first employment. Occup Med (Lond), 22 (Epub ahead of print).

van Schaardenburg, D., Van den Brande, K.J., Ligthart, G.J., et al. (1994). Musculoskeletal disorders and disability in persons aged 85 and over: a community survey. Ann Rheum Dis, 53 (12), 807–11.

Van Tulder, M.W., Esmail, R., Bombardier, C., et al. (2000). Back schools for non-specific low back pain. Cochrane Database Syst Rev, 2, CD 000261.

Van Tulder, M., Koes, B. (2002). Low back pain and sciatica: chronic. Clinical Evidence, 8, 1171–87.

Van Tulder, M.W., Koes, B.W., Bouter, L.M. (1997). Conservative treatment of acute and chronic nonspecific low back pain: a systematic review of randomized controlled trials of the most common interventions. Spine, 22, 2128–56.

Van Tulder, M., Malmivaara, A., Esmail, R. (2000). Exercise therapy for low back pain: a systematic review within the frame of the Cochrane back review group. Spine, 25, 2784–96.

Vargo, N. (2003). Basal cell and squamous cell carcinoma. Semin Oncol Nurs, 19 (1): 12–21.

Varo Cenarruzabeitia, J.J., Martinez Hernandez, J.A., Martinez-Gonzalez, M.A. (2003). Benefits of physical activity and harms of inactivity. Med Clin (Barc), 121 (17), 665–72.

Veglia, F., Vineis, P., Berrino, F., et al. (2003). Determinants of exposure to environmental tobacco smoke in 21,588 Italian non-smokers. Tumori, 89 (6), 665–8.

Verbrugge, L.M., Gates, D.M., Ike, R.W. (1991). Risk factors for disability among U.S. adults with arthritis. J Clin Epideiol, 44 (2), 67–82.

Victor, C.R., Ross, F., Axford, J. (2004). Capturing lay perspectives in a randomized control trial of a health promotion intervention for people with osteoarthritis of the knee. J Eval Clin Pract, 10 (1), 63–70.

Vijan, S., Stuart, N.S., Fitzgerald, J.T., et al. (2005). Barriers to following dietary recommendations in Type 2 diabetes. Diabet Med, 22 (1), 32–8.

Vishvakarman, D., Wong, J.C. (2003). Description of the use of a risk estimation model to assess the increased risk of non-melanoma skin cancer among outdoor workers in Central Queensland, Australia. Photodermatol Photoimmunol Photomed, 19 (2), 81–8.

Volk, R.J., Spann, S.J., Cass, A.R., et al. (2003). Patient education for informed decision making about prostate cancer screening: a randomized controlled trial with 1-year follow-up. Ann Fam Med, 1 (1), 22–8.

Vrethem, M., Voivie, J., Arnqvist, H. (1997). A comparison of amitriptyline and maprotiline in the treatment of painful polyneuropathy in diabetics and nondiabetics. Clinical Journal of Pain, 13 (4), 313–23.

Vrkljan, M., Thaller, V., Lovricevic, I., et al. (2001). Depressive disorder as possible risk factor of osteoporosis. Coll Antroplo, 25 (2), 485–92.

Wabitsch, M., Hauner, H., Hertrampf, M., et al. (2003). Type II diabetes mellitus and impaired glucose regulation in Caucasian children and adolescents with obesity living in Germany. International Journal of Obesity and Related Metabolic Disorders, 28 (2), 307–13.

Waddell, G. (1998). The back pain revolution. Edinburgh: Churchill Livingstone.

Waddell, G., Newton, M., Henderson, I., et al. (1993). Fear-Avoidance Beliefs Questionnaire (FABQ) and the role of fear-avoidance beliefs in chronic low back pain and disability. Pain, 52, 157–68.

Wahle, K.W., Caruso, D., Ochoa, J.J., et al. (2004). Olive oil and modulation of cell signaling in disease prevention. Lipids, 39 (12), 1223–31.

Waki, K., Noda, M., Saaki, S., et al. (2005). Alcohol consumption and other risk factors for self-reported diabetes among middle-aged Japanese: a population-based prospective study in the JPHC study cohort I. Diabet Med, 22 (3), 323–31.

Walker, A.R., Adam, F.I., Walker, B.F. (2004). Breast cancer in black African women: a changing situation. J R Soc Health, 124 (2), 81–5.

Wallace, L.S., Rogers, E.S., Malagon-Rogers, M. (2004). Literacy, medical care, and health status in Tennessee. Tenn Med, 97 (9), 405–6.

Wang, C., Lin, J., Chang, C.J., et al. (2004). Therapeutic effects of hyaluronic acid on osteoarthritis of the knee. A meta-analysis of randomized controlled trials. J Bone Joint Surg Am, 86-A (3), 538–45.

Wang, J., Costantino, J.P., Tan-Chiu, E., et al. (2004). Lower-category benign breast disease and the risk of invasive breast cancer. J Natl Cancer Inst, 96 (8), 616–20.

Wang, J.X., Zhang, L.A., Li, B.X. (2002). Cancer incidence and risk estimation among medical x-ray workers in China, 1950–1995. Health Phys, 82 (4), 455–66.

Wannamethee, S.G., Camargo, C.A., Manson, J.E., et al. (2003). Alcohol drinking patterns and risk of type 2 diabetes mellitus among younger women. Archives of Internal Medicine, 163 (11), 1329–36.

Wannamethee, S.G., Shaper, A.G. (1999). Weight change and duration of overweight and obesity in the incidence of type 2 diabetes. Diabetes Care, 22 (8), 1266–72.

Ward, E.M., Burnett, C.A., Ruder, A., et al. (1997). Industries and cancer. Cancer Causes Control, 8 (3), 356–70.

Watson, P.J., Booker, C.K., Moores, L., et al. (2004). Returning the chronically unemployed with low back pain to employment. Eur J Pain, 8 (4), 359–69.

Watts, R.W., Silagy, C.A. (1995). Meta-analysis and the efficacy of epidural corticosteroids in the treatment of sciatica. Anaesthesia Intens Care, 223, 564–9.

Waylonis, G.W., Perkins, R.H. (1994). Post-traumatic fibromyalgia. A long-term follow-up. Am J Phys Med Rehabil, 73 (6), 403–12.

Wei, E.K., Ma, J., Pollak, M.N., et al. (2005). A prospective study of C-peptide, insulin-like growth factor-I, insulin-like growth factor binding protein-I, and the risk of colorectal cancer in women. Cancer Epidemiol Biomarkers Prev, 14 (4), 850–5.

Wei, M., Gibbons, L.W., Mitchell, T.L., et al. (1999). The association between cardiorespiratory fitness and impaired fasting glucose and type 2 diabetes mellitus in men. Annals of Internal Medicine, 130 (2), 89–96.

Wei, M., Kampert, J.B., Barlow, C.E., et al. (1999). Relationship between low cardiorespiratory fitness and mortality in normal-weight, overweight, and obese men. JAMA, 282 (16), 1547–53.

Weiner, D.K., Ernst, E. (2004). Complementary and alternative approaches to the treatment of persistent musculoskeletal pain. Clin J Pain, 20 (4), 244–55.

Weir, R., Nielson, W.R. (2001). Intervention for disability management. Clin J Pain, 17, S128–32.

Wells, K., Golding, J.M., Burnam, M.A. (1988). Psychiatric disorder in a sample of the general population with and without chronic medical conditions. American Journal of Psychiatry, 145 (8), 976–81.

Wen, L.K., Shepherd, M.D., Parchman, M.L. (2004). Family support, diet, and exercise among older Mexican Americans with type 2 diabetes. Diabetes Educ, 30 (6), 980–93.

Wheatcroft, S.B., Williams, I.L., Shah, A.M. (2003). Pathophysiological implications of insulin resistance on vascular endothelial function. Diabet Med, 20 (4), 255–68.

White, J.R. (2005). Topiramate and weight loss . . . Does it work? Doc News, January, 5.

White, K.P., Harth, M., Teasell, R.W. (1995). Work disability evaluation and the fibromyalgia syndrome. Semin Arthritis Rheum, 24 (6), 371–81.

White, K.P., Speechley, M., Harth, M., et al. (1999). Comparing self-reported function and work disability in 100 community cases of fibromyalgia syndrome versus controls in London, Ontario: the London Fibromyalgia Epidemiology Study. Arthritis Rheum, 42 (11), 76–83.

Whitrow, M.J., Smith, B.J., Pilotto, L.S., et al. (2003). Environmental exposure to carcinogens causing lung cancer: epidemiological evidence from the medical literature. Respirology, 8 (4), 513–21.

Wilcox, S., Brenes, G.A., Levine, D., et al. (2000). Factors related to sleep disturbance in older adults experiencing knee pain or knee pain with radiographic evidence of knee osteoarthritis. J Am Geriatr Soc, 48 (10), 1241–51.

Wilkins, K. (2004). Incident arthritis in relation to excess weight. Health Rep, 15 (1), 39–49.

Williams, M.V., Davis, T., Parker, R.M., et al. (2002). The role of health literacy in patient-physician communication. Fam Med, 34 (5), 383–9.

Willrich, A., Pinzur, M., McNeil, M., et al. (2005). Health related quality of life, cognitive function, and depression in diabetic patients with foot ulcer or amputation. A preliminary study. Foot Ankle Int, 26 (2), 128–34.

Wilson, A., Yu, H.T., Goodnough, L.T., et al. (2004). Prevalence and outcomes of anemia in rheumatoid arthritis: a systematic review of the literature. Am J Med, 116 (Suppl 7A), 50S–57S.

Wilson, W., Ary, D.V., Biglan, A., et al. (1986). Psychosocial predictors of self-care behaviors (compliance) and glycemic control in non-insulin-dependent diabetes mellitus. Diabetes Care, 9 (6), 614–22.

Winningham, M.L. (2001). Strategies for managing cancer-related fatigue syndrome: a rehabilitation approach. Cancer, 92 (4 Suppl), 988–97.

Winton, T., Livingston, R., Johnson, D., et al. (2005). Vinorelbine plus cisplatin vs. observation in resected non-small-cell lung cancer. New Engl J Med, 352 (25), 2589–97.

Woby, S.R., Watson, P.J., Roach, N.K., et al. (2004a). Are changes in fear-avoidance beliefs, catastrophizing, and appraisals of control, predictive of changes in chronic low back pain and disability? Eur J Pain, 8 (3), 201–10.

Woby, S.R., Watson, P.J., Roach, N.K., et al. (2004b). Adjustment to chronic low back pain—the relative influence of fear-avoidance belief, catastrophizing, and appraisals of control. Beh Res Ther, 42 (7), 761–74.

Wolf, F., Anderson, J., Harkness, D., et al. (1997). Work and disability status of persons with fibromyalgia. J Rheumatol, 24 (6), 1171–8.

Wolfe, F., Michaud, K. (2004). Heart failure in rheumatoid arthritis: rates, predictors, and the effect of anti-tumor necrosis factor therapy. Am J Med, 116 (5), 305–11.

Wolfe, F., Michaud, K. (2004). Severe rheumatoid arthritis (RA), worse outcomes, comorbid illness, and sociodemographic disadvantage characterize ra patients with fibromyalgia. J Rheumatol, 31 (4), 695–700.

Wolfe, F., Potter, J. (1996). Fibromyalgia and work disability: Is fibromyalgia a disabling disorder? Rheum Dis Clin Am, 22 (2), 369–91.

Wolff, A.M., Taylor, S.A., McCabe, J.F. (2004). Using checklists and reminders in clinical pathways to improve hospital inpatient care. Med J Aust, 181 (8), 428–31.

Woodhead, A.D., Setlow, R.B., Tanaka, M. (1999). Environmental factors in nonmelanoma and melanoma skin cancer. J Epidemiol, 9 (6 Suppl), S102–14.

Woodman, R.J., Chew, G.T., Watts, G.F. (2005). Mechanisms, significance and treatment of vascular dysfunction in type 2 diabetes mellitus: focus on lipid-regulating therapy. Drugs, 65 (1), 31–74.

Woolf, A.D., Pfleger, B. (2003). Burden of major musculoskeletal conditions. Bull World Health Organ, 81 (9), 646–56. Epub 2003 Nov 14.

Wuesten, O., Balz, C.H., Bretzel, R.G., et al. (2005). Effects of oral fat load on insulin output and glucose tolerance in healthy control subjects and obese patients without diabetes. Diabetes Care, 28 (2), 360–5.

Xiang, H., Stallones, L., Keefe, T.J. (1999). Back pain and agricultural work among farmers: an analysis of the Colorado Farm Health and Hazard Surveillance Survey. Am J Ind Med, 35 (3), 30–6.

Yach, D., Hawkes, C., Gould, C.L. (2004). The global burden of chronic diseases: overcoming impediments to prevention and control. JAMA, 291 (2), 2616–22.

Yamagishi, K., Hosoda, T., Sairenchi, T., et al. (2003). Body mass index and subsequent risk of hypertension, diabetes and hypercholesterolemia in a population-based sample of Japanese. Nippon Koshu Eisei Zasshi, 50 (11), 1050–7.

Yan, H., Sellick, K. (2004). Symptoms, psychological distress, social support, and quality of life of Chinese patients newly diagnosed with gastrointestinal cancer. Cancer Nurs, 27 (5), 389–99.

Yardley, D.A. (2004). Integrating gemcitabine into breast cancer therapy. Oncology (Huntingt). 18 (14 Suppl 12), 37–48.

Yelin, E., Trupin, L., Katz, P., et al. (2003). Association between etanercept use and employment outcomes among patients with rheumatoid arthritis. Arthritis Rheum, 48 (11), 3046–54.

Yin, W., Willard, F., Carreiro, J., et al. (2003). Sensory stimulation-guided sacroiliac joint radiofrequency neurotomy: technique based on neuroanatomy of the dorsal sacral plexus. Spine, 28 (20), 2419–25.

Yong, P.F., Milner, P.C., Payne, J.N., et al. (2004). Inequalities in access to knee joint replacements for people in need. Ann Rheum Dis, 63 (11), 1483–9.

Young, A., Dixey, J., Kulinskaya, E., et al. (2002). Which patients stop working because of rheumatoid arthritis? Results of five years' follow up in 732 patients from the Early RA Study (ERAS). Ann Rheum Dis, 61 (4), 335–40.

Young, B.A., Maynard, C., Boyko, E.J. (2003). Racial differences in diabetic nephropathy, cardiovascular disease, and mortality in a national population of veterans. Diabetes Care, 26 (8): 2392–9.

Yu, H.S., Lee, C.H., Jee, S.H., et al. (2001). Environmental and occupational skin diseases in Taiwan. J Dermatol, 28 (11), 628–31.

Yuyun, M.F., Adler, A.I., Wareham, N.J., et al. (2005). What is the evidence that microalbuminuria is a predictor of cardiovascular disease events? Curr Opin Nephrol Hypertens, 14 (3), 271–6.

Zak-Prelich, M., Narbutt, J., Sysa-Jedrzejowska, A. (2004). Environmental risk factors predisposing to the development of basal cell carcinoma. Dermatol Surg, 30 (2 Pt 2): 248–52.

Zautra, A.J., Smith, B.W. (2001). Depression and reactivity to stress in older women with rheumatoid arthritis and osteoarthritis. Psychosom Med, 63 (4), 687–96.

Zeeb, H., Blettner, M., Langner, I., et al. (2003). Mortality from cancer and other causes among airline cabin attendants in Europe: a collaborative cohort study in eight countries. Am J Epidemiol, 158 (1), 35–46.

Zeegers, W.S., Bohnen, L.M., et al. (1999). Artificial disc replacement with the modular type SB Charite III: 2-year results in 50 prospectively studied patients. Eur Spine J, 8 (3), 210–17.

Zhang, L.F., Zhao, L.C., Zhou, B.F., et al. (2004). Alcohol consumption and incidence of ischemic stroke in male Chinese. Zhonghua Liu Xing Bing Xue Za Zhi, 25 (11), 954–7.

Zhang, S., Hunter, D.J., Forman, M.R., et al. (1999). Dietary carotenoids and vitamins A, C, and E and risk of breast cancer. J Natl Cancer Inst, 91 (6), 547–56.

Zhang, X., Shu, X.O., Yang, G., et al. (2005). Association of passive smoking by husbands with prevalence of stroke among Chinese women nonsmokers. Am J Epidemiol, 161 (3), 213–18.

Zhang, X.Y., Chen, L.H., Guan, Y.F. (2005). PPAR family and its relationship to metabolic syndrome. Sheng Li Ke Xue Jin Zhan, 36 (1), 6–12.

Zhang, Z., Weintraub, W.S., Mahoney, E.M., et al. (2004). Relative benefit of coronary artery bypass grafting versus stent-assisted percutaneous coronary intervention for angina pectoris and multivessel coronary disease in women versus men (one-year results from the Stent or Surgery trial). Am J Cardiol, 93 (4), 404–9.

Zheng, W., Gao, Y.T., Shu, X.O., et al. (2004). Population-based case-control study of CYP11A gene polymorphism and breast cancer risk. Cancer Epidemiol Biomarkers Prev, 13 (5), 709–14.

Ziebland, S., Chapple, A., Dumelow, C., et al. (2004). How the internet affects patients' experience of cancer: a qualitative study. BMJ, 328 (7439), 564.

Author Index

Aaron, L.A., 107
Acton, R.T., 140
Adjadj, E., 195
Ahlbom, C., 195–196
Akechi, T., 224
Akimoto, M., 51
Alavanja, M.C., 183
Albus, C., 147
Aldana, S.G., 165
Aldwin, C.M., 94–95
Allegra, C., 236
Allegrante, J.P., 92
Allen, J.K., 139
Allen, N.E., 190
Almahroos, M., 209
Al-Otaibi, S.T., 220
Altaf, F.J., 186
Amos, A.F., 4
Amouyel, P., 139–140
Andersen, A., 184
Andersen, B.L., 239
Anderson, R.J., 17–18
Andrus, M.R., 10–11
Annas, G.D., 208
Arab, L., 204
Araki, A., 42, 45–46, 50
Archenholtz, B., 80
Ardizzoni, A., 230–231
Armstrong, B.K., 210–211
Arnold, L.M., 107
Aronoff, G.M., 110
Arthur, H.M., 168
Artinian, N.T., 173

Ary, D.V., 50
Asbring, P., 112
Assendelft, W.J., 133
Astin, J.A., 112
Atienza, A.A., 84
Aure, O.F., 133
Austenfeld, J.L., 226
Azizi, E., 213
Azizi, F., 141, 154–155

Backman, C.L., 67, 75–76, 79, 83, 88
Badley, E.M., 70–71
Baecklund, E., 78
Bagga, H., 5, 90–91
Baird, C.L., 94
Bakitas, M., 228
Bakris, G.L., 37
Balagopal, P. 25, 55, 152
Banaszkiewicz, P.A., 126
Barlow, J.H., 83
Baron, J.A., 205
Barrera, M., 228
Barton, M.B., 242
Baselga, J., 234
Bataillle, V., 209–210, 218
Ben-Zur, H., 227
Berger, J.P., 35, 56
Bernard, A.L., 108, 111
Bernstein, J.L., 185, 195
Berto, P., 10, 14–15
Berwick, M., 211
Bhutra, S., 116, 124–126, 128, 133
Biffi, R.G., 228

Subject Index

304 SUBJECT INDEX